KU-784-731

Speech Audiometry
2nd Edition

Edited by
Michael Martin OBE

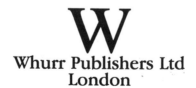

Whurr Publishers Ltd
London

© 1997 Whurr Publishers Ltd
Whurr Publishers Ltd
19B Compton Terrace, London N1 2UN, England

First Edition published by Taylor and Francis Ltd 1987.
All rights acquired by Whurr Publishers Ltd 1990.

All rights reserved. No part of this publication may
be reproduced, stored in a retrieval system, or transmitted in any form or by any means, electronic,
mechanical, photocopying, recording or otherwise,
without the prior permission of Whurr Publishers
Limited.

This publication is sold subject to the conditions that
it shall not, by way of trade or otherwise, be lent,
resold, hired out, or otherwise circulated without
the publisher's prior consent, in any form of binding
or cover other than that in which it is published, and
without a similar condition including this condition
being imposed upon any subsequent purchaser.

British Library Cataloguing in Publication Data
A catalogue record for this book is available from the
British Library.

ISBN 1-897635-12-5

Printed and bound in the UK by Athenaeum Press Ltd,
Gateshead, Tyne & Wear

Contents

Preface to the second edition of Speech Audiometry

It is now some ten years since the first edition of Speech Audiometry was published. During this time there have been significant developments in audiology and these have reflected particularly on the application of speech audiometry.

It has become very clear that the use of speech audiometry for advanced diagnostic purposes has been almost entirely replaced by electrophysiological tests in many countries. However, it must be remembered that not all countries have these advanced facilities and that there remains a place for speech audiometry for diagnostic purposes in these countries.

One area that has made significant progress over the last ten years is that of standards for speech audiometry. The production by the International Electrotechnical Commission of IEC 645-2, Audiometers Part 2 *Equipment for Speech Audiometry* in 1993 has provided a basis for establishing the efficiency of instrumentation and a value for audiometric zero for speech in terms of a pure tone sound pressure level. The title reflects the fact that very few speech audiometers as such are manufactured today, but that many pure tone audiometers have facilities for speech audiometry built into them. The International Organisation for Standardization (ISO) produced ISO 8253-3, Techniques for Audiometry: Part 3 *Speech Audiometry*, (produced in 1994 and published in 1996) which describes standardised procedures for speech audiometry as well as requirements on the recordings used. Both of these developments should go a long way to reducing the inherent variability in speech tests. No attempt has been made on an international basis to standardise the speech test material itself because of the variability that occurs as a result of the nature of speech and language itself.

The development and application of cochlear implant technology over the past ten years has lead to a significant interest in the need to assess the speech recognition abilities of profoundly deaf people. This is reflected in the development of speech test material both for use in the recognition of speech by auditory means alone and by auditory and visual means combined. In more recent times the development of digital signal processing hearing aids has also called for better means of assessing the abilities of hearing impaired people with regard to speech recognition.

The availability of greatly improved recording means, such as the compact disc, has meant that both the reliability of test material and the means to manipulate it has also been greatly improved. This in turn has lead to reassessment of existing material before it has been rerecorded and the development of new material which can be used in interactive ways.

However, the overall shift in emphasis has been for the use of speech audiometry in rehabilitation rather than for diagnostic purposes. It still remains the case that for any hearing impaired person the final arbiter of the success of any treatment or the use of any equipment is the ability to understand speech in an individual. To assess this improvement quantitatively requires the use of some form of speech testing. Developments in this area are likely to move towards more qualitative tests whose results can be expressed numerically. I hope that this second edition of *Speech Audiometry* will bring readers up to date on the progress in this area and provide a marker for future developments.

M.C.Martin
December 1996

Contributors

Stig Arlinger
Department of Technical Audiology, University Hospital of Linköping, S–581 85 Linköping, Sweden

John Bench
School of Communication Disorders, La Trobe University, Bundoora, Victoria, 13083, Australia

Klaus Brinkmann
Physikalisch-Technische, Bundesanstalt, Postfach 3345, D-3300 Braunschweig, Germany

Phillip Dermody
Formerly National Acoustic Laboratories, 126 Greville Street, Chatswood, NSW 2067, Australia

Phillip Evans
Newcomen Centre, Guy's Hospital, London SE1 9RT, UK

Hilary Fuller
Formerly National Physical Laboratory, Teddington, Middlesex TW11 0LW, UK

Stuart Gatehouse
MRC Institute of Hearing Research, Scottish Section, Glasgow Royal Infirmary, University NHS Trust, Queen Elizabeth Building, 16 Alexandra Parade, Glasgow G31 2ER, UK

Roger Green
King Edward VII Hospital, Windsor SL4 3DP, UK

Björn Hagerman
Kungliga Tekniska Högskolan, Teknisk Audiologi, S-100 44 Stockholm, Sweden

Valerie Hazan
Department of Phonetics and Linguistics, University College London, 4 Stephenson Way, London NW1 2HE, UK

John Knight
Formerly Institute of Laryngology and Otology, University of London, Grays Inn Road, London WC1, UK

Barbara Kruger
Audiology and Communication Services, 37 Somerset Drive, Commack, NY 11725–1636, USA

Frederick M Kruger
Kruger Associates Inc, 37 Somerset Drive, Commack, NY 11725–1636, USA

Kerrie Lee
Department of Communication Disorders, University of Sydney, East Street, Lidcombe, New South Wales 2141, Australia.

Mark Lutman
Institute of Sound and Vibration Research, University of Southampton, Highfield, Southampton SO17 1BJ, UK

Paul Lyregaard
Oticon a/s, Strandvejen 58, DK-2900 Hellerup, Denmark

Andreas Markides
The A.M Consultancy on Hearing Impairment, 15 Meadow Close, Whaley Bridge, Cheshire SK12 7BD, UK

Geoff Plant
Audiological Engineering Corporation, 35 Medford Street Somerville, MA 02143, USA

Ken Robinson
MRC Institute of Hearing Research Scottish Section, Glasgow Royal Infirmary, University NHS Trust, Queen Elizabeth Building, 16 Alexandra Parade, Glasgow G31 2ER, UK

Tim Sherwood
National Physical Laboratory, Teddington, Middlesex TW11 0LW, UK

Richard Wright
Consultant, 64 Highgate Road, London NW5 1PA, UK

Acknowledgements

Chapter 11
Preparation of this chapter, and portions of the work reported, were supported by Grants No. DC01166-03, R01 DC00126 and 1 R 43 DC 02 79-01 from the National Institutes of Health.

Chapter 14
Most of the speech developments described in this chapter were conducted while Kerrie Lee was working in the Speech Communication group at the National Acoustic Laboratories (NAL). Several studies have been carried out collaboratively between NAL and the University of Sydney since 1992.

Chapter 1
Basic properties of speech

RICHARD WRIGHT

Many areas of research and clinical practice involve some aspect of speech, and many people are thus expected to have some knowledge of the subject. But what kind of knowledge? Linguistics, phonetics, psychology, acoustics, signal processing, physiology, communication engineering: there is no end to it. It is tempting to assume that one's own innate knowledge will suffice, at least for clinical subjects like audiology. After all, most of us are (given normal hearing and a few other favours) expert in the use of speech — is that not sufficient?

It is not enough when dealing clinically with hearing loss, because we are then intervening in a process which has gone wrong. No mechanical knowledge may be required to drive a car, but we should like rather more when faced with a breakdown. One useful aspect of the multidisciplinary nature of speech studies is that quite a lot of information is available at the introductory level. There are excellent texts to introduce linguistics, phonetics, the physics of sound and of speech, and the basics of psychoacoustics and speech perception.

This chapter will refer to all the above areas at an introductory level, but the reader is referred to Ladefoged (1962, 1982), Denes and Pinson (1963), Fry (1979), Gimson (1980), Rosen and Howard (1990) and Moore (1989) for a more complete introduction. None requires a degree in maths or other prerequisites. They all take the time and space to provide a proper foundation, whereas this chapter is only a summary, a list of findings.

Given a basic understanding at the introductory level, this chapter will try to emphasize two particular aspects of speech:

1. The importance of viewing speech as something very different from a sequence of sounds. It is usual to introduce phonetics with a description of 'the sounds'; this approach leads to many problems. It encourages a view that speech can be adequately described at a

1

single level of analysis. This in turn makes it awkward to introduce linguistics and a hierarchy of descriptive levels. It is then equally awkward to describe prosodic aspects such as stress and intonation. They tend to be introduced as something added to speech more or less as an optional extra or afterthought. This chapter will go very much to the opposite extreme, and will try to cover almost all of speech perception without recourse to a segmental description.

2. The importance of decision making. Speaking and hearing are often treated as opposite ends of a 'speech chain'; articulatory phonetics is often viewed as opposed to acoustic phonetics; but the speaker and hearer are joined in the task of making a set of decisions concerning units at various linguistic levels. Speech perception will therefore be presented in terms of a set of yes/no (or at worst three-way) decisions, and the acoustic characteristics which encode the speaker's decisions and provide the cues to the listener's decisions.

This approach is not meant to be idiosyncratic. Hearing impairment only becomes a problem for speech when decisions about the speech signal begin to be made incorrectly. By and large, many segmental decisions can be incomplete before communication begins to be affected (because they were not necessary for correct decisions at higher levels). This process can only begin to be adequately explained by consideration of a hierarchy of suprasegmental aspects of the decision making involved in speech perception. The point of speech audiometry is to provide a methodology which tests a person's ability to make these decisions.

The speech signal

Periodic and aperiodic waveforms

The physical description of speech usually begins with a consideration of waveforms (Figure 1.1). Speech at this level can be considered as simply a disturbance of the air pressure, a sound wave.

The first distinction to be made concerning waves is whether or not they repeat. A repetitive wave is termed periodic, as shown in Figure 1.1(a). A non-repetitive or aperiodic wave is shown in Figure 1.1(b).

Many interesting physical phenomena have a repetitive aspect, including the idealized vibration of the larynx when used for speech. The resultant periodic waves are essentially different from aperiodic waves, because they are completely described by one repetition (one period). Thus Figure 1.1(a) is a complete description whereas for the aperiodic wave, Figure 1.1(b) the figure is only a portion, an incomplete description.

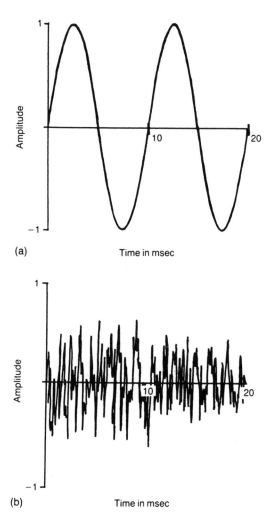

Figure 1.1 Periodic and aperiodic waveforms: (a) an example of a periodic wave, a 100 Hz pure tone; (b) an aperiodic waveform. random noise

Properties of a periodic wave

A periodic wave is characterized by three properties:

1. The period, which is the repetition interval.
2. The amplitude, which is simply the height for the pure tone in Figure 1.1(a) (an exact definition of amplitude can be made for any periodic wave, however complicated the shape).
3. The wave shape (wave form).

The pure tone in Figure 1.2 has a period of 1 millisecond (0.001 second). Thus it repeats 1000 times per second and has a fundamental frequency of 1 kHz. The amplitude shown represents the quietest sound that the normal ear can hear at this frequency. In this case the amplitude has units of length, representing the actual amount of motion of notional small volumes of air. It should be noted that this motion is very small: it is of the order of the diameter of an air molecule!

It is more usual to give pressure rather than amplitude, because pressure can be directly measured. The equivalent pressure is also shown in Figure 1.2.

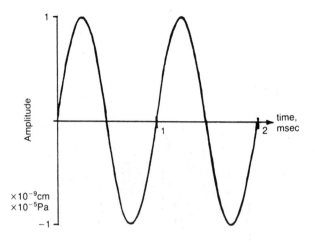

Figure 1.2 A pure tone with a frequency of 1000 Hz, at a level corresponding to the detection threshold for normal hearing

Wave shape and spectrum

The key to formally characterizing a wave form is presented in Figure 1.3, showing how a complicated shape is equivalent to a combination of pure tones, varying in period and amplitude. This principle was developed by the French mathematician (and Utopian socialist) Fourier, ca 1800, and is called Fourier analysis.

Fourier analysis shows that ANY periodic waveform can be represented as a combination of pure tones. Further, the frequencies of the pure tones to be used are specified: it is sufficient merely to use those tones whose frequencies are integer multiples of the fundamental frequency. These tones constitute a Fourier series. The wave shape can be exactly specified in terms of the amplitudes and phases of a set of pure tones. The lowest frequency tone (with period equal to that of the complicated waveform) is the fundamental of the Fourier series. The remaining tones are the harmonics, beginning with the second

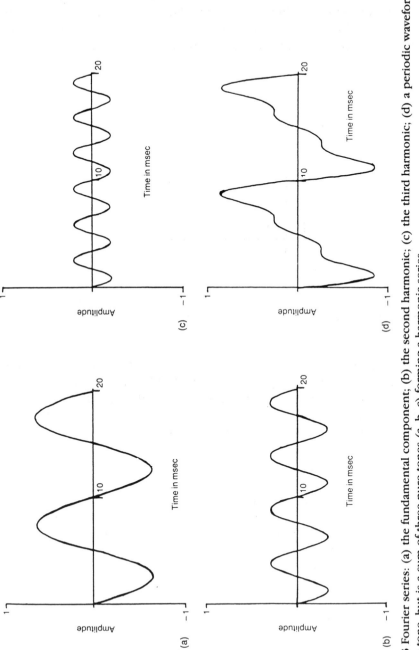

Figure 1.3 Fourier series: (a) the fundamental component; (b) the second harmonic; (c) the third harmonic; (d) a periodic waveform that is not a pure tone, but is a sum of three pure tones (a, b, c) forming a harmonic series

harmonic. This method of representation of waveforms is also called harmonic analysis.

A bar graph can be constructed showing the amplitude of each harmonic of the series, Figure 1.4. This shows the same information as in Figure 1.3, but in a compact way (especially if many more harmonics were to be used). This graph is a line spectrum or discrete spectrum.

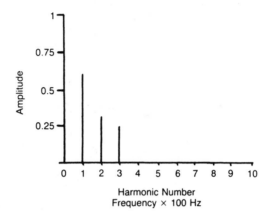

Figure 1.4 The line spectrum for the waveform in Figure 3(d)

Knowledge of the period, the overall amplitude, and the spectrum completely characterize a periodic signal. Further, the period is evident in the spectrum, and the overall amplitude is defined in terms of the individual amplitudes that constitute the spectrum. Thus the spectrum is a complete description of a periodic waveform.

Aperiodic waveforms

Fourier analysis can be extended to non-repetitive signals. A non-mathematical interpretation would be to consider such signals as actually having a period, but one of duration approaching infinity. Thus the fundamental frequency becomes very low (approaching zero), and the lines in the spectrum get very close together. The result is a continuous spectrum, a spectrum that has energy (or could have energy; some frequency regions may make no contribution) at all frequencies. Because it is impossible to draw an infinite number of vertical bars, it is conventional to just draw the tops of the bars. Figure 1.5 shows an aperiodic sound and its continuous spectrum.

It is worth emphasizing that sounds which occur at very low repetition rates can have very high frequency content. Thus although the normal ear is said to reach a lower frequency limit at about 20 Hz, this

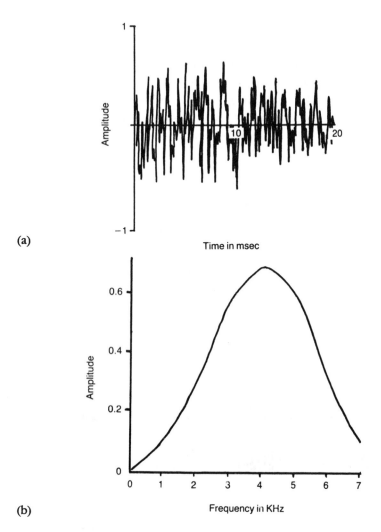

Figure 1.5 Aperiodic signals: (a) a noise waveform; (b) the continuous spectrum of the noise waveform

does not mean that one must slam a door at a frequency greater than 20 Hz in order to be heard. A person may slam a particular door once per day. This is not a very low frequency (one cycle/day) sound, because it is not a pure tone. It can be analysed as an aperiodic signal with a continuous spectrum, and with significant energy at audible frequencies.

Duration

The fact that a waveform can be described in terms of amplitude, period and spectrum has already been discussed. One more dimension is necessary: time. We wish to deal with speech signals, and so must describe signals that are of finite duration: they start and stop.

This involves a compromise with the definition of a periodic signal, and hence with the requirements of Fourier analysis. Speech signals will have a repetitive aspect, but will not be perfectly repetitive because of their finite duration. Thus making a line spectrum from one period of a speech signal is an approximation: a very good approximation for a sustained sound with many similar periods; a poor approximation for a rapidly changing sound which is really not at all repetitive.

Given the above reservation concerning periodic signals, we can physically describe speech signals in terms of their amplitude, period, spectrum and duration. The duration is simply the time from the beginning to the end of the signal involved. If the signal changes over the course of its duration, then properly we need multiple values of amplitude, period and spectrum. A three-dimensional graph of spectrum vs. time could be produced (amplitude vs. frequency vs. time) and this is exactly the information in a speech spectrogram, the basic tool of acoustic phonetics research (Figure 1.6).

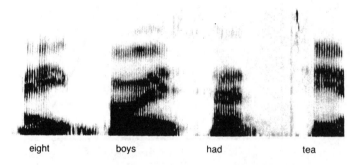

Figure 1.6 A speech spectrogram, a three-dimensional representation of speech. Frequency is the vertical dimension, time is horizontal and the signal level is represented by the amount of darkness. Spectrogram courtesy IBM (UK) Science Centre, Winchester

Psychoacoustics

The human observer is not just like a microphone and a Fourier analysis system. Human response on any physical dimension does not in general uniformly equate to the physical units that describe that dimension. This is the whole subject of psychophysical scaling, and deserves separate study in its own right. We can only summarize the most relevant results.

For each of the physical descriptions so far discussed (duration, amplitude, period and spectrum) we can present an equivalent perceptual description, Table 1.1.

Table 1.1 Physical (acoustic) and perceptual (auditory) descriptions

Physical	Perceptual
Amplitude	Loudness
Period	Pitch
Spectrum	Quality
Duration	Length

Perceptually speech sounds can thus be described in the following terms:

LOUDNESS. There is a proportionality effect to the perception of loudness (and pitch; and many other sensory phenomena): small changes to small signals are as significant as much larger changes to large signals. Thus a change in sensation depends upon the ratio of the stimulus change to the size of the original stimulus. This is not at all the same as a linear response. In a linear system the sensation change (or measurement) depends only upon the stimulus change, and no ratio is involved. Most physical devices (like microphones) are built to have a linear response, and hence differ in a basic way from human auditory perception.

The decibel scale is a way of numerically coping with the wide range of sound levels. Human auditory processing is faced with the same problem, and also solves it by the use of a logarithmic relationship. Thus the decibel scale is an approximation to loudness, the auditory scaling of acoustic intensity.

So decibel steps should represent loudness steps. Indeed, one decibel is approximately the minimum detectable loudness change over a wide range of intensities and frequencies. Although decibels are still a physical measurement, a logarithmic conversion from linear physical measurements, the decibel uses a mathematical relation (the logarithm) which is a good approximation to the perceptual scaling for loudness.

A common problem in hearing impairment is the phenomenon of recruitment, in which a person is abnormally sensitive to changes in sound level. This can be viewed as an alteration to the proportionality constant in the logarithmic scaling such that loudness increases faster than for the normal ear.

PITCH. A periodic sound will produce a sensation of pitch (so will other sounds; this is a complex subject and the reader is referred to Moore, 1989). Pitch is determined mainly by the repetition period.

It is a commonplace error to confuse fundamental frequency with the amplitude of the fundamental component in the line spectrum. This leads to the conclusion that if the amplitude of this component is reduced to zero, then the fundamental frequency is eliminated. People then marvel at the power of human perception in 'recovering' the 'missing' fundamental frequency (as in telephone bandwidth speech).

Simple inspection of the time waveforms can help clarify the issue. Figure 1.7(a) shows a signal and its spectrum; Figure 1.7(b) shows the same signal except the amplitude of the fundamental component is zero. As is evident from the figure, the obvious period is unaltered. Changing the amplitudes in the spectrum will change the quality, not the period. There is no missing fundamental as far as the eye (or the ear) is concerned: the period of Figure 1.7(b) is as evident as that of Figure 1.7(a). Further, even in the spectrum the fundamental frequency is still evident, as the harmonic spacing. In practice, as few as three higher harmonics (such as 17, 18 and 19 in Figure 1.8) are sufficient to produce a clearly evident periodicity (again, clear to the eye in the figure, and clear to the ear as an actual signal).

The basis of pitch in periodicity (NOT in strength of the fundamental of the spectrum) should be borne in mind in any consideration of pitch perception through either an impaired ear or a band-limiting device.

As with loudness, pitch relations are on approximately a log scale. Thus uniform intervals in pitch relate to uniform ratios in frequency. In music this leads to units such as semitones and octaves, which do not represent a fixed step size in physical terms, but rather represent a fixed ratio. Thus an octave is a doubling in frequency, and an octave rise in pitch can occupy a small (from 50 Hz to 100 Hz) or large (300 Hz to 600 Hz) frequency range. Both of these one-octave pitch rises would be perceived as being of approximately the same 'size'.

QUALITY. There is a difference between the sustained sounds produced by two different musical instruments playing the same note (i.e. same pitch, loudness and duration). In music this difference is called timbre but in speech it is called quality. The quality difference depends upon the spectrum, or equivalently the waveform.

For speech sounds, two vowels can be matched for pitch, loudness and duration, but their phonemic category (identity) will be determined by their quality.

LENGTH. Perception of length is not so regular as for pitch and loudness. There is not an accepted psychophysical scale in general use in audiology or phonetics, primarily because it is often unclear in speech just where any particular unit begins and ends (either perceptually or physically). Phoneticians use 'short' and 'long' to represent phonological contrasts (especially for vowels) which may or may not relate to perception of length, and may not be reducible to physical dimensions.

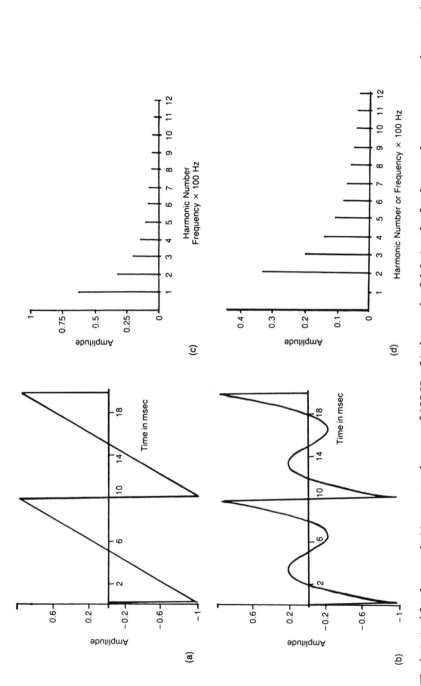

Figure 1.7 The 'missing' fundamental: (a) a sawtooth wave of 100 Hz; (b) the result of deleting the fundamental component — the period is unaffected; (c) the spectrum of (a), consisting of the fundamental and harmonics; (d) the spectrum of (b) — the greatest common divisor of the harmonics is still the 'missing' fundamental

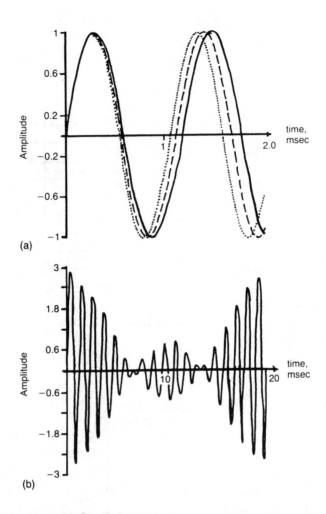

Figure 1.8 An extreme case of periodicity determined solely by higher harmonics: (a) the first cycle of pure tones at 850, 900 and 950 Hz, which are harmonics 17, 18 and 19 of a series beginning at 50 Hz; (b) the sum of the three very high harmonics, with obvious periodicity at 20 milliseconds, corresponding to 50 Hz

Linguistics

Speech is used for communication between persons. It is this role which is considered at the linguistic level.

Communication proceeds by the encoding (at the source) and the decoding (at the receiver) of information. The encoding and decoding consist of specific yes/no decisions operating upon various units that constitute a linguistic hierarchy. As with psychophysics and phonetics, linguistics is a major field of study in its own right. Speech can be analysed for decision making purposes according to the following (simplified!) linguistic hierarchy, summarized in Table 1.2:

The UTTERANCE. An utterance constitutes the largest unit of syntax, which is the system of word-arrangement constraints.

The PHRASE (tone group). Within an utterance, divisions can be made into the major syntactic constituents. Acoustically the divisions may be marked with pauses or changes in fundamental frequency, or may be determined purely by syntactic structure. A defining characteristic of a tone group is that it has within it one main pitch change, called the nucleus of the intonation pattern. As soon as we attempt to divide an utterance into any smaller information-bearing units we must have pitch information, operating within an intonation system. The first decisions made about an utterance (first in terms of the size of the unit which the decision governs) are decisions based upon pitch perception.

Table 1.2 Hierarchy of linguistic units and their associated speech contrasts

Linguistic Unit	Decision System
Utterance	Syntax
Phrase	Intonation
Foot	Stress
Syllable	Vocalic vs. Consonantal
Syllable-part	Manner
Segment	Place

The FOOT (stress group). The next level down requires the identification of stressed syllables, or at the very least the unit of 'stressed and following unstressed syllables', called the foot. Only a stressed syllable can carry an intonation marker (a pitch change), and thus only a stressed syllable can be the nucleus of a tone group. In English, an unstressed syllable MAY (not must; some do not) reduce, and a reduced syllable is shorter in length than an unreduced syllable. There is often also a difference in quality: the vowel in a reduced syllable 'reduces' to /ɪ/ or /ə/.

Thus we see that just to divide an utterance into stress groups requires all of the perceptual dimensions except loudness, although the use of quality may not be necessary for the determination of stress. Rather it should be viewed as a correlate, with duration as the determiner. Similarly, loudness will also be affected (modulated) by stress and intonation patterns, as a secondary effect. Interestingly, when periodicity cues are removed (in whispered speech) intonation patterns can still be conveyed through the use of the secondary cue (correlate) of loudness; duration as a cue to stress is unaffected by presence or absence of periodicity.

The SYLLABLE. The foot is defined as a stressed syllable followed by any number of unstressed syllables. We have indicated that stress on a syllable is determined principally by duration. How is the syllable defined?

A syllable must have one and only one syllable centre, a sound with a vocalic role (a vocoid). Thus a foot divides into syllables, each of which has a centre (a vowel sound or another sound with a vowel role); then anything left over must attach to one or the other (preceding or following; in time) adjacent centres as a syllable margin. A part of the speech signal 'attached' to a following centre is thus syllable initial; otherwise it becomes syllable final.

The SYLLABLE-PART. Conventionally in English a syllable centre is a vowel, and an initial or final syllable margin is a consonant or consonant cluster. Additionally certain consonants may extend their roles to also serve as syllable centres. Thus 'syllable' nasals or /r/ or /l/ are consonantal segments with a role (one level up) as syllable centres.

In English a syllable centre can be a single vowel, diphthong or syllabic consonant. A syllable margin, however, can consist of from zero to three consonants (and very rarely four as in 'twelfths').

It is possible to describe syllable parts without reference to vowels and consonants. From the decision making point of view a syllable centre requires a certain set of decisions about quality, and the margins require different decisions about 'manner'. Only one yes/no decision about each manner type may be 'loaded' onto a given syllable margin. This fact can be used to divide margins and thus divide syllables. This approach will be discussed in detail in the acoustic phonetics section.

The SEGMENT. The lowest-level unit is the individual speech sound. Decisions about speech at this level are phonemic; thus a phoneme is the minimum information bearing unit of the speech signal. It is only at this very lowest level that we encounter the units naively thought of as constituting speech. A wealth of interpretation must be accomplished before decisions at the segmental level are reached. Of course, if only the stylized enunciation of isolated monosyllabic words is considered (as in some types of speech audiometry) then most of the higher levels are completely eliminated. We should at least be aware of what is being thrown away.

Acoustic phonetics

This section will cover the description of speech (in particular, spoken English) in terms of the acoustic consequences of speech production, and the acoustic cues to speech perception. A complete description of speech would cover the many overall characteristics (voice quality, pitch range, rate; speaker sex, class, dialect, nationality) which must be present but which do not encode a message. Thus there are overall features and contrastive features. The contrastive features carry the information, and require the decisions which form production and perception. The contrastive features will be the main concern of this discussion.

This section will attempt to cover every speech decision (from top to bottom) and the associated acoustic cues. As mentioned earlier, it is usual in introductory phonetics to concentrate on speech sound contrasts. Such an approach undervalues the linguistic complexity of speech, and leaves out decisions about syllable structure, stress and intonation. These higher linguistic levels also have contrasts, and are referred to collectively as prosodics or suprasegmentals. To give these aspects their due, this discussion will begin with prosodics and only arrive at segmentals after all the higher levels of decision making have been described.

Prosodic aspects: pitch, length, loudness

The last section endeavoured to show how (at least for English) the whole shape of an utterance and all the perceptual decisions down to the level of the syllable are prosodic, meaning based on pitch and length and perhaps loudness, and not based on spectral quality or anything to do with individual speech sounds.

The first decision about an utterance is the division into tone groups, each with its major pitch change on the nucleus. For simple utterances there will be just one tone group, and one nucleus. The role of the pitch change to mark the nucleus is especially significant, as this will be the most important word in the utterance.

Pitch is primarily determined by the periodicity of the speech signal. In normal speech, median values for fundamental frequency range from about 120 Hz for adult male voices to 180 Hz for adult females and roughly up to 250 Hz for children. Variation about this median in ordinary speech does not usually span much more than an octave, and variation tends to be toward higher pitches. Thus the median is usually near the low end of a person's range. Most people are actually capable of producing nearly a 2 octave range of fundamental frequencies, but for speech they tend to use about an octave located (again) at the low end of their range of possibilities. Within a single utterance a range of half an octave is quite usual, though the variation can be anything from nearly zero (a dull monotone) to an octave or more (extreme emphasis).

The next decision concerns stressed and unstressed syllables. This is an area which has considerable variation from language to language. In English the stress system is rather complex, because two factors are principally involved: pitch and length.

The nucleus is not the only syllable in an utterance which may have a pitch change; other stressed syllables may have a pitch marker (pitch motion). The important distinction is that unstressed syllables can never have a pitch marker.

Furthermore, in English an unstressed syllable may reduce. The vowel duration may be shortened by 50% or more, and the vowel quality may also reduce to /I/ or /ə/.

Thus there are four sorts of syllable:

1. Stressed plus pitch motion.
2. Stressed.
3. Unstressed but not reduced.
4. Reduced.

The clearest distinction is the three-way division between types 1, 2 and 3 together and type 4. Type 1 has a pitch motion, type 4 has short-ened length, and types 2 and 3 are both of full length but without pitch motion.

Many discussions of this subject founder on treating stress as a question of separating type 2 vs. type 3. It is much clearer (and more important for speech perception) to begin with the very much easier separation of types 1 vs. 2 + types 3 vs. 4. Then type 2 vs. type 3 can be put in proper perspective. It is not the first decision to be made regarding stress; rather it is the last. The physical basis of this decision is not well established. According to Ladefoged (1982) it relates to 'effort', but effort can manifest itself in any (or any combination) of the prosodic dimensions.

Typical conversational speech proceeds at 100 to 150 words per minute, or two to three words per second. Thus the syllabic rate is approximately five syllables per second. A stressed syllable marked with a pitch change can typically have a duration of 100 to 200 msec, and could extend to 500 msec or more. A reduced syllable can easily have a duration of less than 50 msec, and in the extreme can reduce to nothing.

Segmental aspects: vowel and consonant contrasts

At the segmental level information in the speech spectrum (and hence the sound quality) becomes important for the first time. Of particular interest is the change of quality with time, as quality on its own provides limited information.

Vowel contrasts

A uniform tube (such as an organ pipe) has the property of resonance; certain frequencies are favoured, others are subject to cancellation. For speech the resonant frequencies (or modes) of the vocal tract are called formants. Vowel perception is based mainly on the position in frequency of the first two formants, F1 and F2.

These two formants determine a two-dimensional space, as shown in Figure 1.9(a), which shows the F1 and F2 values for the vowels of American English. Perceptual studies have shown a close agreement between physical formant measurements and perceptual scaling of vowel similarities, as shown in Figure 1.9(b). Furthermore, the physical and perceptual data bear a striking similarity to the 'vowel quadrilateral' used in the traditional teaching of phonetics, Figure 1.9(c). Thus the vowel quadrilateral closely represents speech perception, although it is conventionally labelled in terms of speech production. Further, the perception is closely linked to the acoustic description of the vowels, not the articulatory description. Thus the real success of the vowel quadrilateral (and the cardinal vowels) in phonetics can be explained: it is a good description of perception, and phonetics teaching is mainly a matter of the training of perception.

Both F1 and F2 can range over about two octaves (adult male F1: 200–800 Hz; F2: 700 Hz–2.8 kHz). Formants can be about 40% higher for adult females, and still higher for children. Unfortunately, each formant does not scale uniformly with vocal tract length, so a child's formants will not be a fixed percentage increase on the adult male values quoted. But one would not expect a child's formants to be more than double those given above. The basic decisions about vowels are:

1. F1 and F2 far apart vs. close together ('front' vs. 'back' vowels).
2. F1 high vs. F1 low ('open' vs. 'close' vowels).

Many of the world's languages can use the above decisions to produce a system using from three to five vowels. In English the perception can be modelled as based on five vowels: a three-way decision on F1 and a two-way decision on F2–F1, which yields six categories. This collapses to five because F2 is constrained when F1 is high.

But English has many more than five vowels! A second decision is added, based upon length, yielding five more vowels (there may well also be quality differences between the 'long', and 'short' members of a pair). Finally, if the formants move slowly, diphthongs are produced of which southern British English has a particularly large number. Interested readers are referred to Gimson (1980) and Lasdefoged (1982) for further details.

In southern British English, perception is aided by constraints imposed upon vowels. Syllables can be divided into open (no syllable-final consonants) vs. closed (ending in a consonant or cluster of consonants). ONLY long vowels can occur in open stressed syllables. In unstressed open syllables the reduced forms /ə/ and /ɪ/ also occur. Thus whether a vowel is heard as long is governed partly by the syllable structure. If it is an open syllable, it will be a long vowel, regardless of

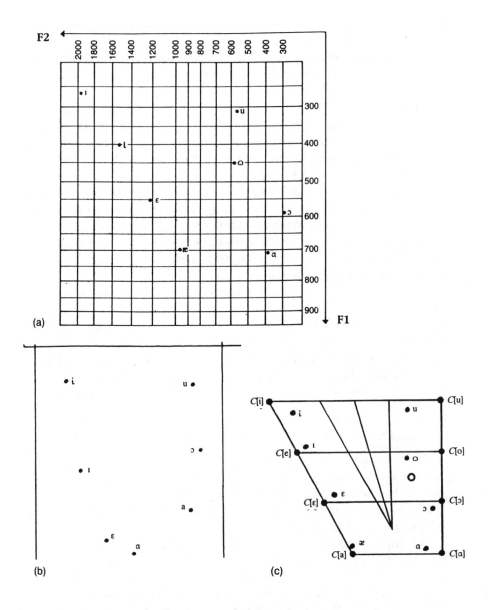

Figure 1.9 Vowel space and the significance of formants: (a) acoustic — the representation of the English steady vowels plotted according to the two lowest resonant frequencies of the vocal tract, F1 and F2; (b) perceptual — the result of judgements of perceptual distances between vowels; (c) phonetic — the vowel quadrilateral used in descriptive phonetics. Figures taken from: (a) Ladefoged (1982), Fig. 8.7; the vowels are for American English. (b) Klein, Plomp and Pols (1970), Fig. 1.5.1; from a study of Dutch vowels. Their figure has been rotated and reflected about the central axis. (c) Gimson (1980), Fig. 6; data on American vowels from Ladefoged (1982, Fig. 4.2) have been added

the actual acoustic properties of the vowel itself. This is one example of the many ways in which the sounds of speech are really a question of larger units (the syllable) and the whole system of contrasts

Consonants contrasts

Consonants are by definition those sounds occurring in the syllable margins. It is conventional to divide consonants according to place and manner (of articulation) and voicing. This section will extend this description to the acoustic consequences of the place, manner and voicing taxonomy.

Voicing principally refers in articulary terms to laryngeal activity, the presence or absence of vibration of the vocal cords. The acoustic consequences of the place is ideally a periodic or aperiodic waveform. The actual acoustic cues to voicing depend upon the consonants involved (stops or fricatives or affricates), syllable stress, syllable position and whether or not the consonant is part of a cluster. Manner categories are shown in Table 1.3.

Table 1.3 Manner categories

Manner	Speech Sounds
Stop	p t k b d g
Fricative	f θ s ∫ v ð z ʒ h
Affricate	t∫ dʒ
Nasal	m n ŋ
Approximant	w j r l

Place refers to the main place of constriction within the vocal tract, as shown in Table 1.4. These categories are the main positions for English, working from the front of the mouth to the back. For detailed phonetics more places and multiple articulatory gestures may actually be involved, but those given will suffice for a discussion of the system of contrasts.

Table 1.4 Place categories

Place	Speech Sounds	Examples
Bilabial	p b m	pie, buy, my
Labiodental	f v	face, vase
Dental	θ ð	thin, then
Alveolar	t d n s z	to, do, new, Sue, zoo
Palato-alveolar	∫ ʒ t∫ dʒ	shy, measure, church, judge
Velar	k g ŋ	back, bag, bang
Laryngeal	h	hooray, Henry

Syllable initial consonant contrasts

Decoding of consonants within the syllable-initial margin is considerably simplified by a very strong constraint: only ONE yes/no decision is
required for each manner possibility for the whole cluster, and ONE
voicing decision for the whole cluster. For instance, a cluster AS A
WHOLE is either nasal or non-nasal. There is no possibility of combin-
ing nasals into clusters to require two or more decisions about nasality.
The same simplification applies to all the manner contrasts, and to
voicing. Thus a syllable initial consonant cluster (as a whole) is either:

1. Nasal or not.
2. Fricative or not.
3. Stop or not.
4. Approximant or not.
5. Voiced or voiceless.

Further there are usually only one or two and at most three initial
consonants, and their sequence is subject to further strict constraints.
The result is that, although there are about 24 consonants, there are
nowhere near 24 x 24 x 24 = 13,824 possible clusters involving three
consonants. In fact there are less than 10 (some variation according to
dialect); they all begin with /s/, the second consonant is a voiceless stop,
the third is an approximant, and nearly half of the stop + approximant
pairs are not allowed (/tl/, /kl/, /pw/ and /tw/). Now these five manner
and voice decisions can be discussed in turn.

NASAL. The main acoustic cue to nasality is the presence of a relatively
strong nasal formant at about 300 Hz. The F1 for the related non-nasal
articulatory configuration is eliminated, and F2 and higher resonances
decay more quickly because of the extra loss through the nasal tract.
This extra loss can also be described as a widening of formant band-
widths and a reduction of formant amplitude (see Ladefoged, 1962 for
a discussion of loss and bandwidth).

FRICATIVE. Acoustic cues to frication, on the other hand, lie in the
frequencies above 1 kHz, and spreading as high as 8 to10 kHz for /s/.
Frication is the audible consequence of air turbulence at a constriction.
This signal is aperiodic, though it may be added to a periodic signal
from the larynx in the case of voiced fricatives. In either case, the presence of random noise above 1 kHz will be the cue to frication.

STOP. A stop has a temporal cue, an abrupt interruption or gap in the
signal. This definition is sensible for words within an utterance, but not
for the beginning of an utterance. Although no gap as such occurs in this

position, the release from vocal tract closure is still cued by the abrupt onset (half a gap!), the rapid energy rise as the syllable begins. Also associated with stops is rapid formant motion as the vocal tract moves from an obstructed to a non-obstructed shape. In particular, F1 will rise. The change in F2, though ultimately of great significance, is related to place, and so can be ignored for the purposes of manner decisions.

An affricate is acoustically a stop with a slow release, so the gap is followed by frication produced at the same 'place' as the closure (homorganic fricative).

APPROXIMANT. An approximant is vowel-like but with slowly varying formants (but not so slow and not with the same pattern of motion as for diphthongs).

VOICING. Voicing in syllable initial position is complicated. There is no voicing contrast for nasals and approximants. Similarly many clusters have no voicing contrast. Fricative + stop is always 'voiceless', regardless of the actual articulation or acoustic manifestation. Similarly fricative + nasal has a 'voice less' fricative. All that really remains are single stops, and stop + approximant clusters; even here a voicing contrast may not be required except on stressed syllables.

For unconjoined stops and stop + approximant clusters, on stressed syllables, in syllable-initial position, one must consider acoustic cues to voicing. The cue is generally characterized by voice onset time (VOT), which is the asynchrony between release of the closure and initiation of larynx vibration. In English the sounds /b,d,g/ begin to have laryngeal vibration at about the time the constriction opens (is released), or shortly (less than 25 milliseconds) thereafter. If larynx vibration does not begin until well after release (well over 25 milliseconds) the sound is categorized as a /p,t,k/.

The same holds for stop + approximant, except that the VOT may become very long indeed and an entire /r/ or /l/ (for instance) may be produced without laryngeal vibration (as a voiceless fricative). The perception of this difficult contrast (a few milliseconds either way from 25 milliseconds) is aided by concomitant effects: larynx activity produces low frequency (below 1 kHz) spectral content, so the tilt of the spectrum is a cue. Lack of low frequency energy means there is little excitation for F1, so absence (cutback) of F1 is a related cue.

Syllable final consonant contrasts

Syllable final contrasts start off by following the same simplification as for syllable initial: only one manner and voicing decision for the whole cluster. Unfortunately this is then complicated by the affix system in English which can add markers for plural or possessive (/s/, /z/, /Iz/) and for past tense and past participle (/t/, /d/, /ɪd/). Only one voicing decision still must be made, because these affixes 'agree' for voicing; but multiple fricative and stop combinations are introduced. Also longer sequences are possible (up to four), and fewer constraints upon combinations.

One simplification, however, is that the approximant possibilities are reduced to just /r/ or /l/ in English, and reduced even more (though with a compensatory increase in diphthong possibilities) to just /l/ in some dialects (non-rhotic; no /r/ sound).

The basis for fricative and stop decisions is essentially as for syllable initial position. For nasality (in clusters) and voicing, however, the decision has much to do with the preceding vowel.

NASALITY. A vowel preceding a cluster involving nasality will itself be nasalized, and this will acoustically be cued by the 'nasal' formant at about 300 Hz and a general widening of the other formants. Whether an actual nasal consonant is produced is less important. 'Granted' will be heard the same whether pronounced /grãntɪd/ or /grãtɪd/. Of course if the pronunciation changes to /grãnɪd/ then the nasal consonant must occur; but then it is no longer a consonant cluster. One might even say that the vowel always carries the nasality information, and the /n/ is only required to mark the syllable as closed.

VOICING. The syllable final voicing contrast is almost a misnomer, because the periodicity of the signal during the final portion of the syllable is somewhat irrelevant. The strong cue is the length of the preceding vowel: long for voiced, short for voiceless. The syllable initial VOT and the syllable final vowel length decisions are both temporal; thus decisions about the time domain must be made correctly in order to properly decode the 'periodicity' distinction voiced vs. voiceless.

Differentiation within a manner group: place contrasts

Speech perception is now almost complete. Given all the decisions about prosodic shape and stress pattern and syllables and syllable structure and the decisions about which manner categories are involved in consonant clusters, only differentiation within a manner group remains. This differentiation consists of place distinctions. It deserves note that there are strong visual place cues. In fact, the visual cue can be stronger than the acoustic cues for bilabial stops (McGurk and Macdonald, 1976).

At this lowest level the decisions are made which finally unambiguously decode the 'sounds' of English. These decisions do not 'recognize' sounds; they decide amongst a few alternatives. Once all the decisions about the structure of a syllable margin have been made (manner and voicing contrasts) only decisions within a manner group (roughly, decisions as to place) remain.

Stop: /ptk/ or /bdg/.
Nasal: /mnŋ/ (just /mn/ syllable initially).
Approximant: /wjrl/ (just /rl/ or just /l/ syllable finally).
Fricative: /fəsʃ/ /vðzʒ/ (/h/).
(affricate: /tʃ/ /dʒ/).

Affricate manner could be treated as detecting stop followed by fricative.

The status of /h/ requires discussion. It is only possible syllable-initially, has no voicing contrast, and is acoustically similar to a fricative but produced by 'aspirant' turbulence at the larynx rather than fricative turbulence at another constriction. In articulatory and phonological terms it might be considered a separate manner, but for perception it is close to the other sounds produced by turbulence, the fricatives. So decoding /h/ can be considered part of the determination of place, along with /fəsʃ/ (presenting an asymmetry in that it has no voiced counterpart, owing to laryngeal place).

The differentiation within these groups will now be discussed in detail.

STOP. The F2 transition must now be used. Bilabial /pb/ lower F2, alveolar /td/ raise it. Because actual place of articulation varies according to the neighbouring vowel for /kg/ (closure may occur along the hard palate rather than at the velum), the acoustic cue for /kg/ is modified by vowel context.

These transitions are among the most difficult cues in speech. The durations can be less than 50 msec, and the amplitude is low, 30 dB or more below the level of an adjacent vowel.

NASAL. The same F2 transition cue as used for stops will separate /m/ from /n/. Syllable final /ŋ/ has the same variation according to neighbouring vowel as has /kg/. There is no syllable initial /ŋ/.

FRICATIVE. The sibilants /sʃ/ /zʒ/ and non-sibilants /fə/ /vð/ have a sizeable amplitude difference. The voiceless non-sibilant fricatives are the weakest of the sounds of English, roughly 30 dB below the loudest vowel sounds. Separation by amplitude and voicing leaves the four pairs listed above.

All that remains is the decision within these pairs, which is mainly cued by the frequency at which the noise energy is concentrated. For the sibilants, /s/ and /z/ will have appreciable energy between 4 and 8 kHz, whilst /ʃ/ and /ʒ/ will have a lower frequency concentration. This distinction is very much a matter of a contrast between relatively higher and relatively lower; absolute values vary greatly across speakers.

Similarly, the dental fricatives /θ/ and /ð/ will have a higher frequency concentration of energy than for /f/ and /v/.

Finally, the aspirant /h/ does not have a characteristic energy concentration, and this fact becomes its distinctive cue. The energy will be determined by vocal tract shape, thus making the spectrum for /h/ very much conditioned by any associated vowel. Indeed in whispered (all aspirant) speech, the /h/ is not really distinguishable from a neighbouring vowel in purely acoustic terms.

In all cases fricative energy is mainly above 1 kHz, and in many cases, as mentioned, the sound is quite weak. Thus problems with fricatives provide an early warning system for hearing impairment.

As with stops and nasals, visual cues are useful for partly differentiating fricatives: /θ/ and /ð/ are clearly different from /f/ and /v/; and liprounding is a cue to /ʃ/ and /ʒ/ vs. /s/ and /z/.

APPROXIMANT. In general, the approximants have an amplitude somewhat below that of vowels. This is especially true for /r/ and /l/. A strong cue for /r/ is provided by F3. In a spectrogram a very clear dip in F3 is observed for an intervocalic /r/. Another clear cue to /r/ is liprounding. Both /r/ and /l/ produce a lowering of F2, though the significance of this effect varies according to the vowel involved (vowels with a high F2 are affected more than those with a low F2).

The 'semivowels' /w/ and /j/ are similar to diphthongs, with two differences:

1. Formant motion is faster (though still slower than for stop and nasal transitions).
2. Formant motion is greatest at the beginning of the sequence (a /w/ or /j/ followed by a vowel), whereas for diphthongs the motion is faster toward the end.

Note that cue (2) can only be used (in English) because /w/ and /j/ are restricted to syllable initial position.

With completion of the place decisions the decoding of the speech signal is complete.

Speech perception

Auditory space

The implications for speech perception are a main concern in hearing loss. It is common in audiology texts to summarize certain acoustic properties of the speech signal on a sort of audiogram (level vs. frequency), with areas marked out for the various categories of speech sound. A typical diagram is Figure 1.10.

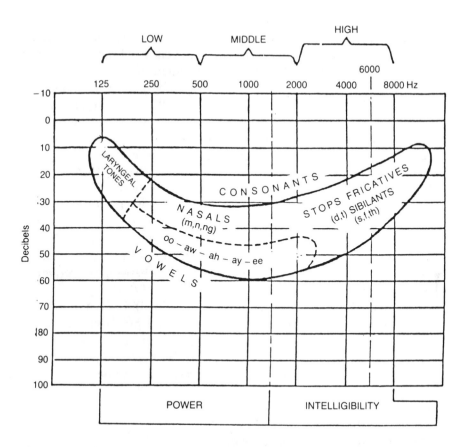

Figure 1.10 The frequency components of English speech sounds. Auditory space, from Ballantyne (1970) Deafness, 2nd Edn J & A Churchill Ltd.

Such a chart is informative but incomplete. It is a map only of the short term spectral content of speech superimposed on the auditory dimensions of response to the level and frequency of pure tones. It provides mainly a summary of the parts of 'auditory space' involved in vowel contrasts and place/manner decisions.

Pitch detection is usually neglected, or consigned misleadingly to the part in auditory space occupied by the 'laryngeal tone'. As has been discussed, strength of the fundamental is not the determiner of pitch, and a more informative diagram would show pitch related information as dependent upon the entire spectral content of the signal, although a voiced sound would ordinarily have most of its energy below 1 kHz.

The real problem with conventional auditory space, for pitch perception and generally for all of speech processing, is that the time dimension is neglected. Speech perception depends upon a three-dimensional auditory space (amplitude vs. frequency vs. time), and the conventional diagram is just a slice through this space. The time we selected for

Figure 1.10 is at the short time end of the complete picture. Consideration of a time dimension is particularly relevant to pitch perception and sensorineural hearing loss, because of the existence of a temporal mechanism for frequency discrimination.

Audiologists are familiar with the frequency selectivity along the basilar membrane within the cochlea. Hair cell loss or other damage impairs the capabilities of this frequency analyser. Stronger signals must be used to get a response. Minimum detectable frequency change is increased. The rate at which frequency changes can be followed is reduced. Finally, frequency selectivity is reduced (Moore, 1989).

But pitch judgements for speech do not have to depend upon this 'place mechanism' of frequency analysis, as a temporal mechanism is available for signals up to at least 1 kHz. Similarly, the various durational aspects of speech contrasts can also be handled by temporal processing. These temporal capabilities are not essentially properties of the cochlea, as is the place (on the basilar membrane) mechanism of frequency discrimination.

Figure 1.11 shows normal frequency discrimination. It is a plot of the minimum detectable change in the frequency of a pure tone as a function of frequency. Such a minimum change is referred to as the Just Noticeable Difference (JND). For auditory frequency discrimination, there are essentially two quite different areas on the graph:

1. Discrimination for frequencies below 2 kHz is nearly constant at about 2–3 Hz.
2. Discrimination above 2 kHz follows a ratio scale. The JND is a fixed ratio of about 0.2% of the frequency.

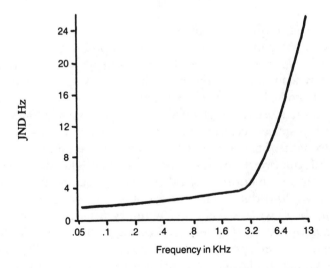

Figure 1.11 Frequency discrimination

The difference in slope for the two regions reflects the difference in mechanism. The implication for hearing impairment is that low frequency temporal processing, including the entire range for human voice pitch, may continue when place processing is lost.

Temporal processing

The only decisions that have no temporal aspect are those relating to vowel quality. Even for vowels, we can only establish (in English) five categories before we must consider the time dimension for 'short' vs. 'long' and for diphthongs. Everything else directly involves time.

PROSODIC SHAPE. The first decisions require pitch and pitch motion to determine the major parts of the utterance, called tone groups. The pitch itself depends upon the temporal mechanism (periodicity) of pitch detection. The periods involved for the human voice range from 20 msec down to 2 msec. The minimum detectable change in period can be deduced from Figure 1.11, but is presented directly in Figure 1.12.

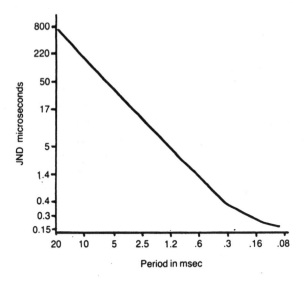

Figure 1.12 Period discrimination

It can be seen that the changes in period required to detect a frequency shift are relatively large at low frequencies (and large periods), whereas they are small at high frequencies (small periods). At 2 kHz a JND of 4 Hz represents a change in period of 1μ second. Obviously a temporal mechanism needs to be extremely accurate to work at 2 kHz, and would have to be impossibly refined for higher frequencies. Thus it is very reasonable for the place mechanism to take over for the higher frequencies.

The size of a tone group can vary from a single syllable ('No!') to very many words ('I THOUGHT it was Miss Scarlet in the library with a piece of pipe').

INTONATION. The patterns of pitch change (and related loudness and duration changes) operate at the phrase or tone group level. Divisions may be made within a tone group, though this becomes very much a matter of the 'school' of intonation theory to which one adheres. The important fact is that intonation patterns never operate below the unit of the syllable. Thus the fastest motion we should expect (in terms of frequency change per unit of time) is about an octave over the duration of a single syllable (probably several hundred msec for so large an intonation marker). Ordinarily pitch motion will be rather less emphatic, and have lower rates of change.

STRESSED SYLLABLES. Stressed syllables have been defined in terms of their length and ability to carry an intonation marker. A syllable is roughly 100 to 500 msec. Durational differences between stressed and unstressed syllables are usually quite clear; a two-to-one ratio is typical.

SYLLABLES. Defining the syllable is fraught with difficulties. The easy case is a vowel surrounded by stops. The utterance /bebebeb/ is clearly three syllables, and each syllable division is marked by a 30 dB amplitude change over as little as 30 msec. At the difficult end are words like "power", and words in which only the approximants /wrlj/ divide the vowels. For such words there may be no amplitude changes, but there will still be a change of spectrum vs. time, occupying something like 50 to 100 msec in the ordinary case. The hearing impaired person can be expected to have most difficulty with these spectral cues to syllable division.

VOICING. Voicing is the name for the contrast in English between two groups of stops and fricatives which otherwise have identical place and manner. The actual acoustic cues involve periodicity, spectral balance, and vowel length. These decisions are made only once per syllable margin (consonant cluster). Allowing for the open syllables and for those syllables not involving stops and fricatives, there is as a rough average one voicing decision per syllable. The duration of the cues themselves, however, can be very brief: 30 msec VOT difference between a definite /p/ and /b. Vowel length differences for syllable-final voicing will be roughly twice this long, or more.

MANNER CONTRASTS. As with voicing, there is only one decision per syllable margin for each of the possible manners. So again the decisions are progressing at something like the syllabic rate, though there can be two stops or fricatives in a syllable final cluster (because of suffixes). The manner cues thus can be thought of as occupying the roughly 50 to 100 msec slot that we have allowed for syllable margins, and in worst case will be half that length. Manner cues tend to depend mainly upon lower frequencies, below 1 kHz. The exception is frication, which is characterized by random noise above 1 kHz.

PLACE CONTRASTS. Place contrasts operate at the segmental level, and thus have multiple decisions per syllable margin. The decision making is simplified by various phonological processes. Elision (deleting segments) and assimilation (making adjoining segments agree for place) reduce the number of place decisions. Thus though one might expect at worst to make five or six (or possibly seven) place decisions for a single syllable, the average is probably again something like one per syllable margin.

Place cues are the shortest speech cues, principally involving 20–50 msec transitions in the second formant. These cues will be in the 1 kHz to 3 kHz region, and will be transitions from or to low amplitudes for stops and nasals. Cues to fricative place will be more spread out, from 1 kHz up to 8 kHz or so, but will also be of low amplitude, as much as 30 dB less than the centre of a stressed vowel. These temporal considerations are summarized in the three-dimensional auditory space diagram, Figure 1.13.

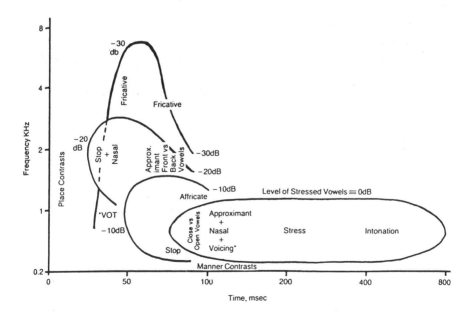

Figure 1.13 Auditory space-time

How to use speech in speech audiometry

Two important questions about various approaches to speech audiometry are: (1) the kind of speech to be used and (2) the kind of results to be collected. The various answers produce a range of possibilities, which will be considered in turn.

Speech detection and recognition threshold

The simplest possible approach is to:

1. Dispense with all the linguistic levels except the very lowest and simply use isolated monosyllables.
2. Ignore all questions of structure. Do not score anything about phonetic type or context. Just score items as right vs. wrong.
3. Ignore confusions between perception and production: the person taking the test 'simply' says what he or she hears. These are called open response tests, because the set of allowed responses is open rather than closed.
4. Ignore all problems of constraints upon perception and production. Ignore differences in probability of various sounds and sequences; ignore the general tendency to 'grasp after meaning', to prefer a known word to a nonsense word. Ignore the difficulty of producing non-English sequences, even if they were perceived.
5. Do not enquire into what the person hears. Simply concentrate on the acoustic level at which the sounds begin to be heard (speech detection threshold, SDT), or the level at which sounds are heard with a specified accuracy (such as 50% correct; speech recognition threshold, SRT). This approach concentrates on questions of level rather than questions of speech, which is convenient for reducing speech audiometry to something like pure tone audiometry.

Speech audiogram

The next simplest form of speech audiometry is to make all the simplifications just mentioned, with the exception of testing at various discrimination levels. A graph can then be made of percent correct vs. presentation level, as in Figure 1.14. In psychophysics such a graph is called a discrimination function, but audiology uses the term speech audiogram.

A speech audiogram improves upon a simple SDT or SRT measurement in that it recognizes that speech is more complicated than pure tones, and hence there are more questions to ask than simple detection threshold. But all the speech audiogram actually tests is multiple thresholds rather than single thresholds. The whole approach still reflects a preoccupation with levels.

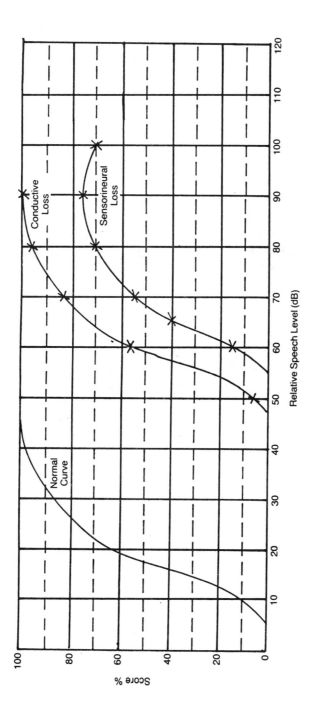

Figure 1.14 Speech audiogram with the format recommended by the British Society of Audiology published in the British Journal of Audiology Vol. 9, 1975. A 20% change in score is equal to a 10 dB change in level. The shape of the normal curve will depend upon the speech material used. The other two curves illustrate the results from two people one with a conductive hearing loss and the other with a sensorineural loss

Closed response tests

The problems of interaction of production with perception, and the constraints of the language involved are largely overcome through 'multiple-choice' tests (see Stevenson and Martin, 1977 for a review). The subject selects from a small set of allowed responses. The selection is usually made by marking a response sheet. A written response simplifies the test, eliminating problems of speech production on the part of the person taking the test (and of perception of that production). Special 'pointing to picture' responses have been used with children.

Closed response tests were originally developed to assess the intelligibility of speech transmission systems (the rhyme test and its descendants; Hawley, 1977).

A very important benefit of closed response tests is control over 'errors'. The key to behavioural tests is to restrict the subject just to those decisions being investigated. With only a few error possibilities it becomes possible to analyse errors rather than simply to accumulate them. Such diagnostic tests (DRT:Voiers, 1977; FAAF:Foster and Haggard, 1984) can then be used to add a qualitative aspect to the audiometry. Such tests not only quantify the impairment, but point to specific problem areas.

Continuous speech tests

The concept of linguistic levels and their associated constraints can be introduced through the use of continuous speech, sentences and paragraphs. Unfortunately, continuous speech adds a whole new set of problems; responses can now be even more variable than for single words, scoring becomes almost impossible, and it is hard to control the difficulty level of materials.

Again, it improves matters greatly to use closed response tests. One particular development (the SPIN test; Kalikow et al., 1977) really only extracts one bit of information out of the whole linguistic structure: how the same acoustic item is perceived in a highly constrained sentence (high predictability) vs. a marginally constrained sentence (low predictability). Much research involves linguistic constraints, but very few clinically appropriate tests exist.

Synthetic speech tests

Systematic and detailed investigation of auditory space-time requires the use of synthetic stimuli. Much basic research has been performed, but little of direct clinical application. However the advent of the microcomputer and the proliferation of speech synthesis devices at much lower cost than was the case 10 years ago eliminate the main technical difficulties with the use of synthesis.

Synthetic speech adds the missing dimensions to a speech audio-gram. With synthesis an experimental continuum can be explored step-by-step. The result is a comparison with normal performance on a single acoustic cue to a single speech contrast. Thus in a methodical way the whole pattern of contrasts can begin to be tested. Further, the fact that synthetic speech requires a control computer can be turned to advan-tage and the stimuli can be computer generated according to the subject's response pattern. These adaptive tests can be made compara-tively efficient.

Further, synthetic speech allows a form of speech audiometry which can be made suitable for use with the profoundly deaf, with persons who score at chance level on conventional speech tests. Such testing is very relevant to the screening of candidates for tactile and electrical prostheses, such as cochlear implants and wearable vibrotactile stimula-tors (Fisher et al., 1983; Pickett et al., 1983; Hazan and Fourcin 1985; Hazan, chapter 10, this volume).

There are many difficulties with speech audiometry. Several have just been mentioned, and other chapters of this book will raise further prob-lems. But we point to these problems in order to find solutions. It should be of great interest for the reader to see how the remaining chap-ters in this book attempt not just to find problems, but to solve them.

Chapter 2
Towards a theory of speech audiometry tests

PAUL LYREGAARD

By and large speech audiometry is empirically based, which is not surprising given that our knowledge of the factors mediating speech intelligibility is rudimentary, particularly when a hearing impairment is involved. The present chapter outlines the framework of a theoretical approach to speech audiometry which, although incomplete in detail, nevertheless may be helpful, particularly for the development of new tests. The theory was developed in the wider context of speech intelligibility tests, for the purposes of handling the difficult problem of the international standardization of such tests. It largely draws on work performed at The National Physical Laboratory in Teddington (Lyregaard, Robinson and Hinchcliffe, 1976).

Even if our knowledge of the detailed mechanisms of speech perception were profound, this would not imply that a theory of speech audiometry were readily available; this is partly due to the fact that a large number of practical factors also affect speech audiometry (e.g. manner of presentation, response technique, scoring method and interpretation of results), but perhaps more importantly, that the purpose for which speech audiometry is used in the audiological clinic is unclear. It would appear that speech audiometry is mostly being used as a general-purpose test, for such purposes as differential diagnoses, assessment of social handicap, monitoring rehabilitation progress and hearing aid fitting. Needless to say it is highly inconceivable that one single test can be optimum for such diverse uses.

Inevitably, therefore, it is necessary to discuss some of the factors involved and how they affect the outcome of speech audiometry tests. Following this discussion the framework of a theory will be introduced, and its consequences discussed. The presentation will by and large be limited to monosyllabic words, since this is the most common type of material in use.

The rationale for speech audiometry

Carhart (1951) has defined speech audiometry as follows:
The technique wherein standardized samples of a language are presented through a calibrated system to measure some aspect of hearing ability.

Lyregaard et al. (1976) offer the following definition:
Speech audiometry means any method for assessing the state or ability of the auditory system of an individual, using speech sounds as the response evoking stimuli.

These definitions are broadly similar, and they both emphasize that the purpose of speech audiometry is to assess the auditory system. Speech audiometry forms a subgroup within the more general domain of speech tests, and the basic principle involved is illustrated in Figure 2.1: selected speech items, e.g. words, are presented through an electroacoustic system to the listener, who in turn indicates what was heard; these responses are compared to the original material, and the percentage of correct responses is taken as the test result. In speech audiometry this test result would then typically be compared to results obtained in similar test conditions for a group of normal hearing individuals. Test validity hence requires that all factors other than the test subject be held constant. The auditory system of the individual test subject is therefore, as mentioned previously, the object under scrutiny. As illustrated in Table 2.1 other uses of speech tests appear when the focus of attention is shifted to the other system components shown in Figure 2.1.

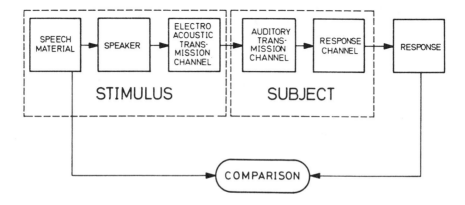

Figure 2.1 Block diagram of the major components/variables in speech audiometry

Speech audiometry tests are notoriously difficult to specify and standardize. What, then, is the rationale for using them in the first place?

Table 2.1 Examples of areas in which speech tests are used

Independent Variable	Typical Areas of Utilization
Speech material	Linguistic research (grammar, semantics) Phonological research
Speaker	Phonetic research (articulation) Diagnosis of articulatory disorders Speaker identification research Speech synthesizer assessment
Electroacoustic transmission channel	Speech transmission systems Speech distortion and noise interference Acoustic environment in halls, offices, etc. Hearing aid design
Auditory transmission channel	Assessment of auditory handicap Monitoring audiometry Test of occupational fitness Monitoring improvements in the auditory training of hearing handicapped Diagnosis of auditory dysfunction Research in hearing and neurophysiology
Response channel	Psychological research (motivation, association, memory, etc.)

In other words, what are the advantages likely to accrue in speech audiometry, as compared with simpler audiometric tests? The answer is by no means clear-cut, given that speech audiometry is used for a variety of purposes. Partly it boils down to the fact that speech signals, being highly complex, are representative for sounds in daily life, that speech comprehension is an important human faculty in society, that the speech test situation is readily understood by test subjects and finally that the human auditory system is believed to be peculiarly geared to perception of speech. Speech audiometry has, in other words, a very high degree of face validity.

General factors in speech audiometry

Speech recognition scores are affected by a large number of factors, and it is inconceivable that one would ever be able to establish a model dealing with all these. If feasible, such a model could, in an analytic formulation, be stated as:

$$R = f(a,b,c \ldots)$$

where R is the recognition score, and a,b,c . . . represent the different factors. Factors in this context are all parameters that in one way or other affect the result, such as the number of test items (e.g. words) in a list, the number of phonemes per item, the linguistic competence of the listener, and the level and spectrum of background noise. Some factors may be virtually unquantifiable, e.g. the degree of mismatch between the speaker's and the listener's dialect. Consider the following reformulation:

$$R = f(a) \cdot g(b) \cdot h(c) \ldots$$

where one assumes that factors do not interact, and their effects are therefore independent of each other. While this simplification is probably not accurate in detail, the information available at present does not include interactions.

In considering the generation of a new speech test one is, implicitly or explicitly, forced to take decisions on all the relevant factors, and this is of even greater importance when comparing the merits of different tests.

A few preliminary comments on speech perception in general may be useful. Speech perception is here regarded as a pattern recognition process where the listener hears (perceives) certain acoustic cues and selects an 'appropriate' category in which the item 'fits'. Here the operative word is 'appropriate'. Thus this selection is based not only on acoustic/phonetic factors, but also on syntax, semantics and overall context. The choice, in other words, is governed by expectations, and the fewer cues the acoustical image provides, the more do expectations determine the response. It is this effect which can induce a listener to believe that their name has been called out in what turns out to be only ambient noise, one's own name being a stimulus with high expectation. But note that even this strong 'halo' effect may be overridden; in speech audiometry the listener's name is virtually never among the responses given, because they 'know' that in a formal testing procedure this particular stimulus is very unlikely. What constitutes an 'appropriate' response must therefore be seen in the light of all information, explicit and implicit, available to the listener.

Note also that recognition is regarded as a categorization process, thereby implying some underlying continuum, namely the multidimensional set of acoustic parameters. Consider, for instance, the listener engaged in a phoneme recognition task. Within limits, a speaker can vary the articulation of a phoneme but still elicit the correct response. In acoustical terms, one can appreciably vary the parameters (duration, formant frequencies, formant transitions) whilst maintaining the correct response, whereas a larger variation will cause the sound to resemble some other phoneme, and the response to change accordingly. A phoneme therefore corresponds to a subspace of the phono-acoustic space that is needed to describe the stimulus. This is illustrated in Figure 2.2, where for simplicity only two phono-acoustic parameters are included. Whereas each point in the plane in principle corresponds to a particular phone, the listener would, on hearing a phone, categorize it into one of a small set of phonemes (possibly with some ambiguity near the boundaries). In phonetic terms variations within such a subspace are known as allophonic variations, and point towards the important distinction between a phonetic and phonemic description of utterances; the phoneme is an abstract concept, related to semantics, whereas its many possible realizations (phones) are the physical manifestations.

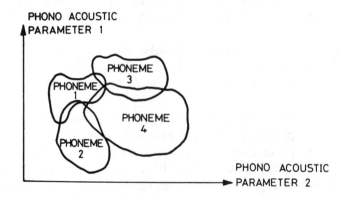

Figure 2.2 Illustration of the phonemic categorization process in speech perception

Factors related to the test material

The test material consists of speech stimuli (items). Whether these items should be described in phonetic or phonemic terms is uncertain. Initially we will therefore consider the phonemic aspects, and subsequently the ramifications of the acoustic realization of the material.

But first a few remarks on the nature of items and lists, and their characteristics. An item is a response-evoking stimulus, typically a syllable, word or sentence. Quite apart from whether we consider the item to be a linguistic element or one of its many acoustic images, the term 'item' is used in a somewhat ambiguous way in the literature of speech tests. In fact it may refer to at least four different concepts, as suggested below:

ELEMENT OF INTEREST (or independent variable). For instance we might be interested in the effect of varying a phoneme, but nevertheless present words (containing the phoneme) to the listener.

STIMULUS ELEMENT. If, for instance, the elements of interest are words, they will occasionally be inserted into sentences (called carrier sentences), whereby the physical stimulus becomes a sentence rather than a word.

RESPONSE ELEMENT. Although frequently the listener is asked to repeat or identify the stimulus as heard, certain experiments will call for other types of response. The example mentioned above might for instance require the listener to respond only with the inserted word, not the whole sentence.

SCORING ELEMENT. Even when the response is in the form of a sentence one may opt to score certain key words only, rather than the whole sentence.

Where these distinctions are of minor importance we shall simply use the word 'item'. Items may be construed as the fundamental unit of speech tests, just as an isolated tone burst is the fundamental unit in pure-tone audiometry. But just as presenting a pure tone once will not yield a statistically satisfactory result; one is forced to present a speech test item again and again until the statistical variation on the compounded score is reasonably low. Unfortunately, repeated presentation of a speech item is not a viable method, because memory effects will render the result meaningless.

The alternative commonly employed is to select a number of *different* items, all within the speech material to be considered, and to present each item of this subset once. If all items are equal with respect to the relevant properties, this subset (list) will yield a compound result (score) equivalent to that which would have been obtained if a single item could have been used again and again (Lyregaard, 1973).

A list is thus the set of items necessary to obtain a stable score for the conditions imposed (e.g. speech level, masking noise). In this respect it is akin to the set of pure-tone stimuli necessary to obtain an estimate of threshold at a given frequency. Because we may want to compare scores for different imposed conditions, several lists may be needed, all with exactly the same properties; thus, irrespective of the particular set of conditions, scores obtained from any of the lists should be equal, save for random fluctuations. In summary, the list concept is based on:

1. Statistical stability of scores (implying that items must be repeated, or a set of items presented).
2. Human memory (implying that items in the list must be different).
3. Interchangeability of lists (implying that lists must have equal relevant properties in all test conditions).

For some purposes these fundamental requirements are supplemented by others, for example, that the speech material should be representative of everyday speech. Given a frame of items and lists as described above, a strategy for filling in the frame (i.e. selecting the items) is needed. This problem divides into two; from which population should the items be sampled?, and which method of sampling should be employed?

Selection of speech material

The type of material to be used would be one of the following, or a combination thereof:

Phonemes.
Syllables.
Words (mono-, bi- or polysyllabic).
Sentences.

These categories are not mutually exclusive, and there may be difficulties in defining their boundaries. It is of importance to bear in mind that the material to be selected is spoken rather than written. The differences between written and spoken English can be rather large, particularly in more colloquial forms, and the syntactic structures proper to written English are often distorted in the spoken language, where prosodic features in part perform the role of syntax.

Selection of speech test material entails consideration of the following factors:

REDUNDANCIES. Phonemes are the least, sentences the most redundant type of item; the less choice among alternatives, the more redundant are the items. This is reflected in the shape of the intelligibility curves for different types of items (Lehmann, 1962), suggesting that the higher the redundancy, the fewer the acoustic cues needed to recognize the stimulus. A test using sentences will therefore partly measure a hearing deficiency at the peripheral level, and partly a combination of linguistic competence and general cerebral function.

SCORING OF RESPONSES. Responses to phonemes, and to some extent syllables, are difficult to score in the absence of a phonemic transcription system familiar to the average patient. At the other end of the scale, sentences are equally difficult to score because a correct response would be one showing that the sentence was understood even though not repeated verbatim, minor errors in adverbs, prepositions, etc. being irrelevant. Attempts have been made to do this in immediate appreciation tests (Richards, 1973) and more oblique scoring methods have been devised in telephonometry, based on the time required for a complete information transfer to be accomplished, e.g. the reproduction, by the listener, of geometrical designs (Richards, 1973).

RELATION TO 'EVERYDAY' SPEECH. There is little doubt that, in terms of 'face validity', sentences (and possibly words) would rank high as prospective speech test material, and that results so obtained would be more easily related to speech hearing performance than would be the case with syllables or phonemes.

TEST DURATION. This plays an important role in clinical audiometry, and in this respect long items such as sentences are inefficient compared with other types of item, for a given target variance (reliability) of the compound test score. In other words, a given number of sentences will require much longer measurement time than would the same number of words, but the information yielded by the test does not increase in the same proportion.

Arguably the most important factor is that of redundancy. As stated by Fry (1961), the more specific the items, the more the test results will be predictable from the pure-tone audiograms, and thus reflect a measure of peripheral hearing. Conversely, linguistic competence and intelligence will substantially affect results of tests using more complicated items such as sentences, and the test will become a measure of both peripheral and central hearing processes. Various attempts have been made to control this redundancy in speech test materials. Telephone engineers, for example, have for a long time used logatoms to test electroacoustic systems. Logatoms are artificial words which, on the basis of their phonemic composition, could well have been meaningful words but in fact are not, at least in the language in question. Examples of the consonant-vowel-consonant (CVC)-C-type are 'GAV' and 'NED'. Quite a different approach has been used for the assessment of room acoustics, using artificial sentences consisting of real words linked together in syntactically satisfactory but meaningless sentences.

In the face of such conflicting requirements most designers of speech audiometry tests have opted for a compromise, in the form of monosyllabic meaningful words (CVC).

Selection of test items

Having selected the type of material, it is then necessary to sample the items actually to be used in the test. Sampling is the principle utilized when one needs to measure a property of a large number of objects (the population), but can only manage to measure a few of them; the technique is to select a few hopefully representative objects such that, if the whole population had in fact been measured, the results would be rather similar to those obtained from the sample. Obviously the larger the sample, the better the fidelity. If one has no prior knowledge of the properties of items in the population, the selection (sampling) should be random, implying that all items have the same probability of being selected. Under these circumstances probable deviations on measures, as compared to the 'true' measures, can be estimated by standard statistical methods. On the other hand, if one already possesses some prior knowledge of the parameters to be measured, a more economical stratified sampling scheme may be adopted, generally leading to the sampling of a subgroup within the population rather than the whole population, but the statistical methods needed to estimate the results and their relation to population values may then not be as simple as before.

In what way does the choice of a particular sampling scheme affect the speech test?

Provided the population to be sampled is reasonably wide, the choice will make little difference to the test results per se, but results will, at least on the face of it, only be valid for the subgroup from which the sampling has been done. (In a series of tests using medical students as listeners and medical phraseology as items, a drastic change of scores occurred once the listeners realized the subgroup from which samples had been drawn (Quist-Hanssen, personal communication). Thus too narrow a sampling can lead to entirely false results.) Thus any imposed phonemic balance scheme will not necessarily affect the scores, but only the validity of these as measures of some general speech-hearing ability.

The purpose for which the test is intended therefore becomes important, and the relevant distinction is primarily between assessment of communication ability and diagnosis. Clearly the sampling aspects as stated above are crucial for speech tests for communication, results from such tests being ultimately used to assess a person's ability to hear and understand a spoken language. By contrast, such considerations are irrelevant for diagnostic speech tests because the merits of tests for diagnostic purposes must be evaluated in terms of ability to differentiate between different disorders. In this case items are to be selected so as to optimize a diagnostic distinction, irrespective of whether they correctly reflect the linguistic/phonetic properties of the parent population from which they are sampled. By way of example, assume that a particular disorder results in poor discrimination of the fricatives /s/ and /ʃ/ (as in SEE and SHE). In this case a sensitive test would consist of items containing a large proportion of fricatives, whereas if items had been selected on a basis of phonemic balance, the fairly small proportion of fricatives would diminish the diagnostic sensitivity for the disorder in question. Thus a good diagnostic test may prove unsuitable for assessing the ability to perceive speech in general and vice-versa.

Although hypothetical, this example illustrates that item selection is linked to the purpose of the test, and that the current practice of demanding phonemic balance in diagnostic speech test materials may well result in a test of poor diagnostic sensitivity. In the following we examine in detail two frequently used selection criteria, namely phonemic balance and familiarity.

Phonemic balance

This is normally, but erroneously, termed phonetic balance (or PB for short). It is realized by a test material having a phonemic composition equivalent to that of everyday speech, that is, the different phonemes should appear in the test material with the same relative frequencies as in everyday speech. The rationale is as follows: if the listener was totally unable to perceive a particular phoneme that occurs infrequently in normal everyday speech, the handicap he/she experiences is not as severe as it would have been had the phoneme been a more common one. In effect one may consider phonemic balance as a weighting:

$$S = W_1 S_1 + W_2 S_2 \ldots + W_i S_i \ldots + W_N S_N$$

where S is the total score, W_i the weighting factor for the i-th phoneme, S_i the score obtained for the phoneme i, and N the total number of phonemes. A score obtained in such a test would be analogous to a cost-of-living index, in that a loss (or price increase) is weighted according to how often it occurs (or how many pence the average family spends on the item in question). A number of points regarding PB should be mentioned.

Although phonemes in context differ markedly in respect of their sequential affinities, PB is normally based on a simple count, as if the phonemes occurred in isolation.

The very strong sequential and semantic constraints in normal words or sentences diminish the relevance of PB. In a way this is fortunate, because PB is not easy to achieve except in submorphemic material.

Phonemic (or phonetic) balance may be thought of as a relation between parent population and test material. In fact the same concept is relevant at the next stage, namely between test material and list. For speech audiometry, test lists are regarded as interchangeable if each has the same phonemic balance. We should term this *phonemic equalization* as opposed to *phonemic balance*. Assuming that the principle of phonemic balance is accepted, there remain two factors to resolve, namely:

Selecting a suitable phonemic alphabet.

Determining the relative occurrences of the phonemes in the parent population.

It may be useful at this point to reiterate the essential difference between phonemic and phonetic elements. Roughly speaking, phonemes are abstract concepts related to semantics; phonetic elements (phones), on the other hand, are articulatory/acoustic manifestations of phonemes. Thus, a particular phoneme can manifest itself as a number of different phones, all of which would be interpreted as the same phoneme. To test whether two phonetically different elements relate to different phonemes, one must insert the two alternatives in all possible words of a language. If, in any word, the substitution of one phonetic element for the other results in a change of the semantic content of the word, the phonetic elements must belong to two different phonemes. Otherwise they would be regarded as allophonic variants of the same phoneme.

A common phonemic inventory is thus a prerequisite for communication, whereas differences in the phonetic inventory, such as are found between different dialects of a language, will not necessarily impede communication. According to our fundamental view of speech perception, it is phonemic rather than phonetic balance that is relevant.

Fortunately this makes for simplification, in that there are far fewer phonemic than phonetic elements to take into account, and a given phonemic balance is likely to yield an effect independent of the listener's dialect. In a given language phonemic elements are common, whereas phonetic elements may vary, for instance on a geographical, demographical or even idiosyncratic basis. If two different languages are compared, both phonemic and phonetic inventories may differ, thus inhibiting international work in this field. In fact the situation can be even more perplexing, as when two phones are phonemically distinct in one language, but not the other. By way of example the words MAN and MEN are readily distinguished by persons whose native language is English but not, for example, if it is Dutch.

The question of a suitable phonemic inventory is not as simple as it may seem. Whereas the consonants are fairly well defined, vowels give rise to considerable disagreement, to some extent related to dialectal differences. Likewise phoneme clusters are subject to arguments, centred on such questions as whether the consonant clusters /ltʃ/ and /dʒ/ should be regarded as a single phoneme or not; whether diphthongs are to be regarded as single phonemes, and if so, how many diphthongs should be included in the phonemic alphabet; whether more complex clusters like /ndl/ as in 'HANDLE' and /str/ as in 'STRUG-GLE' should be admitted.

There is no simple answer to these questions, because phonemes (or rather phones) do not occur as individual units, but in an articulatory or acoustic stream, linked together in such a way that they interact, mainly due to the limitations of the articulatory musculature. This interaction is called coarticulation, and its effect is to smooth out the distinctiveness of phones, thus making the distinction between single phones and clusters a matter of arbitrary decision. Tables 2.2 and 2.3 show a phonemic alphabet found suitable for standard British English (often termed RP, or Received Pronunciation). American English deviates from this in respect of the vowels.

Table 2.2 Frequency-of-occurrence of consonants in British English, from Fry (1947) and Denes (1963)

Consonant	Fry (%)	Denes (%)
n	12.47	11.67
t	10.56	13.84
d	8.46	6.88
s	7.91	8.38
l	6.02	6.08
ð	5.86	4.93
r	5 77	4 56
m	5.30	5.42
k	5.08	4.77
w	4.62	4.23
z	4.05	4.10
v	3.29	3.05
b	3.24	3.43
f	2.95	2.85
p	2.93	2.91
h	2.40	2.75
ŋ	1.89	2.05
g	1.73	1.91
ʃ	1.58	1.16
j	1 45	2 52
dʒ	0.99	0.85
tʃ	0.67	0.61
θ	0.61	0.98
ʒ	0.16	0.08
TOTAL	60.78	60.73

As regards the frequency of occurrence of phonemes there are at least a dozen different counts to choose from, mostly based on American English. A comparison of these counts has indicated that consonant frequencies are fairly stable (Wang and Crawford, 1960), and that vowel/consonant ratios are typically 2/3. Differences in the counts are mainly due to the following:

Different material (conversations, texts, plays, dictionaries).
Exclusion of certain parts of the material, e.g. exclamations, articles).
Dialect in which the material is recorded.
Differences in phonemic inventories.
Random sampling error.

Table 2.3 Frequency-of-occurrence of vowels in British English, from Fry (1947) and Denes (1963)

Vowel	Fry (%)	Denes (%)
ə	27.39	23.03
i	21.24	21.02
e	7.57	7.16
ai	4.67	7.25
ʌ	4.46	4.25
ei	4.36	3.81
i:	4.21	4.55
ou	3.85	4.45
a	3.70	3.89
o	3.49	3.90
o:	3.16	3.06
u:	2.88	3.62
u	2.19	1.95
a:	2.01	1.97
au	1.56	1.97
ə:	1.33	1.70
eə	0.87	1.10
iə	0.54	0.73
oi	0.36	0.22
uə	0.15	0.36
TOTAL	39.22	39.27

Tables 2.2 and 2.3 include two counts of particular relevance to British conditions. Both are based on 'phonetic readers' and southern British English, and they both make use of the same phonemic inventory. One set is based on some 17,000 phonemes (Fry, 1947), the other on 72,210 phonemes (Denes, 1963). Even accepting that such counts are in fact representative of the parent population, practical implementation can lead to difficulties. Consider, for illustration, the construction of CVC monosyllables:

1. The most frequently occurring vowel is the unstressed e (/ə/, as in CONSERVATION), however this vowel is virtually never found in monosyllabic words.

2. The phoneme counts are averages over all words and also over all positions in a word. But in fact the distributions of initial and final consonants are unequal (French et al., 1930), e.g. no English word ends on /h/, or begins with /ŋ/.

3. Given that phonemic equalization of lists is needed, and only a rather limited number of words per list is contemplated (say 10–50), the very infrequent phonemes will not be represented at all. This, however, is probably not a serious problem because PB word scores could be obtained by weighting the responses on individual phonemes in lists with equal distribution of phonemes (isophonemic lists), rather than use PB lists. Using this method each phoneme need in principle only occur once in a list, and all of them could be included.

In conclusion it appears that there is sufficient information available to ensure an approximate phonemic balance of English speech material. However, it is suggested that phonemic balancing is irrelevant for diagnostic purposes, and that its precise fulfilment for communication purposes is questionable, except perhaps for 'nonsense' material.

Familiarity of material

Whereas the question of phonemic balance has little bearing on the actual test, but is possibly important for the interpretation of results, the familiarity of speech material is important for both test and interpretation. The notion of familiarity is rather vague, and implies that the more one is acquainted with a stimulus, the more readily will one recognize it. In order to quantify the familiarity of a word, the assumption is often made that it is equivalent to the frequency with which a person has been exposed to the word, and that this in turn is approximated by the frequency of occurrence of words as found in a corpus of word material, sampled so as to ensure a good coverage of written or spoken material (e.g. Table 2.4).

Table 2.4 Selected word counts in English

Reference		Source	Language	Total Sample
Thorndike and Lorge	(1944)	Literature, magazines, etc.	American	4,500,000
Carrol et al.	(1971)	School texts	American	5,000,000
French et al.	(1930)	Telephone conversations	American	80,000
Howes	(1966)	Interviews	American	250,000

The work of Black (1952), Howes (1957), Pollack et al. (1959), Owens (1961) and Savin (1963) indicates that uncommon words have a lower intelligibility than common words, everything else being equal. The size of the effect, in terms of shift of SRT from common (2000 ppm) to uncommon words (1 ppm), is estimated at 15 dB (Howes, 1957). If, however, subjects are acquainted with the words before or during the experiments, no word-frequency effect is found (Pollack et al., 1959). In the studies cited the measured word-frequency effect has been somewhat confounded by intervening factors. Thus, there is a correlation between word length and word-frequency effect, likewise phonetic similarities between correct and alternative response are of importance.

In practice most speech tests have, to a greater or lesser extent, allowed for the word-frequency effect. Normally very uncommon words are excluded from the test material, and sometimes the very common words are also omitted. In the testing of communication equipment it is common practice to familiarize the listeners with the test material prior to the start of the experiment. Tests based on a forced-choice methodology are insensitive to the word-frequency effect. Although familiarity (or, at least, frequency of occurrence) of the test words clearly has an effect on intelligibility, that in itself is no impediment to diagnostic speech audiometry, provided the effect is equal for all patients. Certain groups of patients (persons with minimum scholastic aptitude, children, and persons for whom English is a second language) will, however, tend to exhibit deviant frequency-of-occurrence effects, leading to depressed intelligibility scores that have no relation to their auditory capacity, and therefore confounding the diagnostic test. The difficulty is largely remedied if lists are composed of fairly common words only.

Selection of speaker

The final factor to be considered in relation to speech material is the speaker. In many ways this is the most difficult to deal with, as it is all but unquantifiable. It is a serious impediment to standardization in that a listener may obtain different scores if the same list is read by two different speakers (Asher, 1958). Probably the best known example of this is the two different recordings of the PB-50 lists, by Rush-Hughes and Hirsh respectively. Not only do these two recordings give significantly different scores for normal listeners (difference 10–20%), but this difference is increased for listeners with sensorineural hearing loss (Carhart, 1965).

Male and female voices are sufficiently different to cause differences in intelligibility scores for the same material and listener, and, as one might expect, such differences are aggravated if the speech signal is low-pass filtered before presentation (Hirsch et al., 1954).

It has been suggested that there is an element of familiarization on score differences due to different speakers; in other words there is a 'tuning-in' period during which one may become accustomed to the peculiarities of a particular voice. A difference has been found where scores obtained with lists read by the same person throughout are compared with scores from lists where each word was read by a different speaker (Creelman, 1957). However, the effect is rather small, consistent with a phonemic rather than a phonetic mode of perception. The problem might be more serious if the speaker and listener have vastly different dialects, although there are ways of overcoming such difficulties. This is achieved merely by recording the material in a 'dialect' typical of broadcasting speakers, and subsequently pruning the material of any items that are sensitive to dialectal differences, either on phonetic, grammatical or semantic grounds. No doubt proliferation of radio and television will gradually erode dialectal barriers, at least for the listener, even though dialects persist in direct communication regionally. Nevertheless full generality is probably not achievable and speech audiometry scores should therefore always be interpreted with caution if the listeners are of foreign origin.

Even a single speaker will not articulate words in precisely the same way on different occasions. Scores obtained by the same listeners, lists and speaker, but recorded on different occasions, yield differences of up to 10% (Brandy, 1966).

Statistics of speech audiometry scores

The purpose of a list in speech audiometry is to provide convenient subsets of the total test material, each allowing the estimation of a score under the specified test conditions. By transmitting different lists at different speech levels one can determine sufficient points to estimate the intelligibility curve, provided the lists are interchangeable.

There remains the problem of deciding how many items, N, each list should contain. Essentially this is trade-off between precision and test duration. Test duration is linearly related to the number of items per list, and the relation between precision and N is found as follows (Lyregaard, 1973):

Assuming, for simplicity, that every word in the list has the same probability (p) of being perceived correctly by a listener, then the intelligibility score (i.e. the number of words perceived correctly) is a stochastic variable (I), the distribution of which is binomial. This distribution is discrete, and, as illustrated in Figure 2.3, the dispersion depends on the value of p. The probability of obtaining a score of S words is:

$$\Pr \{I = S\} = (N/S)\, p^S\, (1 - p)^{N-S}$$

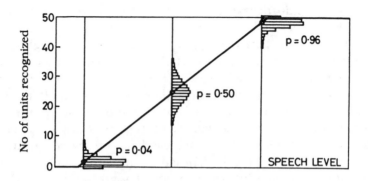

Figure 2.3 Illustration of the binomial distribution of list scores (N = 50)

Figure 2.4 gives the equivalent cumulative distribution for 50-word lists. Although the exact distributions could similarly be derived for lists containing other than 50 words, the method is clearly cumbersome. A closer inspection of Figure 2.4 reveals that, if extreme values of S and p are avoided, the distribution is approximately gaussian (corresponding to straight lines on the plot), with a mean value of n·p, and a standard deviation of $(N·p· (1 - p))^{1/2}$.

This standard deviation is plotted in Figure 2.5, as a function of p. Using the gaussian approximation it is possible to estimate the number of words required to achieve a given precision (Figure 2.6). It is apparent that the statistical fluctuation is quite substantial in speech audiometry, and moreover that fairly long lists are required to bring it down to an acceptable level.

In practice every word in a list does not have the same probability of being recognized, and the simple binomial distribution must therefore be substituted by the more general *subnormal binomial distribution*. In this case a simple analytical expression is not feasible, but it appears (Lyregaard, 1973) that, if the distribution of *probabilities* is not too wide, the dispersion will only be slightly less than the one pertaining to the simple binomial.

There are ways of approaching the statistics of speech test data other than that given above. One such method effectively abolishes the list concept (Barfod, 1973). If test words are selected at random from a large dictionary of words, then the resultant distribution will be strictly binomial, even if the items have different recognition probabilities (Barfod, 1973; Lyregaard, 1973). At present the technical means of presenting words in a random order are, however, not generally available in routine clinical testing.

A good approximation to the variance of the subnormal binomial distribution is given as:

$$V(I) = N[E(p) (1 - E(p)) - V(p)]$$

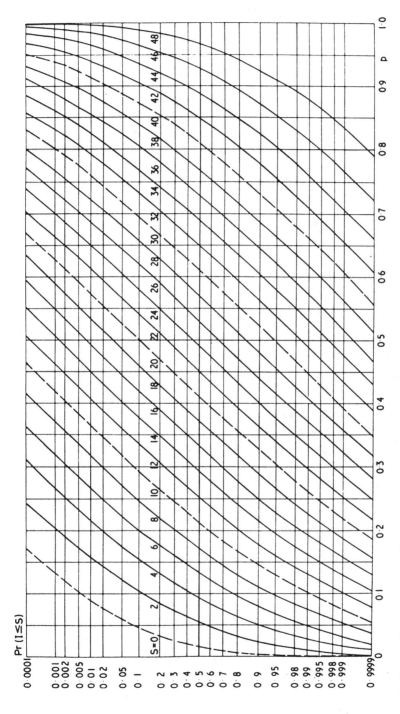

Figure 2.4 Cumulative binomial distribution from N = 50. Note that the ordinate is gaussian. There is for example a probability of 0.1 (10%) of obtaining a score of 20 or less correct words when p = 0.5

QUEEN MARGARET COLLEGE LIBRARY

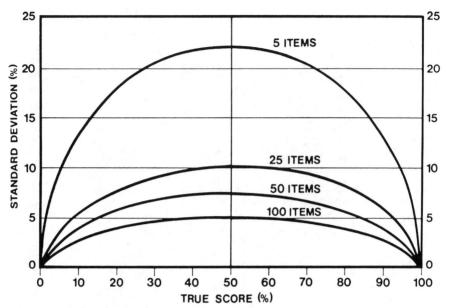

Figure 2.5 The standard deviation of a list score (in %) as a function of the mean score, for various items per list. A binomial distribution is assumed

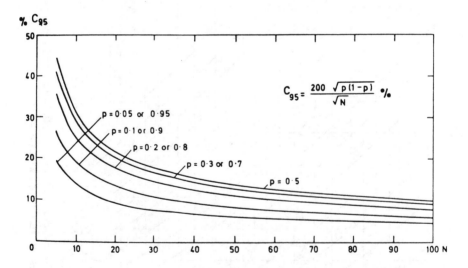

Figure 2.6 The 95% confidence interval (in %) for the binomial distribution, as a function of number of items per list

where E(p) and V(p) are the mean and variance respectively of the probability distribution (Kendall and Stuart, 1958). Clearly a large dispersion of probabilities will tend to narrow the confidence limits; however, this is inevitably accompanied by a loss of information obtained (Lyregaard, 1973). Therefore this method of increasing reliability of scores is not attractive.

However, two other methods are in current use to achieve increased reliability; if the list items consist of monosyllabic CVC words, one might choose to score responses in terms of phonemes rather than words. On the face of it the number of scoring items would be multiplied by three and thus, for the same time and effort, yield a three times smaller variance of the intelligibility score. This interpretation would be correct provided the number of degrees of freedom were in fact multiplied by three, but in general the advantage will be less than threefold due to sequential constraints between phonemes. As an example, take the word MOUTH/mauð/. If the final consonant and one of two remaining phonemes have been determined, only one English monosyllable will fit, and therefore the third phoneme conveys no new information. In this case the number of degrees of freedom is 2 rather than 3. Thus the effective number of degrees of freedom for phoneme scoring is higher than for word scoring, but not as high as the number of phonemes.

Word and phoneme scores will in practice differ, the latter typically being 20% higher, as shown in Figure 2.7.

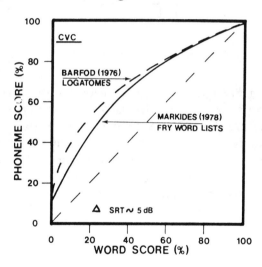

Figure 2.7 Average relation between word and phoneme scores for CVC monosyllables

The primary objective of speech audiometry is usually considered to be the determination of the *recognition curve*. This is conveniently done by determining list scores corresponding to different speech levels, and estimating the curve from these points, as illustrated in Figure 2.8. If the form of the curve were known beforehand, and therefore only a single point were needed to fix its position in the I–L diagram, the list scores could be compounded to yield an uncertainty estimate substantially better than each list score would yield on its own.

If, on the other hand, absolutely nothing were known about the curve, no such improvement would occur. In practice the situation is somewhere between these two extremes, although there is no general agreement on how well the form of the curve is known.

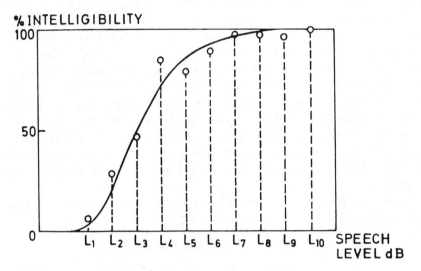

Figure 2.8 Illustration of the speech recognition curve

American practice tends towards considering the curve determined except for two parameters, so that two measurements are sufficient. These measures are the SRT and the maximum recognition attainable, the latter conventionally considered to occur at a speech level 30–40 dB higher than the threshold. European practice favours a determination of the whole curve, thus making fewer assumptions about its form. These assumptions are unfortunately difficult to quantify even for normal hearing. Consider, for example, the most elementary assumptions:

(a) $I(L) \rightarrow 0\%$ for $L \rightarrow -\infty$.
(b) $I(L) \rightarrow 100\%$ for $L \rightarrow \infty$.
(c) $dI/dL \geq 0$.
(d) Absence of 'fine structure', i.e. the curve is 'smooth'.

Here b) and c) are of doubtful validity and certainly violated in sensorineural cases.

This analysis presupposes that the recognition curve is indeed the result we seek to determine. Clearly any decision on the length of a list depends on what one sets out to determine, but having made such a decision, an estimate of reliability, and hence length of test, may be made.

Theory of speech audiometry

Consider the following question: What responses are to be expected in speech audiometry, when words are used as stimuli, and the listeners are instructed to repeat what they believed they heard? Is it perhaps possible to predict the actual responses recorded in speech audiometry, rather than solely how many correct and how many incorrect? If so it might be hoped that deviations from expectation would be of clinical interest, indeed useful in assessing rehabilitational progress, and therefore worth clarifying; furthermore such knowledge would allow one to assemble new word lists according to a clear rationale rather than on the more or less random basis normally adopted. The latter would in turn enable speech materials more sensitive than at present to be assembled, because each single word would be 'pulling its weight' rather than perhaps being redundant.

Table 2.5 tabulates the responses obtained for the stimulus word NUN /nʌn/, in a typical speech audiometry situation involving listeners with normal hearing. All the different responses obtained are listed in the first column, with the responses most similar to the stimulus word at the top, and the most dissimilar ones at the bottom. The five different data columns (A,B,C,D,E) refer to different level and masking conditions; for present purposes they may be considered simply as defining a generalized speech level axis, the level ascending from A to E. At first glance there is not much of a pattern to be seen, but closer examination reveals that, whereas the vastly dissimilar responses occur only at low speech levels, the more similar responses are found at low as well as at high speech levels. This trend is generally seen in all speech audiometry data, and the pattern of probabilities of words being responded, vs. speech level, is as shown in Figure 2.9. At high speech levels, 100% correct responses are obtained (disregarding distortion effects at excessively high levels, or a sensorineural hearing impairment), and as the level is decreased a few error words start intruding, these tending to sound fairly similar to the stimulus word. As the speech level is decreased further, more and more different words occur, and these tend to have less phonetic similarity to the stimulus word. At very low levels one approaches a condition of random choice amongst a very large number of alternatives, most of them without much resemblance to the stimulus word. The latter does, however, assume that listeners are forced to respond; failing that the probability of not getting a response at all will quickly dominate.

A few other observations concerning word response patterns are worth noting. Whether or not the listeners are instructed in what type of material to expect, their responses will nearly always be of the type used. In other words, if the words presented are monosyllabic, the responses will be predominantly monosyllabic words, even if listeners

ers are asked to respond to just that part of the word they actually heard. Furthermore responses will seldom if ever include uncommon words. Finally, in using monosyllabic words, it is observed that errors in one of the consonants are much more frequent than errors in the vowel.

Table 2.5 Responses to the word 'NUN', classified according to the type of phoneme error (column 2), the bottom two rows indicate no-response and total number of responses respectively

Response	Type			Group		
		A	B	C	D	E
NUN	111	2	11	5	3	5
NUMB	110	1	1	2	3	–
RUN	011	2	4	3	–	–
HUN	011	–	1	–	–	–
ONE	011	–	1	–	–	–
NINE	101	–	1	–	–	–
NOW	100	–	1	–	–	–
AGAIN	001	1	–	–	–	–
BONE	001	–	1	–	–	–
LINE	001	–	1	–	–	–
MUM	010	–	1	2	–	–
COME	010	–	2	–	–	–
YOUNG	010	–	–	1	–	–
LUNG	010	–	–	1	–	–
LOVE	010	1	–	–	–	–
ENOUGH	010	1	–	–	–	–
RUNG	010	1	–	–	–	–
THUMB	010	1	1	–	–	–
DRUG	010	1	–	–	–	–
UP	010	1	–	–	–	–
DANCE	000	–	1	–	–	–
LONG	000	–	2	–	–	–
ROW	000	1	–	–	–	–
FILL	000	1	–	–	–	–
WRONG	000	2	1	–	–	–
LAMP	000	1	–	–	–	–
MORE	000	–	2	1	–	–
–	–	5	2	1	–	–
		22	34	16	6	5

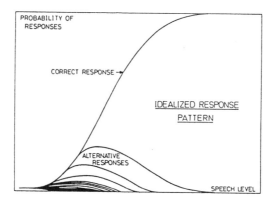

Figure 2.9 Illustration of the pattern of correct/incorrect responses, as a function of speech level

To generalize these observations based on experiments conducted with monosyllables, errors in speech audiometry seem to have the following properties:

They nearly always have the same number of syllables as the stimuli.
They tend to be phonetically similar to the stimuli, particularly at high speech levels/favourable listening conditions.
They are meaningful words, and predominantly common ones.
Consonants are more easily missed than vowels.

It therefore seems that the probability of word B being mistaken for word A depends on (a) how common word B is, (b) how similar words A and B are phonetically and (c) whether word B is a viable response word, given the knowledge the listener has regarding the test.

All these effects are well-established in the literature, but, with a few exceptions, they have been investigated separately, although they will always coexist. A suitable model must take them all into account.

The model

For a given listener and a given recorded word material, presented in fixed acoustical conditions, the probabilities of different responses are conveniently described by a word confusion matrix (WCM) as shown in Figure 2.10.

This matrix gives the probability of obtaining a response W_j for the stimulus W_i. As we shall mainly consider the free-response situation (which is the most normal in speech audiometry, but unfortunately also the most difficult to deal with theoretically), W_j may be any conceivable word, whereas W_i is restricted to the words contained in the word material. If we can assume that the probabilities are time-invariant and

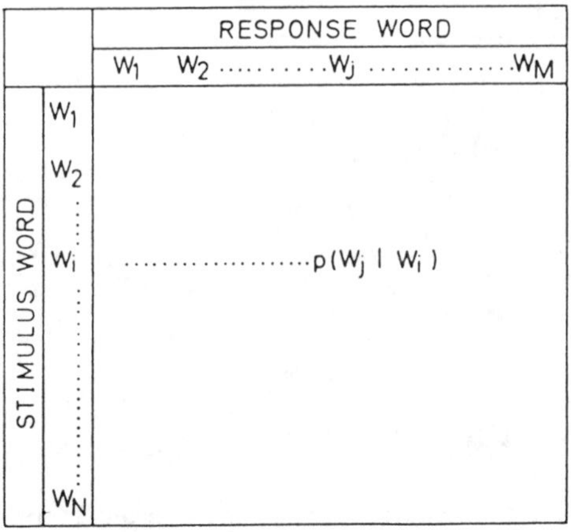

```
              ┌──────────────────────────────────────┐
              │              RESPONSE  WORD           │
              │  W₁   W₂ ........ Wⱼ ............ Wₘ   │
```

WORD CONFUSION MATRIX

Figure 2.10 Word confusion matrix (WCM), indicating the probability of word W_j being responded when the stimulus is W_i. The WCM depends on the test conditions, particularly the speech level

statistically independent, the WCM furnishes a complete description of the speech audiometry test (Lyregaard, 1973). Obviously the probabilities are normalized, hence:

$$\sum_{j=1}^{M} p(W_j \mid W_i) = 1$$

and the expected (i.e. mean) test score is:

$$E\{1\} = \sum_{i=1}^{N} p(W_i \mid W_i)$$

However, bearing in mind that the number of response alternatives is in principle equal to the number of words in the English language, this probability matrix is too large to be of any use, let alone to be determined experimentally. Therefore simplification is called for, and it is proposed to consider only monosyllabic words, both as stimuli and responses. To simplify the problem further we will consider each probability as a product of three independent probabilities:

$$p(W_j \mid W_i) = \alpha(W_j \mid W_i) \cdot \beta(W_j \mid W_i) \cdot \gamma(W_j \mid W_i)$$

where α reflects the influence of acoustic factors, β the linguistic factors and γ the phonetic factors. Briefly they may be described as follows:

α is the probability of obtaining a response at all, and depends therefore on such acoustic factors as speech level and/or signal-to-noise ratio, but also on the methodology. Thus in a forced-response situation α will always be unity. In the free-response situation it will depend on the speech level and thus the stimulus word in question, but not on the response word. In fact we hypothesize that it will be equal to the psychometric function of the word, regarding the word as a physical stimulus (i.e. the probability that the listener will hear the word). The α-curve therefore depends on the definition of speech level. Indeed, one might argue that an optimum method of measuring speech level in speech audiometry is one that ensures that α is similar for all words.

Just as α takes account of the response probabilities in respect of the acoustic characteristics of the stimuli, ß deals with the linguistic properties. Words (at least in one's native tongue) are perceived as entities rather than on a phoneme-by-phoneme basis. Therefore recognition may be regarded as a matching of the incoming acoustic/phonetic pattern with stored word images, and the question of which images are available, and even how available they are, becomes important. The availability or expectation is accounted for by ß, and it may be thought of as the probability that a given word appears as response in the limit where no input stimulus at all is presented. Clearly the expectation is affected by any explicit or implicit limitation of choice, and in this sense ß depends on the method used. Even if two words were both allowed as responses, and they were exactly alike in terms of acoustic/ phonetic features (as could be achieved with homophones such as BEAR and BARE), we would not expect their probabilities to be equal. This has been described as the frequency-of-occurrence effect, which asserts that, on average, uncommon words have a lower probability of recognition than common words. Evidently ß will depend on the response word and the listener, but not on the stimulus word or speech level. Experiments with the frequency-of occurrence effect seem to suggest that listener-to-listener differences are not large and we shall therefore, as an approximation, disregard listener variations. The estimation of ß can then be based on frequency-of-occurrence data (Lyregaard, 1976), as shown in Figure 2.11.

The γ-factor describes the phonetic similarity (and thus the 'confusibility') of the stimulus and response word. As it depends on both stimulus and response it forms a matrix of the same dimensions as the WCM. However, by introducing the following simplifications: (1) that phonetic similarity is the same as phonemic similarity, meaning that the abstraction of a word can be considered rather than its physical manifestation, and consequently that speaker-to-speaker variations may be disregarded, and (2) that consideration can be limited to monosyllabic stimuli and responses of the CVC-type, one can write:

$$\gamma = p(W'|W) = p(C'_1 V' C'_2 | C_1 V C_2) = p(C'_1 | C_1) \cdot p(V'|V) \cdot p(C'_2 | C_2)$$

on the assumption that the latter probabilities are uncorrelated. Due to well known sequential constraints (Shannon, 1948) this assumption may not appear warranted; however, since a large proportion of phoneme combinations do not form meaningful words in English, their contribution to the overall phoneme correlations may be disregarded if only meaningful responses are considered.

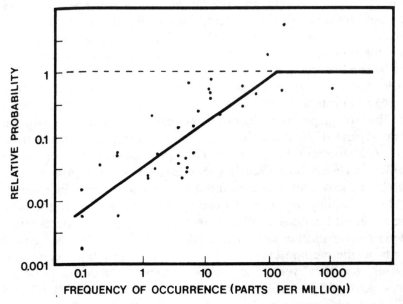

Figure 2.11 Estimate of ß, based on the frequency of occurrence of words. Data obtained in an open-choice speech audiometry test using homophones (Lyregaard, 1976)

The simplification achieved by the delineation above is substantial, as the phoneme confusion matrices are of a manageable dimension (typically 20×20). But some difficulties remain, for instance the extent to which consonant clusters should be regarded as single phonemes; also vowel probabilities are intrinsically higher than consonant probabilities, due to the higher speech level of vowels relative to consonants. These problems are tractable, but further experimental evidence is necessary in order to resolve them.

Interpretation of model

Although some of the factors still remain to be quantified, it is possible to consider implications of the model qualitatively.

Free response

If the stimulus is a common word (high ß), and there are no other common words nearly similar to it, then the intelligibility curve of this word will approximate the psychometric function (α). In fact the psychometric function is the limiting curve for any recognition curve, and if all words in a list approximate it we should expect a good agreement between average pure-tone thresholds and SRT.

If, on the other hand, there are many alternatives with a high degree of similarity to the stimulus, and especially if the stimulus is an uncommon word, pure-tone audiometry and speech audiometry results will not agree. In other words the α-curve describes the intelligibility when the only possible response is the stimulus word, and the extent to which this curve deviates from the actual recognition curve is an indication of the number and degree of 'intrusion' of erroneous responses. It is precisely this deviation which the ß-and γ-factors describe, and which accounts for the difference between pure-tone and speech audiometry. The excess loss of recognition is not due to the listener not hearing the word, but due to their confusing them with likely alternatives.

Forced choice

Here the model is simplified because both α and ß are constant (the listener is forced to respond, and the alternatives are known). Therefore a forced choice technique will essentially limit speech audiometry to depend on the phonetic factor. Here the form of the recognition curve for each item, and thus for the whole list, can be dramatically modified simply by manipulation of the alternatives/foils allowed.

Limited free response

An explicit or implicit limitation of acceptable responses will change the listener's expectations, thus ß for response words outside the limits will be zero. The net effect is a shift of the recognition curve towards lower speech levels (nearer to the α-curve), a shift that is observed when for instance digits are used as words.

Discussion

Pending experimental evidence, the ramifications of the model presented here can be summarized as follows, bearing in mind that only CVC-monosyllables have been implicated.

It provides a framework for a rational interpretation and comparison of different methodologies, and an understanding of the results obtained. Because responses are, in a statistical sense, predictable, there is a vast fund of information available in speech audiometry, namely the deviations from predicted errors in response. This information is even available in currently used tests without extending the test duration, but it is at present discarded.

In assembling new speech audiometry materials, or modifying already existing ones, the model allows one to select words such that error intrusion is controlled, thereby ensuring that the words have a prescribed distribution of correct-response probabilities. In particular it is possible, without resorting to extensive experimental work, to ensure approximately equal probabilities throughout the list, thereby avoiding words that do not contribute any information to the list scores. The model is particularly useful in selecting foils in the forced-choice method; without having to resort to experimental work one can predict the most probable alternatives, and thus ensure a maximally sensitive test.

It seems plausible that auditory disorders may be interpreted in terms of the factors of the model. Thus a conductive hearing loss will only affect α. A sensorineural loss may be interpreted as consisting of a conductive loss component and a 'distortion'; whereas the former only affects α, the latter will only implicate γ. Whether or not specific types of 'distortion' lead to specific confusion patterns remains to be investigated; if it were so, more discriminating speech tests would clearly be feasible. The ß-factor is implicated in cortical disorders such as aphasia and to some extent in presbyacusis.

The model also has good prospects for the difficult question of international standardization of speech tests. The main problem here is to ensure that materials prepared in different languages are in fact equivalent, and this could be managed by specifying the probability factors discussed here. Such specifications could then be translated into words and word lists in each language. Such an approach is still some way off, but certainly appears to be feasible.

Chapter 3
Speech tests in quiet and noise as a measure of auditory processing

MARK E LUTMAN

Understanding of speech is fundamental to verbal communication and depends on many characteristics of the auditory system. This chapter aims to describe the more important aspects of auditory performance which are necessary for satisfactory speech processing and how these are affected by hearing impairment. The chapter also outlines methods which are commonly used to assess speech intelligibility in the individual and how the measures thus obtained may be used to estimate the disability or handicap experienced.

A model of speech processing

The ability of the ear to unravel the complexities of speech depends on many aspects of hearing, including sensitivity as measured by the pure-tone audiogram. Much interest has been focused on the role played by *frequency resolution* (the ability of the ear to detect a target signal at one frequency in the presence of a competing sound at a different frequency). Some of this research is reviewed briefly in a later section in this chapter. Information has also become available to implicate *temporal resolution* (the ability to resolve detail in the waveform envelope of a signal), *suppression* (the increase in threshold at one frequency due to presentation of a sound at an adjacent frequency) and *intensity discrimination* (the ability to distinguish between two similar sounds at different intensities). It is known that all of these properties of audition are influenced adversely by hearing impairment, particularly of the sensorineural type.

In order to develop a tractable model of speech processing, Plomp and Duquesnoy (1982) have simplified the above by lumping all of the above characteristics, other than sensitivity, under a category termed *distortion*. Their model expresses speech performance in terms of different levels of sensitivity and distortion. A series of experiments were undertaken to validate the model in which speech intelligibility was measured at various intensity levels. The measure of speech intelligibility they used was the speech intensity required for 50% correct score on sentences when presented together with a competing noise. Measurements were made at various noise levels in order to plot the speech level as a function of the noise level. Using decibel scales, if the speech were to be correctly identified at a constant signal-to-noise ratio (SNR), the plotted function would be a straight line with a slope of 45 degrees. Figure 3.1 illustrates the form of the relationship that was found in four groups of subjects categorized respectively as (i) normal sensitivity, normal distortion, (ii) normal sensitivity, increased distortion, (iii) reduced sensitivity, normal distortion and (iv) reduced sensitivity, increased distortion.

All of the curves are flat at the left-hand side. This is due to the effect of absolute threshold. Obviously, the speech must be above absolute

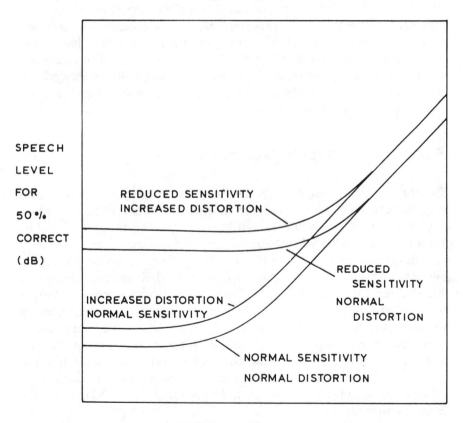

Figure 3.1 The form of relationship found in four groups of subjects when categorized by sensitivity and distortion

threshold to be heard, independent of noise level, and the speech levels at which the flat portions of the curves occur are strongly influenced by threshold sensitivity.

Once the noise level exceeds a certain point, the curves increase in slope to the predicted 45 degrees. The effect of distortion in both sensitivity groups is to uniformly shift the curves upwards by a few decibels. Expressed in another way, increased distortion results in an increase in the SNR required for correct identification, regardless of intensity level. Notice also that the curves of groups (i) and (iii) and of groups (ii) and (iv) converge at the higher intensities. Thus, at high intensities the only determinant of speech intelligibility is distortion; sensitivity is not a factor as long as the speech is audible.

Relationship between speech intelligibility and pure-tone sensitivity

The model described above was obtained under experimental conditions using subjects who had been selected to form discrete groups for the purpose of the study. Such neat groupings seldom occur in practice and there is a wealth of data on speech intelligibility in which the effects of sensitivity and distortion were hopelessly confounded. In the vast majority of studies, no measures of distortion had been made, but it is well established that most aspects of distortion are correlated with sensitivity. Typically such studies have measured speech reception threshold (SRT) and/or discrimination score (DS) for speech-in-quiet, although a smaller number have used speech-in-noise. Noble (1978) has extensively reviewed this literature. As a very general rule fairly high correlations have been found (circa 0.8) between SRT and auditory sensitivity and slightly lower correlations (circa 0.7) between DS and sensitivity. Best correlations with SRT are generally obtained when sensitivity is averaged over frequencies in the 0.5–4 kHz range.

When speech is presented with noise, the correlations tend to be somewhat lower (e.g. Festen and Plomp, 1983; r = 0.38) but not in all studies (e.g. Tyler and Smith, 1983; r = 0.84). Presumably the direct effect of sensitivity is removed for speech-in-noise and the correlation reflects an indirect relationship mediated through distortion.

The relationship between speech intelligibility and sensitivity has been used as the basis of formulae for predicting speech performance from the pure-tone audiogram. Much attention has been focused on the relative weights that should be attached to each audiometric frequency in the formula, although such an exercise can be misleading. The frequencies that correlate best with the speech identification scores are highly dependent on the test materials used (frequency spectra of speech and noise) and may not be the same for different materials, as pointed out by Haggard et al. (1986). For example, if all subjects had noise-induced hearing losses, there would be little variance in sensitivity at 500 Hz amongst the subject group, leading to a low correlation between speech performance and sensitivity at 500 Hz.

Studies of self-reported speech disability in the general population are not prone to the same biases and Lutman et al. (1987) suggest that the actual choice of frequencies in the range 500 Hz to 4 kHz in a prediction formula does not influence its accuracy very much. Averages including sensitivity at 500 Hz, however, were very slightly better correlated with self-reported disability than those composed only of the higher frequencies.

Relationships between speech intelligibility and measures of distortion

Several studies have shown that frequency resolution is related to speech test performance (e.g. Leshowitz, 1977; Bonding, 1979; Dreschler and Plomp, 1980). With respect to temporal resolution, Tyler et al. (1982) have shown an effect, whereas Festen and Plomp (1983) did not. In all studies of this type, subjects tend to vary in auditory sensitivity, frequency resolution and temporal resolution, as well as in age, and all of these factors tend to covary. Therefore, it is extremely difficult to identify whether one parameter is fundamentally related to speech performance, or simply varies with another parameter that is fundamentally related (so-called collinearity).

Lutman and Clark (1986) have attempted to account for such collinearity and have shown that in hearing aid users with sensorineural hearing impairment, age and sensitivity at 2 kHz are sufficient to account for the variation in performance in a speech-in-noise task, without the necessity to include frequency and temporal resolution measures. This does not mean that the distortion parameters are unimportant; rather, that they can be predicted by the measurement of sensitivity. A factor that has not been investigated adequately is the dependence of the form of any relationship between distortion measures and speech performance on the severity of the hearing loss. It might be expected that different factors would be important in normal and mildly impaired subjects than in moderately or severely impaired subjects. In fact (Lutman, 1987) suggest that frequency resolution is the major factor for mild impairments; and sensitivity at 2 and 4 kHz and temporal resolution are most important for moderate impairments.

Effects of type of hearing loss on speech discrimination

The dependence of speech-in-quiet and speech-in-noise scores on pure-tone sensitivity and measures of distortion has already been described.

A further factor is whether the hearing loss is primarily conductive or sensorineural. From a database of conventional speech-in-quiet test results, Gatehouse and Haggard (1987) obtained word identification scores for a heterogeneous clinical population with sensorineural, conductive and mixed hearing losses. They derived iso-performance contours plotted against axes of mean air-conduction threshold and mean air-bone gap. For a given air-conduction threshold, increasing air-bone gap was associated with poorer performance at all but the highest intensities used for speech (i.e. peak SPLs of 95, 100 and 105 dB). Thus, the presence of a conductive impairment led to worse discrimination for a given air-conduction hearing loss when the speech was at low and moderate speech intensities. It was only at speech intensities at and above 95 dB that sensorineural losses exhibited worse discrimination.

These authors argue that their findings result from recruitment in the sensorineural cases which has the beneficial effect of conferring greater loudness on supra-threshold signals, compared with non-recruiting ears having equal loss of sensitivity at threshold. At the very high intensities (and as a consequence of the speech audiometry procedure, predominantly in the more impaired ears), the greater distortion accompanying a sensorineural impairment becomes the over-riding factor.

Effects of age and socio-economic group

It is normally extremely difficult to separate the effects of age and socio-economic group on speech test performance from the effects of hearing loss, since they tend to be heavily confounded. However, there are indications that age and manual vs. non-manual occupation per se have effects in the expected direction (greater age and manual occupation associated with poorer performance), as described by Davis (1983).

Summarizing the information presented so far, it can be stated that sensitivity and distortion factors interact in a complex fashion to determine speech intelligibility. Sensitivity measures alone can predict speech intelligibility nearly as well as a combination of sensitivity and distortion measures, although the predictive accuracy is not high, particularly for speech-in-noise. Other parameters not included under the umbrella of sensitivity and distortion also affect intelligibility, such as type of hearing loss, cognitive factors and aspects of central processing including those reflected by age. Thus, there is a need to measure speech performance directly which cannot be met by other tests of auditory dysfunction.

Objectives of speech testing

Theoretically, it is possible to design speech tests to measure any specific aspect of auditory processing. However, other than those used for diagnostic purposes, speech tests are generally intended primarily to be representative of everyday speech used for communication and the tests aim to give an indication of disability. Studies of the relationship between self-reported disability and speech tests have often found a poor correspondence, even when using speech-in-noise tests which would suggest themselves as preferable to speech-in-quiet tests for this purpose. Nonetheless, speech testing gives the most practicable performance measure of disability and avoids the difficulties, inherent in self-report methods, of personal opinion and bias.

The use of speech-in-noise tests has an additional advantage over speech-in-quiet tests when testing a heterogeneous population of subjects. The SNR of the test can be set to achieve a suitable range of scores in advance. This means that the absolute level of the materials can be set at a moderately high intensity which is easily audible to all subjects (within reason). In this way, it is possible to reduce or avoid the problems of 'ceiling' and 'floor' effects where the score obtained by a subject is curtailed by the 100% or 0% absolute limits available.

Choice of materials for assessing speech processing ability

Some experimental studies of communication systems or speech processing have used isolated phonemes or nonsense syllables. These items have the advantage of minimal semantic content, thus effectively eliminating differences between subjects in education and vocabulary. However, it requires considerable training to achieve stable performance on the tests and they are not really suitable in a clinical context.

At the other extreme, running speech contains all the semantic, contextual and prosodic features of everyday speech and therefore has great face validity as a material for disability measurement. Nonetheless, it also requires some training for the subject to repeat running speech and it is difficult for the tester to score responses accurately. The most common compromises used in practical clinical tests are lists of either single words or sentences. The latter have greater external validity for representing everyday situations, but they are more difficult to incorporate into tests because of the limitations imposed by grammar and syntax. Also, sentence materials tend to have a steep psychometric function (i.e. the curve relating score to intensity or SNR). This latter characteristic makes sentences more suitable for a speech-in-noise task where the SNR can be pre-set to a level that achieves the desired level of performance and avoids 'ceiling' and 'floor' effects.

Word lists are not subject to the influence of cognitive factors in the subject's use of context and syntax to determine the correct response, as are sentences. This may be an advantage or disadvantage, depending on the purposes of the test. For all types of materials, the efficiency of the test depends on the relative difficulty of items within the test. Ideally, all items should be equally difficult and therefore none will be redundant. Clearly, if an item is significantly easier than others, it will nearly always be identified correctly by all subjects and thus not contribute any information. A corresponding effect occurs if an item is relatively more difficult than the remainder. A great deal of pilot work is necessary to obtain an efficient set of materials that are appropriate to the subjects with whom it is intended to use the test. Speech-in-noise tests require the selection of a suitable noise. In general, this should have significant energy at all frequencies present in the speech signal. Typically, a noise may be generated to have a frequency spectrum which approximates the long-term spectrum of the speech. Alternatively, the voice of another speaker or several speakers may be used. When speech from several speakers is amalgamated to form the noise it is referred to as 'speech babble' or 'cafeteria noise'. When the speech signal and noise have different frequency spectra it is difficult to define the SNR in any meaningful way. For example, if the difference in dB between the overall level of the signal to the overall level of the noise is taken, this may differ quite markedly from the SNR in any specific frequency band. It is usually the most advantageous band signal-to-noise ratio that determines intelligibility, and thus the overall SNR may not relate at all well to intelligibility. Because speech is a spectro-temporal code, containing information in both the frequency and the time domain, the temporal structure of the noise is also a factor. Steady noise is less likely to mask the amplitude modulations of speech than a noise with similar amplitude modulations to those in speech. Therefore either 'babble' or amplitude modulated noise tends to have a greater masking effect than steady noise. Furthermore, modulated noise has a relatively more deleterious effect on intelligibility than steady noise in subjects with a sensorineural hearing loss (Tyler and Smith, 1983). These authors also showed that a sentence-in-noise test using modulated noise was more highly correlated with self-reported disability than the same sentence lists, against a background of steady noise with the same frequency spectrum as the modulated noise.

Whatever speech or noise materials are used, calibration and setting of levels is extremely important. For speech-in-noise tests, variations in SNR of as little as 1 dB can have marked effects. Therefore, accurate documentation of the levels used for each subject is essential. It is most important that descriptions of SNR define exactly what has been measured as there are no accepted standard methods available. More specific details of equipment and calibration are covered in chapter 5.

Method of subject response and scoring

For identification tests, the subject may simply repeat or write down what they have heard. In clinical practice it is common for the subject to repeat what they have heard and for the tester to score the response. This means that the tester must be able to hear the subject clearly, either directly or using a microphone/amplifier system. Scoring (and instructions to the subject) must take account of the possibility that subjects may be lax in their use of plurals or tenses in their reply, even though they may have correctly understood the item.

When the speech test offers a limited set of alternative responses (e.g. four alternatives in a four-alternative-auditory-feature (FAAF) test), scoring may be by pencil and paper using a pro-forma worksheet completed either by the subject or the tester. In the latter case, given that the alternatives in such closed set tests usually sound very similar, there is a possibility of the tester mis-hearing the response. Alternatively, electronic or computer-recorded scoring using push-buttons may be used. Clearly, closed set tests in this general format require that the subject can read, although an equivalent two-alternative-picture-pointing version has been used for children.

Adaptive speech-in-noise tests

It is virtually impossible to design a fixed SNR test that will cater for a wide range of patients without ceiling or floor effects. For example, using the SIiN test that involves sentences against a background of noise, an SNR that gives scores in the region of 80% in normal ears is unusable in patients with hearing impairments greater than about an average of 45 dB because they score less than 20%. Increasing the SNR would cause some of the normal subjects to reach the ceiling of 100%.

One method of overcoming this problem is to adjust the SNR adaptively during the test to achieve a predetermined level of performance (e.g. 50% correct or 71% correct). This approach has been used conventionally for speech-in-quiet tests to measure the SRT. For speech-in-noise, Plomp and Mimpen (1979) have developed a test that uses a fixed level of noise. The signal is composed of Dutch sentences that are presented initially at a relatively high intensity. If the subject repeats the sentence correctly, the speech intensity is reduced. When a mistake is made, the speech level is increased. This procedure continues and it is possible ultimately to estimate the intensity at which a 50% correct score is reached for the given noise level. Thus, the outcome measure is the SNR for 50% correct.

A similar principle is used in the adaptive version of the FAAF test that involves a closed set of single syllable words, each trial having four alternatives. The adaptive test has been described by Lutman and Clark (1986) and involves a fixed level of speech and a variable level of noise, both speech and noise having the same long-term frequency spectrum. The criterion level of performance can be pre-set, levels of 50 and 71% being used in practice.

In general, adaptive speech-in-noise tests have the advantage of widespread applicability in a clinical context and some control of error patterns and would seem to be a favourable choice for assessment of speech processing ability.

Error patterns

For most speech tests, it is possible to score the type of error as well as simply whether or not the item was identified correctly. For example, the error might be plosive instead of fricative, as in 'pan' instead of 'fan'. Tests such as the FAAF have been designed to contain specific contrasts between alternatives within a single trial and therefore give the opportunity to test for specific error types. Thus, scoring of the test can be focused on analysis of the error patterns as well as the overall performance. These data can be used to infer how information from different regions of the frequency spectrum is being used.

In general, errors of place of articulation (e.g. the contrast between 'gay', 'day' and 'bay') are sensitive even to mild hearing impairment or noise masking. Place of articulation information is carried predominantly in the higher frequencies. Manner of articulation (e.g. the contrast between 'tick', 'lick' and 'pick') and voicing (e.g. 'bay' vs. 'pay') are relatively robust. As a consequence, in speech-in-noise tests, subjects scoring highly will probably be making only place of articulation errors, whereas those scoring poorly will be making all types of error. An advantage of adaptive testing when comparing individuals is that subjects will all tend to be making similar error types. The disadvantage is that this limits further analysis of error type.

Lip reading

Hearing and lip reading are elegantly complementary (Summerfield, 1983). The place of articulation information in speech (e.g. 'gay', 'day', 'pay') which is so easily removed by hearing loss or masked by background noise is most easily inferred from lip reading. Additionally, the timing information obtained from a combination of lip reading and hearing provides extremely useful (audio-visual) cues, as exemplified by the relative onsets of lip opening and voicing in 'mole', 'bole', 'pole'.

Audio-visual tests involving lip reading are difficult to devise for a heterogeneous population because they are extremely prone to floor and ceiling effects.

Despite these difficulties, audio-visual tests of speech identification have seemingly a high face validity for disability assessment, but require further research to support this contention.

Practical speech tests

The following are some of the speech test materials used in the UK that are potentially available for measurement of speech processing using English (not American) speakers.

Speech-in-quiet

Arthur Boothroyd word lists (Boothroyd, 1968). Fifteen lists of 10 consonant- vowel-consonant (CVC) words isophonemically constructed. Normally scored as phonemes correct out of 30. AB(s) recordings have 'standard British southern' pronunciation using a male speaker.
BKB sentence lists for children. Twenty-one lists of 16 sentences, each list containing a total of 50 key words to be scored. Restricted to vocabulary of partially-hearing children (Bench and Bamford, 1979). Recorded by female speaker with southern English accent.

Speech-in-noise

Sentence-identification-in-noise SIiN. Based on BKB recordings against modulated noise. Noise has the same long-term spectrum as speech and is modulated with the same amplitude envelope.

Two example sentences from the SIiN test follow. Scoring is based on key words which are in capitals (based on BKB word lists).

The BATH TOWEL was WET
The MATCHES LIE on the SHELF

Four-alternative-auditory-feature (FAAF) test. Four-alternative-forced choice test based on a vocabulary of 80 CVC words in 20 sets of four, composed like rhyme tests on the binary feature principle. Items presented in the carrier phrase 'Can you hear . . . clearly' and against a steady noise background with the same long-term frequency spectrum as the speech. Male speaker with resonant voice and 'standard British southern' accent. Scoring may be total correct or by error types. Computer program assists in analysis of error types.

Two example trials from the FAAF test follow.

BAD	BAG	BAT	BACK
GAB	DAB	TAB	CAB

Two-alternative-picture-pointing tests. Described by Haggard, Wood and Carroll (1984). Recording of 48 CVC words, against a background of steady speech-spectrum-shaped noise, by a female speaker with a north Midlands regional accent using vocabulary of 24 minimal pairs, each pair differing only in the initial phoneme. Illustrates corresponding to the 48 words allows forced-choice picture-pointing response suitable for use with 5-year-old children. Scored as percent words correct.

Audio-visual tests

Four-alternative-disability-and-speechreading-test (FADAST). Similar in principle to the FAAF test, but recorded on Sony U-matic video cassette and displaying head and shoulders of speaker. No carrier phrase is incorporated, but visible cues warn of onsets of words. Four alternative responses also displayed as caption and differ in vowel as well as either initial or final consonant.

Two examples from the FADAST follow.

HEEL	SEAL	HAIL	SAIL
SUCK	SUNG	SACK	SANG

Chapter 4
Speech tests as measures of auditory processing

STUART GATEHOUSE and KEN ROBINSON

Speech is an acoustical signal which carries its information via a rapidly changing relationship between frequency, intensity and time. The normal auditory system contains the inherent ability to identify, process and code these salient cues. It of course follows that any degradation in the auditory system's ability to perform these functions may lead to a decline in the hearing impaired listener's ability to understand speech in certain listening situations. This chapter aims to review our current understanding of the impact of hearing impairments on our ability to understand speech, and considers the properties that speech material and a speech test should include when its primary aim is to assess the level of and improvements in hearing impaired speech identification abilities. This, by the nature of the exercise, cannot be realistically divorced from the application to which the practitioner aims to direct the speech assessment procedure.

Determinants of speech processing ability

Over the last decade or so, the audiological literature has seen attempts to describe and determine the ways in which various aspects that accompany sensorineural hearing impairment can affect the ability of a hearing impaired listener to process speech. The most obvious way in which this can occur is by a loss of access of the system to speech information due to a loss of threshold sensitivity — that is, parts or perhaps all of the speech signal may simply not be audible. Where the decrease in audibility overcomes the high redundancy in speech (which certainly predominate for favourable listening conditions), then a decrease in speech identification performance will be observed.

To a very good approximation it is likely that, for a simple attenuation (that is, a pure conductive hearing loss), then the loss of speech information will be directly and simply related to the level of hearing impairment as a function of frequency. Because of some of the non-linearities which accompany a sensorineural hearing impairment this relationship may be more complex (Gatehouse and Haggard, 1987), with an abnormal growth of loudness above threshold (clinically referred to as *recruitment*) potentially leading to an increase in the information available to a sensorineural hearing impaired listener compared to an equivalent conductive hearing loss. However, it is well established that the distortions which usually accompany a sensorineural hearing impairment (in terms of the auditory system's abilities to process cues located in both the frequency and time domains) are material in the presence of such an impairment. The debate that has occurred concerning the relative impact of such factors in relationship to the impact of losses of audibility has been intense but ultimately relatively uninformative. For example, the simplified model of speech processing put forward by Plomp and Duquesnoy (1982) with its attractive formulation of a component of loss of sensitivity and a component of distortion has not necessarily resolved matters.

Other experimenters have attempted to assess the validity of this model via the relative contribution of audibility (Humes et al., 1986; Dubno et al., 1989; Wilde and Humes, 1990; Humes and Roberts, 1990). The fundamental problem arises because of the high correlation between the non-linear distortions that occur in sensorineural hearing loss and the degree of the sensorineural hearing loss itself. Thus it has been extremely difficult to decouple the different components from the model and to document the extent to which the distortion component of Plomp's model determines performance for listeners with sensorineural hearing impairment. It is certainly the case that even from the most fervent adherents of such a model, the measures of the distortion component are modest when decoupled from the impairment level.

This should in no way be taken to undermine the importance of these distortions, but rather to highlight the sterility of the debate, because of their high correlations with measures of loss of audibility via the audiogram itself. In theory, it would be possible to conduct experiments to compare the residual speech identification abilities under a variety of conditions in a group of normal hearing subjects and in a group of sensorineural hearing impaired subjects for whom the 'losses of audibility' had been perfectly alleviated — assuming of course that one knew how to achieve such alleviation in the presence of a non-linearity such as abnormally rapid growth of loudness. It should be noted that the early experiments which attempted to overcome problems with lack of audibility merely by raising the level of all of the frequency components of speech were unlikely to achieve their aim because of the way in which a sensorineural hearing impairment (and its supra-threshold decrements in loudness) varied as a function of frequency.

Audibility of speech

If measures are taken of an individual's ability to understand a speech signal in quiet or a speech signal in noise, there will be some degree of correlation with the pure-tone audiogram (the threshold sensitivity of the system), which would appear to be able to range from high values, particularly in quiet, to lower values when the speech is presented in a background of noise. A large part of these variations can be regarded as purely procedural, resulting from the conditions of presentation, the levels of presentation, the frequency spectra of the speech and the variance in the sample of the thresholds that are used to perform the correlations (see e.g. Haggard et al., 1986). The audiological literature has again seen a somewhat unproductive debate as to the combination of frequencies from the clinical audiogram which can be best used to correlate with, and therefore predict, speech identification abilities. Because of the procedural effects, these are always unlikely to generalize across subject samples and different speech materials.

Speech is a signal that changes rapidly in intensity, frequency and time. For any given speaker in a particular listening environment, speech may be characterized by its average level in dB sound pressure level (SPL). This is the average root mean square level at which speech is heard at any given distance from the speaker. It is generally accepted that normal conversational speech in a quiet background achieves a level of some 60 to 65 dB SPL at a distance of 1 m from the speaker and that this may range in intensity from 50 to 80 dB SPL over a range of quiet to loud speech for different communication circumstances. Thus the average level over which a listener (and hence a hearing aid) could be reasonably expected to perform could range on average from 50 dB SPL to approximately 80 dB SPL, though this of course will depend upon individual speakers and listening circumstances.

It is also important to realize that for example while average conversational speech may achieve an overall level of some 62 dB SPL, for any given speaker this is only an average level, and an utterance such as a sentence will contain some elements which are louder and some elements which are quieter than this overall average. It is usually accepted that across a range of speakers, the peaks in speech can be some 12 dB greater than the average and the quieter components of speech some 18 dB less than the average. Thus for any given range of speech, the individual elements can vary by some 30 dB. Table 4.1, columns 2–5 (computed from Pavlovic, Rossi and Espesser, 1990) show the contributions of the different frequency bands to speech at a variety of overall levels (vocal efforts). It can be seen that speech has greater intensity at low rather than high frequencies. The table also shows the

Table 4.1 The distribution of energy as a function of frequency for a number of vocal efforts and the relative importance of frequency bands to the intelligibility of conversational speech

Frequency band (Hz)	Overall level 63 dB SPL (normal effort)	Overall level 68 dB SPL (raised effort)	Overall level 75 dB SPL (loud effort)	Overall level 82 dB SPL (shout effort)	Band importance for average speech
	Mean dBSPL	Mean dBSPL	Mean dBSPL	Mean dBSPL	
100–200	31	34	34	28	0.01
200–300	34	38	41	42	0.02
300–400	34	38	43	47	0.03
400–510	34	39	44	48	0.04
510–630	33	39	45	50	0.04
630–770	30	37	45	51	0.04
770–920	27	35	43	51	0.04
920–1080	25	33	42	51	0.04
1080–1270	23	32	41	49	0.05
1270–1480	22	30	39	49	0.05
1480–1720	20	28	37	47	0.05
1720–2000	18	26	35	45	0.06
2000–2320	16	24	33	43	0.07
2320–2700	13	22	30	40	0.07
2700–3150	12	21	29	39	0.06
3150–3700	11	19	27	37	0.06
3700–4400	9	16	25	34	0.06
4400–5300	5	12	19	29	0.06
5300–6400	3	9	15	25	0.05
6400–7700	1	6	12	22	0.02
7700–9500	0	3	9	18	0.00

effect whereby, as an individual raises vocal effort (remember that one reason for raising vocal effort will be increases in background competing noise), the increases in the low frequency energy can be relatively modest, while increases in high frequencies can be observed in an attempt to make sure that the relatively less intense high frequencies are not physically masked by the more intense low frequencies.

So far, this discussion has concentrated purely on the physical distribution of the elements of speech without any consideration of their contribution to intelligibility. Speech is made up of different phonetic and phonemic structures, some of which can be thought of as relatively low frequency, relatively intense elements (e.g. vowel sounds), and others which can be characterized as relatively less intense, relatively high frequency components (such as consonants). Unfortunately the information content of speech does not equate directly with the energy content of speech, and in particular the high frequency less intense consonant sounds can be of greater importance for understanding speech than the relatively less intense lower frequencies. This is also illustrated in Table 4.1, column 6 (from Studebaker, Pavlovic and Sherbecoe, 1987) which shows the band importance to the understanding of speech of the different frequency components for an average conversational speech over a number of speakers and number of different languages. The table illustrates quite clearly that speech contains important information for intelligibility at frequencies, say, above 4 kHz which are not usually considered important for hearing aid fitting. Certainly, when frequencies in the 2–4 kHz region are taken into account, the band importance functions show how much of the speech signal is likely to be degraded by inattention to the high frequency components. This consideration of the physical properties of speech in terms of its distribution as a function of level and frequency and the importance to speech intelligibility of different frequencies has important consequences for the effects of a sensorineural hearing loss, first on the audibility of speech and second on its intelligibility.

These considerations concerning the range and spread of intensities and frequencies contained in a speech signal lead directly to an understanding of how different configurations and degrees of hearing loss can affect the understanding of speech. It becomes evident that relatively small deficits at the high frequencies can lead to parts of the speech spectrum not being available to the impaired auditory system, and that as the overall level of the hearing loss increases for conversational speech, a hearing loss of 45 dB HL leads to substantial elements of the speech spectrum, including the more intense low frequencies, becoming unavailable.

At this point it becomes possible to construct a rule for the major role of a hearing aid and that is to 'make the speech spectrum to the largest possible extent available to the impaired auditory system without being uncomfortably loud'. There are a number of aspects to this rule that deserve consideration. The first of these is, what is 'the speech spectrum?' Different individuals will experience different auditory environments and hence will place different demands upon the auditory abilities. It is normal in considering hearing aid fittings to take the speech spectrum at normal conversational speech levels, usually around 65 dB SPL. However, it is certainly the case that the auditory range of acoustical stimuli will be outside this, and this has implications for more detailed fitting of hearing aids both in groups and across individuals which will be considered later in the chapter.

The second point of consideration is the amplification that is required to make the speech audible, but not uncomfortably loud. It would be relatively easy to prescribe (and using modern technology to deliver) amplification that makes the entire speech spectrum above threshold. However, it is an almost inevitable consequence of sensorineural hearing loss that, while thresholds are elevated, the ear suffers from what is commonly termed 'clinical recruitment'. This is an abnormally rapid growth of loudness such that, while substantial deficits at threshold may be present, the upper end of the dynamic range (often characterized by the threshold of uncomfortable loudness) is elevated only marginally, if at all. Thus there is a limited dynamic range available, into which the speech spectrum can be mapped. It then becomes the task of the hearing aid, having identified the speech spectrum of interest, to provide sufficient amplification to convert the speech spectrum from below threshold to the range of audibility without reaching uncomfortable listening levels.

Earlier in this chapter we considered the degree to which a speech spectrum might be above threshold and the relative importance of the different frequency bands in speech. It is possible to combine these considerations into a single number called the *articulation index*, which varies from 0 to 1. An articulation index of 0 indicates that none of the speech spectrum is available to the auditory system, while an articulation index of 1 indicates that all of the speech information is available for processing by the auditory system — i.e. this is a measure of audibility of speech. Note that the articulation index is not a measure of the intelligibility of speech. Audibility is concerned with how much information is available for processing by the auditory system, intelligibility is the degree to which the auditory system can make use of the information. The articulation index has a history of application to both hearing aid selection and evaluation (Studebaker, Pavlovic and Sherbecoe, 1987; Pavlovic, 1988, 1990; Berger, 1990; Fabry and Van Tasell, 1990; Rankovic, 1991) and in its later manifestations contains many elements appropriate to sensorineural hearing loss, such as masking of one speech band by another and distortions due to excess amplification.

Although still in its infancy as a detailed evaluation tool, the aided articulation index as a single simple outcome measure in the performance domain could find application in clinical practice. Although the articulation index has its critics on theoretical grounds (such as inclusion of group data to derive some of the modifying weights such as measures of upward spread of masking, desensitization, etc.) it has been shown to perform well across large numbers of subjects and offers a degree of face validity and freedom from procedural effects that simple relationships to pure tone sensitivity lack. Given the increasing emphasis in audiology of measures of suprathreshold function as opposed to measures of performance at or close to threshold (which might bear little relationship to everyday performance) there is a case for the wider use of such concepts. The ready availability of small scale computing systems would suggest that the arithmetical overheads of taking on the increased complexity of computation are unlikely to be an overwhelming burden.

What the articulation index model attempts to measure is the extent to which the information in a speech signal is available to the impaired auditory system for further processing, and the ways in which losses of sensitivity can impact upon that. There are few people who will attempt to argue that each and every auditory system (be it from a normal hearing subject or from an individual with sensorineural hearing impairment) contains the same inherent ability to process the cues that are presented to it. Therefore, workers have concentrated on extensions of the audibility model which attempt to identify factors (often labelled 'proficiency factors') associated with processing ability that can encompass other aspects of auditory performance (perhaps based on temporal processing) or may derive from the individual's underlying linguistic skills. Such extensions are of some theoretical interest, but for information to be applied to clinical populations are as yet insufficiently stable and sensitive. It is argued here however that the concepts underlying the articulation index procedure and the ways that it can be applied to speech materials with different spectral and phonetic loadings and presented at different levels from different speakers can and will find ready application in clinical settings.

Applications of speech measure to diagnosis and management

While there will remain diagnostic applications of behavioural tests in audiology, this chapter suggests that the emphasis on such applications will continue to decline as further imaging and electrophysiological techniques for functional assessment are developed. This chapter suggests therefore that the primary applications of speech testing in audiological practice will concentrate on the assessment of communication problems experienced by hearing impaired listeners, and the extent to which a management or intervention has been able to overcome those problems. Thus ideally a speech test aims to assess auditory disability and the extent to which that disability has been reduced by intervention.

Choice of speech materials

Natural speech usually occurs during a discourse between two individuals, and in such circumstances the length of a speech message is usually at least at the sentence level. Few conversations consist of the exchange of monosyllabic words. Thus the objectives of our testing drive the choice of speech material towards procedures which attempt to be as relevant as possible, and to mimic as many of the characteristics as possible, of natural conversation. Such circumstances of necessity become difficult to control, difficult to standardize and may as a consequence lack the analytical balance and power that, for example, single word or nonsense syllable presentations contain. Thus there is a tension between the desire to perform a test that is as 'relevant' or as 'natural' as possible, and the desire to perform a test that provides as much useful information as possible. It is because of these competing requirements that the number and types of speech test have blossomed over the years. This review does not attempt to identify individual tests but rather classes of tests, and to point out some of the potential advantages and disadvantages of these.

At one end of the continuum it is possible to construct a speech test employing stimuli consisting of a series of nonsense syllables with a construction of vowel-consonant-vowel (for example, the utterance ABA). One such test in use in the UK is the 12 intervocalic consonant test (EPI Group, 1986). There can of course be many such utterances that can be constructed to have specific phonemic confusions which are known to load upon particular speech contrasts, which themselves may be known to require particular frequency and/or temporal information. At this analytical end of the spectrum it is usual to present a particular speech item and to offer the subject a number of potential response alternatives, thereby enabling the experimenter to analyse the types of phonemic errors that a subject might make.

Such an assessment can be extremely powerful in attempting to determine an individual's specific auditory abilities. For example a new type of hearing aid which attempts to provide usable information from 6 to 10 kHz may be under assessment. The speech test can then be configured to provide phonetic contrasts and confusions that require the information between 6 and 10 kHz to be available to the listener and to be processed by them. Thus such an assessment procedure could determine (a) whether subjects can make use of the information in the 6 to 10 kHz region and (b) what are the subject characteristics and hearing aid fitting procedures that can capitalize on this. Of course, the weakness of such an approach lies in the fact that making the 6 to 10 kHz band available to the listener may have little or no impact upon their auditory disability and handicap in everyday life.

Moving further along the continuum from 'analytical' to 'real', we now encounter the use of single word tests. These themselves can take a variety of forms but usually divide into open set tests (where the subject is presented with a single word and is asked to identify that word, usually by repeating it) and words which come from a closed set (which, as in the previous example, can contain specific confusions). An example of the former is the set of ABS word lists used in clinical speech audiometry in the UK (Boothroyd, 1968) and an example of the latter is the four-alternative-auditory-feature (FAAF) test (Foster and Haggard, 1979) which carries the predominant consonant confusions of the 12 intervocalic consonant test (EPI Group, 1986) forward to single words, and embeds them in a carrier phrase. Thus even within a single word test, choices can be and have to be made concerning the degree of analytical complexity.

As the complexity of the speech message is allowed to increase, the next step is to encounter sentence material. In sentence testing, the subject's task is usually to repeat back what is heard, and then according to a particular scoring scheme a number of key words in the sentence are scored as either correct or incorrect. Because of the very nature of sentence materials, they are more problematic to standardize for equal difficulty, and because of their greater linguistic relevance are less likely to be able to be repeated at regular intervals. They do however offer the distinct advantage that they can give some global measure of a hearing impaired individual's ability to integrate all of the aspects of auditory ability into a single measure of performance, with some potential relevance to functioning in everyday life.

There are of course many variants on sentence material that aim to include some of the advantages of both lower level analytic procedures, and the more realistic aspects of disability. For example Hagerman and Kinnefors (1995) have constructed sentence material that is derived by rotating a closed set of key words and is therefore potentially reusable without the necessity to generate large bodies of sentence material for which large scale normalization data is required for their validity to be assured. In North America, sets of sentences have been constructed (the SPIN test; Kalikow, Stevens and Elliot, 1977) for which the last word in the sentence is either highly predictable (HP sublists) or has a low predictability (LP sublists) from the preceding carrier phrase, whilst containing the same phonetic difficulty across the lists, in an attempt to include at least some aspects of non-auditory (perhaps linguistic) abilities into the assessment procedure (see e.g. Schum and Matthews, 1992).

Individuals concerned with the assessment and management of profoundly deaf patients (often those who participate in cochlear implant work) have attempted to move beyond the sentence level and to assess the extent to which an intervention or device can be used to facilitate communication (which in this particular application would probably include information available from lip reading). Although the literature on connected discourse tracking (where the procedure measures the rate at which information can be transferred from the speaker to the listener) has identified a number of methodological problems, it is likely that, with technological advantages to control and standardize the modes of speaking and the repair strategies available, these procedures will become more robust. However, at present their application has been mainly restricted to individuals with severe and profound impairments, although extensions into hearing aid selection have been studied to some degree (Cox and McDaniel, 1984).

There has, however, been a recognition that there is potentially more to understanding speech than measures of simple segmental intelligibility, i.e. how many syllables of a word, words in a list, or words in a sentence the subject is able to identify and repeat. Gatehouse (1993) has argued that an important component of auditory disability can be regarded as the listening effort that a subject has to expend to do the decoding that leads to correct identification of a speech signal. This effort will depend on the nature of the hearing impairment and on listening conditions. There have been attempts by investigators (see e.g. Baer et al., 1993; Gatehouse, 1994) to use response times to determine 'ease of listening'. Here the rationale is that the more rapidly one performs a task, then the more easily one has achieved the endpoint — thus shorter response times will indicate greater ease of listening and therefore reduced perceptual effort.

These investigators have argued that this approach not only offers the possibility of making components of speech more audible to hearing impaired listeners, but may also lead to a reduction in the amount of effort that they have to expend to identify speech. Certainly, at an anecdotal level, hearing impaired subjects often report exhaustion and tiredness at the end of a day during which they have had to 'listen hard' for some reason or other. An example which is perhaps closer to home arises from the use of second languages. Those readers who have a second language (however imperfect their schooling in it may have been) will be well aware of the difficulties and degree of concentration that are required when they find themselves overseas.

Although the application of such response time measures is in its infancy, there is some evidence (Baer et al., 1993) that such measures can distinguish between various hearing aid processing strategies that are difficult to separate on the basis of simple segmental intelligibility, and also that measures from response times (Gatehouse, 1994) show superior correlations with aspects of self-reported disability and handicap than do measures of simple segmental intelligibility.

Adaptive testing and testing in noise

Most hearing impaired listeners (certainly those with mild and moderate impairments) are able to function quite well in circumstances where the acoustical conditions are well managed — usually where the background of noise is not excessive or the environment excessively reverberant. When individuals present for management they usually complain of difficulties in noise. While deficits in quiet for realistic levels of conversational speech can be demonstrated when people present for management (hearing impaired individuals usually overcome such difficulties by manipulating the acoustical environment to the detriment of family and friends), current generations of hearing aids are usually successful in providing enough of the (highly redundant) speech signal so that speech identification abilities in quiet for hearing impaired listeners are returned close to those levels enjoyed by normal hearing listeners.

Thus speech tests in quiet are often inadequate and insensitive measures of the relative efficacy of different management options. While current generations of hearing aids are of limited effectiveness in backgrounds of noise, they do provide some benefits, and it remains a goal of audiological management to provide superior benefit in listening circumstances with competing noise. Thus the addition of a noise background to a speech signal as part of a test procedure aims on the one hand to overcome the ceiling effects of testing in quiet (where all subjects can do rather well once audibility has been compensated for), and on the other hand attempts to set up the assessment for management under the circumstances in which the listener is having the most difficulty.

The choice of noise can be important, and again there is a tension between noise backgrounds that have a highly deterministic structure and can be analytically controlled, and those which are more representative of everyday listening environments. If the choice leans towards the analytical end of the continuum, it may be required to assume rigorous control over the spectrum of the noise (perhaps equating it with the either long or short term spectrum of the speech signal) and the temporal properties of the noise (should it vary coherently or incoherently with the speech signal), whilst towards the 'realistic' end of the continuum the competing noise might take the form of other talkers (e.g.

babble) rather than a signal with highly deterministic properties. Again the decision has to be taken on the basis of the objectives of the testing (for a more complete discussion of competing noise structure see Cox et al., 1991; Cox, 1993).

Adaptive testing has a long history of providing robust tractable information for audiological testing (see e.g. Levitt, 1971) which might not be available using a method of constant stimuli, in which the presentation conditions are fixed and performance is expressed as percentage correct, etc. In adaptive testing the conditions are manipulated (usually either the signal level is increased or decreased, or the noise level is increased or decreased) so that performance at a particular level is ascertained (often at the 50% level via a one-up, one-down tracking procedure, or at the 70.7% level via a two-up, one-down tracking procedure).

One of the potential advantages of adaptive testing is that it is less open to the floor and ceiling effects observed when testing under fixed conditions, when the range of hearing impairment in the subjects to be tested is substantial. For example, it would be difficult to configure a presentation level and fixed presentation of signal-to-noise ratio appropriate for both individuals with normal hearing and for those with 70 dB hearing loss, without producing a situation in which normal hearing listeners score almost perfectly and individuals with 70 dB hearing loss score either zero or at chance. It should not however be assumed that adaptive testing can always overcome such floor and ceiling problems, because some of the considerations regarding the audibility of the speech signal in the first instance may come into play. If the speech signal is substantially inaudible then improving the signal-to-noise ratio will not improve performance past a certain point. However, with the advent of more readily available computer systems and programmable equipment for experimental control, the more robust nature of adaptive testing is becoming available in many clinical and evaluation settings.

Principles underlying the choice of a speech test

It would be theoretically possible to take each of the sets of speech materials and procedures currently available for either clinical or research purposes and to evaluate the utility of each for a variety of purposes. However, such an exercise would rapidly become outdated and would be relatively uninformative about the underlying principles that lead to such decisions. The final section in this chapter attempts instead to establish a number of principles that should be borne in mind when attempting to select a set of speech material for a particular purpose. These criteria are predominantly concerned with the assessment of speech materials for the evaluation of the impact of hearing impairments and of the extent to which these impairments can be alleviated by suitable management, but could be generalized to other applications such as diagnostic strategies, if required.

The speech material should be configured in terms of its acoustic and phonetic content to be appropriately sensitive to the impairments under study.

This may seem an obvious point. A test might be appropriate for the assessment of the impact of mild high frequency hearing impairments upon speech perception abilities (examples here could be the FAAF test (Foster and Haggard, 1979) or a nonsense syllable test such as those developed in North America, for example, Levitt and Resnick, 1978; Dubno and Dirks, 1982; Humes et al., 1987). Here the material is constructed to rely upon speech contrasts that revolve around consonant comparisons, which are known to lie predominantly in the less intense high frequency areas of the speech spectrum. However sentence material which was loaded heavily on vowel identification might well not be appropriate and could well prove insensitive to the impairment of interest. It cannot be assumed of course that a sensitive test for one purpose is a sensitive test for another.

A further example could be the assessment of candidates for stapedectomy and the benefits of intervention, where the primary impairment consists of a predominantly low frequency conductive hearing loss. Here the FAAF test that was previously appropriate for the assessment of high frequency sensorineural hearing impairment would be quite inappropriate. Given that it is maximally sensitive to thresholds in the 2 to 4 kHz region it would not necessarily distinguish between a 35 dB low frequency conductive hearing loss and a 65 dB low frequency conductive hearing loss. The material only varies predominantly in the initial or final consonant with little or no information on discriminating power carried by the root vowel.

When assessing an intervention, the speech material should have acoustic and phonetic content which is appropriately sensitive to the form of the intervention.

This is an extension of the previous criterion. It would obviously be highly inappropriate to assess the impact of a hearing aid intended to amplify the speech frequencies between 5 and 10 kHz using material which was predominantly constructed of, and sensitive to, the frequencies below 2 kHz. A null result is almost guaranteed. However, inspection of the literature on using speech tests as evaluation tools yields many examples of the use of insensitive and inappropriately structured experiments which, while not as extreme as the above example, do follow its logical thread.

Given the experimental design and an effect size that it is desired to assess, the speech test should be capable of detecting such an effect size in the requisite number of subjects.

This is a general design principle that is accepted by everybody in the research arena. However, when configuring tests for clinical practice or in the evaluation of devices in field trials, little attention may be paid to the discriminatory power of the speech material under consideration (contributions elsewhere in this volume outline some of the statistical and experimental considerations which underlie the concept of discriminatory power, and a useful review may be found in Lipsey, 1990). This is a particularly severe limitation when in clinical practice the number of subjects under study is, in fact only one, and hence the requirement is to assess the success of management or the relative success of alternative managements in a single individual. In an apparent paradox, the demands of a clinical test are in fact much more stringent than those of a research based environment, where group data may be sufficient to answer the question of interest rather than attempting to identify an optimal management for an individual.

The speech material, any competing noise, and presentation level should be sufficiently representative of everyday acoustical conditions.

It is possible to identify highly artificial and stylized speech assessment procedures for use in the laboratory whose relationship to hearing disabilities and handicaps in everyday listening circumstances is either unknown or unlikely to be appropriate. If the aim of a laboratory assessment (whether it is for clinical practice, evaluation or research purposes) is to derive a surrogate measure of impact upon everyday auditory function, then it must be demonstrated that the speech assessment procedure, and any changes in the performance of the speech assessment procedure, should bear at least some relationship to appropriately structured measures of disability and handicap in everyday life. This does not of course mean that the speech test can only be validated against any self-report system, rather that the self-report system must itself be appropriately structured — an absence of a correlation with a particular hearing disability handicap scale does not necessarily invalidate the speech material.

The acoustical and procedural aspects of the speech material should be sufficiently specifiable as to allow replication of the results on different sites.

This is a general principle of experimental and clinical design but nonetheless worth restating given the wide divergence of presentation conditions, spectra, etc., used in current practice.

Conclusion

This chapter has attempted to outline some of the shifts in current thinking concerning the assessment of the auditory system's ability to process speech, with particular regard to their application in the assessment of degradation in performance following a sensorineural hearing impairment, and the degrees to which this may be alleviated by forms of management. It is the authors' belief that if the requirements of clinical practice impose time limitations, for example if only some 10 minutes can be devoted to the acquisition of speech identification measures, then surrogate measures of audibility are likely to provide as much information of a potentially more robust nature than specific speech tests, given the variability in speech measures and the time that has to be devoted to their acquisition if stable and sensitive results are required.

Chapter 5
Equipment for speech audiometry and its calibration

TIM SHERWOOD and HILARY FULLER

Introduction

The basic requirements for speech testing are a source of speech, a means to control the level of the speech received by the patient and a record of the patient's response. At its very simplest level, a test may be performed by asking questions in a quiet, a normal or a loud voice, to which a patient will provide an appropriate answer if enough is heard for the question to be understood. Such a speech test has many uses, but it does not warrant the name 'speech audiometry' since there is too little control over both the level of the speech reaching the patient and the amount of the stimulus which has to be understood for a response to be made.

The term 'speech audiometry' is reserved for a test in which a representative sample of speech is presented to the patient under measurable conditions and the response is given in a form which indicates how much of the stimulus has been understood. In speech audiometry, it is necessary to be able to measure the stimulus, to measure the response and to relate the two to those of normal hearers and to groups with known pathologies. At all stages the emphasis is on control, measurability and reproducibility.

It is because of the need to measure and control the stimulus that, whether for live-voice testing or for tests using pre-recorded material, speech audiometry usually makes use of an audiometer or an independent amplifier to feed the stimulus signal to the patient via earphones or a loudspeaker.

Figure 5.1, derived from Lyregaard et al. (1976), shows the information flow in a speech audiometry test in which the result is a recognition curve constructed by comparing the stimuli and responses at different measured levels of presentation. The choice of equipment to perform such a test is wide and its selection will often be determined by what is

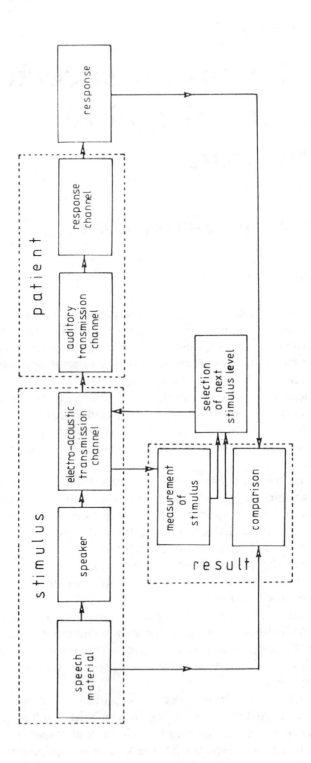

Figure 5.1 Information flow in a speech audiometry test

already available. Some of the considerations that might play a part in equipping a speech audiometry test facility are outlined here together with the measurements and calibrations which are needed to ensure that the test results have meaning and can be compared with those made at other centres.

Work through the IEC Electroacoustics Working Group on Audiometers has provided equipment standards for pure-tone audiometers (IEC 645 Part 1, 1992) and more recently speech audiometers (IEC 645 Part 2, 1993). IEC 645 Part 1 details the requirements for pure-tone audiometers in terms of the performance of each component module. Many of these modules are common to speech audiometers but speech as a signal source is not specified within this part of the standard. IEC 645 Part 2 specifies the requirements for an audiometer where speech is used as a signal source (to avoid duplication this part only lists the required clauses from IEC 645 Part 1), but does not specify the speech material to be used for test purposes or the required acoustic properties of the test room.

The Medical Devices Directive 93/42/EEC came into effect on the 1st January 1995. If an audiometer meets the requirements of IEC 645 it will in the main meet the 'Essential Requirements' of the Directive. The areas of difficulty are those with EMC and potential cross infection from transducers.

IEC 645-1 Clause 5.4.5.1 gives requirements for EMC which are not in keeping with the current generic EMC requirements. The measurements required in IEC 645 were introduced at a time when little was known about generic methods of testing for EMC. Audiometers present special problems in terms of EMC measurements due to the length of the transducer leads and the very low signal voltages at the output of the audiometer. In view of this it has been proposed that instead of measuring the immunity of audiometers, the environment in which they are used should be specified. This would compare with the requirements for maximum background noise levels in audiometry.

Audiometers

Many audiometers are designed so that they can be used for speech tests as well as for pure-tone audiometry. If this is the case the audiometer will be equipped with a wide-band masking facility and a speech or audio channel which will accept the signal from a tape recorder or microphone.

The masking is used to ensure that when one ear is tested, there is no significant contribution caused by a more sensitive non-test ear picking up the test signal by bone conduction or cross hearing. The noise provided will consist of weighted random noise having a spectrum level that is constant from 100 Hz to 1 kHz and a fall of 12 dB per octave from 1 kHz to 6 kHz cutting out the unnecessary energy at the high frequencies. For research purposes, a masking noise is sometimes used which conforms exactly to the spectrum of the voice speaking the test words, but the use of such masking requires non-standard equipment and for most applications the broad-band masking noise facility built into audiometers is quite adequate.

The calibration of audiometers should form an important part of the routine of any test centre. Although a full workshop test, adjustment and re-calibration of the equipment will be necessary if the audiometer develops a major fault, routine checks and calibrations should be made in the clinic at regular intervals. If the audiometer has to be sent out of the clinic to the manufacturer or to a specialized laboratory for routine calibration, the inconvenience is likely to prove a substantial barrier to this important activity. It would be a great advantage, therefore, if each clinic had either the equipment necessary to carry out its own audiometer calibrations or had access to a mobile calibration service visiting at regular intervals.

Since speech audiometry is usually carried out using a facility on a pure-tone audiometer, all of the checks recommended to ensure that the audiometer is working correctly are applicable to the speech audiometer. Some of these checks should be carried out at weekly intervals (or more frequently) and do not require any specialized equipment. For example, the audiometer and its ancillary equipment can be checked visually for any signs of damage or wear, ensuring that the correct earphones are used with the audiometer and that they and their headbands are in good condition. Recommended procedures for routine checks and subjective tests on pure-tone audiometers are given in Annex E of the OIML document R104 (1992) all of which are applicable to speech audiometers. Making use of the fact that one of the best means of checking the audiometer is the audiologist's own ears (if they are normal), the output of the audiometer can be checked approximately by listening to all frequencies at a hearing level of 10 dB or 15 dB.

Listening at high levels, all of the functions of the audiometer, including the speech circuits, can be checked to ensure that there are no distortions, clicks etc., whilst listening at low levels the equipment can be checked for hum and for breakthrough between channels. It is also possible to check the quality of the tones and speech signal, which should not change when masking is introduced, and the attenuators, which should operate over their whole range without introducing mechanical or electrical noise.

Objective calibration of the audiometer, which does require special equipment, should ideally be carried out every 3 months and should comply with IEC 645 Parts 1 and 2. The minimum equipment which would be needed is as follows:

- Precision sound level meter (IEC 651 (1979) Type 1).
- Octave or 1/3 octave filter set.
- IEC 318 artificial ear or IEC 303 reference coupler (dependent on type of earphone used).
- Appropriate measurement microphone (IEC type WS2P or type LS1P).
- Mechanical coupler (artificial mastoid) only required for bone conduction measurements.
- Digital frequency meter (audio frequency range).
- Oscilloscope.

The aspects of the audiometer performance which should be measured, include the frequencies of the pure-tone signals, the output of the earphones and bone vibrators, the levels of the masking noise, the attenuation steps and the harmonic distortion of the whole system. For speech audiometry, the accuracy of the level indicator should also be checked, together with the performance of any ancillary equipment such as a tape recorder. Table 5.1 lists the British Standards and their IEC and ISO equivalents which are relevant for the calibration of audiometers.

Table 5.1 Standards relevant to the calibration of audiometers used for speech audiometry

British Standard	IEC Standard	ISO Standard	Topic Covered
BS EN 60645-1: 1995	IEC 645-1: 1992		Audiometer specification (Pure tone)
BS EN 60645-2: 1995	IEC 645-2: 1993		Audiometer specification (Speech)
		ISO 8253-1: 1989	Audiometric test methods (Pure tone)
		ISO 8253-2: 1992	Audiometric test methods (Sound field testing)
		ISO 8253-3: 1996	Audiometric test methods (Speech)
BS 2497: 1992		ISO 389: 1991	Audiometric zero (Air conduction)
BS ISO 389-3: 1994		ISO 389-3: 1994	Audiometric zero (Bone conduction)
BS 4009: 1991	IEC 373: 1990		Mechanical coupier for the calibration of bone vibrators
BS 4668: 1971	IEC 303: 1970		Acoustic coupler for the calibration of audiometric earphones
BS 4669: 1971	IEC 318: 1970		Artificial ear for the calibration of audiometric earphones

Tape recorders

There are considerable advantages in using recorded speech rather than the live voice for audiometric purposes. The use of a recorded stimulus ensures that the test material is always the same and allows the editing of the master recording, so as to approach the ideal of a set of test materials of equal difficulty which give reproducible recognition curves. The original speech audiometry test lists were recorded on 78 rpm records, but these have long ago been discarded in favour of tape recordings and more recently compact discs (CDs).

The advent of the domestic hi-fi market means that the required electronic specifications for suitable tape recorders and more recently CD players for speech audiometry use, will easily be met by any good domestic equipment. The tape recorder should be capable of handling the dynamic range of speech (about 30 dB), it should have an output impedance which is matched to the input impedance of the audiometer, a harmonic distortion of less than 1% and the flattest possible frequency response over the major speech frequencies (250 Hz to about 4 kHz). The frequency response characteristic of the whole system (i.e. audiometer and tape recorder), measured at normal audiometric test frequencies shall not deviate by more than ±5 dB from that measured at 1000 Hz. In practice none of these requirements are very severe. The impedance will cause no problems as the audiometer speech channel will have been built to accept a signal from a tape recorder and many recorders have a good dynamic range with a very flat frequency response and low distortion well beyond the range needed for speech reproduction.

Cassette recorders, when they were first introduced, gave relatively poor performance compared with reel to reel devices, but with the introduction of noise reduction systems, better quality tape and, more recently, digital audio machines, they are now capable of excellent performance. Many of the recorded lists which were originally only available on 1/4 inch tape have now been transcribed onto cassettes, with the result that the audiologist is now free to choose from a very wide range of equipment. Robustness, convenience, ease of use and cost all play an important part in the selection of the right recorder, and a survey of the National Health Service audiology clinics in the UK showed that approximately half of the clinics used cassette recorders for speech audiometry (Fuller and Moss, 1985).

The performance of the tape recorder or CD player should be measured when the audiometer is calibrated, but as with other audiometric equipment, listening to the quality of its output provides a useful day-to-day check that nothing is seriously wrong. The frequency response, harmonic distortion and for tape recorders, the tape speed should be checked during routine calibrations or after major repair,

IEC 94 (1968). In addition, the tape heads should be cleaned regularly by gently wiping them with a cotton bud impregnated with pure alcohol or a proprietary head-cleaning fluid. The frequency with which this will be necessary will depend on the extent to which the recorder is used and on the quality of the tape, as some tapes shed more oxide coating than others, but it should become part of the regular routine of equipment care in the clinic. Because there is no physical contact with the disc in a CD player, the equipment needs less routine cleaning, but care should be taken to ensure that the discs are dust-free when inserted into the player.

Measurement of word levels

For the audiologist using pre-recorded material, the level for the presentation of a word list to the patient can easily be set using the calibration tone recorded at the beginning of each list or at the beginning of the whole tape or disc. Once the level of the tone is set, adjustments to the level of the whole list are made with the audiometer attenuators which are, in turn, checked as part of the audiometric calibration procedure.

For those who are practising live voice testing or are recording new test material, however, the measurement of the levels of the individual words is important and is by no means a simple matter because of the nature of the speech signal. A plot of amplitude against time for a single word (see Figure 5.2) shows the difficulty.

It can clearly be seen that most of the acoustical energy of the word is in the vowel, yet much of the information is in the consonants and, in addition, the vowel has a very short rise time which might affect the measurement made. The problem is not quite as great as it might at first appear because there is a natural pattern to the relationship between the different phonemes of a word and this will not be broken as long as the speaker does not deliberately try to distort the word by, for example, speaking more 'clearly' than usual.

Fuller and Whittle (1982) made a study of the measurement of word levels for audiometric purposes. They took as their criterion, the speech detection threshold (SDT) that is, the level at which the listener can just detect the stimulus is present, but cannot recognize the word, and investigated which of a number of different physical measures gave the best prediction of the subjectively determined SDT for normal hearing subjects. They included a wide range of instruments and measures in their study, including the VU meter, peak programme meter (PPM), measures of total energy, the peak level, the RMS level measured with fast and slow meter characteristics and the maximum impulse level. The difficulties between the predictive ability of the different measures was comparatively small, but the correlations jumped from 0.7 to 0.9 when the A-weighting

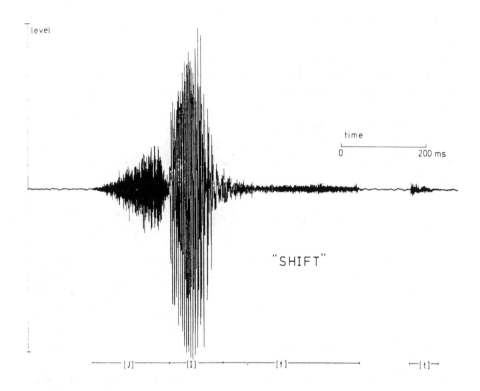

Figure 5.2 Amplitude (instantaneous voltage) plotted against time for the word 'SHIFT'

was added to each of the measures. Brady (1971) also made a study of the measurement of word level and showed that there was considerable variability in measurements made with a VU meter by non-expert observers.

This work suggests that whilst the VU meter, which is the indicator usually fitted to an audiometer, gives an adequate objective measure of the subjective level of the word, it would be better to use a meter which is more easily read. A meter giving an RMS fast reading and with the ability to switch in A-weighting would be a better choice for this purpose.

When recorded lists are being prepared, it is possible to avoid total reliance on measurement of the levels of the words and to produce lists which have been subjectively equalized. The technique is to make a first recording with an experienced speaker using equal vocal effort or feedback from a monitoring meter to get the levels approximately equal. An iterative process is then begun, testing normal hearing subjects close to threshold, to determine which items of the list are particularly easy or difficult to perceive. The levels of these words are then adjusted by lowering those of the easy items and raising the difficult ones until the words are all of approximately the same difficulty. In a similar manner the different word lists of a set can be examined to ensure that the whole corpus of recorded material is homogeneous.

The process of selecting material and setting the recorded levels of individual words by subjective testing is tedious and demands considerable investment of time, but if the resultant material is to have widespread use, the effort is well worthwhile. Hood and Poole (1977) spent considerable time studying one set of British recordings (Medical Research Council, 1974) and found that they were able to improve them markedly by adjusting the levels of the words. In the USA, Hirsh et al. (1952) made a classic study using subjective measurements during the development of the Central Institute for the Deaf lists and this led to reduction in the total number of test items from 84 to 36. Similarly Markides (1978a) performed a normative study on a set of recordings of the British Boothroyd lists (Boothroyd, 1968) recorded at Southampton University. This led to three of the 15 lists being omitted from the final tapes because they gave results which were significantly different from the other members of the set, but it meant that the rest of the recordings could be confidently used as a coherent set.

The final step in the preparation of recordings for use in speech audiometry is to preface each set with a calibration tone which can be used to set up the audiometer and to check the level of reproduction of the word lists. The duration of the tone should be sufficient to allow ample time for the adjustment of the audiometer, which means that it should be at least 60 seconds long. In practice, if the recordings have been edited so that the lists in a particular set have been equalized, it is unlikely that there would be any advantage in recording a separate calibration tone before each list. The stability of the equipment should be more than adequate to allow for a complete test for both ears to be made, and a tone before each list would only be an encumbrance to the audiologist.

ISO 8253-3 gives the following requirements for what shall be on recorded speech test material:

a) the speech test material
b) a calibration signal of duration not less than 60 seconds, the calibration signal should be either a weighted random noise, e.g. as specified in IEC 645-2, a 1/3rd octave band of noise centred at 1kHz or a frequency-modulated tone at 1kHz having a bandwidth of at least 1/3rd octave
c) signals for testing the overall frequency response of the speech audiometer consisting of 1/3rd octave bands of noise centred at the preferred 1/3rd octave frequencies in the range 125 Hz to 8000 Hz

d) signals for testing harmonic distortion consisting of 250 Hz, 500 Hz and 1000 Hz with a duration of at least 60 seconds each and having a peak level corresponding to the highest peak level of the recorded test material

It is important that care should be given to the choice of the recorded level of the calibration tone and to its relationship to the recorded level of the word lists. Ideally, the calibration tone should either be recorded at the mean level of the words or should bear a fixed relationship to it. The definition of the mean level will be dependent upon the method which has been used to equalize the constituent parts of the word lists, but as an example, if it is the peak levels of the words which have been equalized, it would be advisable to record the calibration tone at a level of 3 dB below the peaks.

ISO 8253-3 gives two methods for specifying the level of the speech test material. The material shall be equalized either according to the 'Equal speech level method' or the 'Equal reference speech recognition threshold level method'. The former requires that the speech test material shall be equalized on the basis of all the test material having equal sound pressure level while the latter requires that each test item has an equal recognition threshold. Because of the significant differences between the two methods it is important that the method used for determining the level of the speech test material is clearly stated in any information provided with the recorded material. The relationship between the level of the speech signal and the calibration signal has also to be stated.

Two factors need to be balanced in choosing the recording level used; the need to avoid the possibility of overloading the amplifier by having too high a level and the danger that if too low a level is used, problems may arise through the introduction of excessive background noise. The available dynamic range will vary with equipment which is being used, but a good compromise would seem to be to record the calibration tone at such a level that, when the hearing level control on the audiometer is set to zero, the level produced by the calibration signal is 20 dB SPL.

Earphones

In contrast to the choice of speech source, where the hi-fi market provides highly suitable equipment, the choice of earphones for speech audiometry should properly be confined to those designed specifically for audiometric applications. The performance figures quoted by the manufacturers for domestic circum-aural earphones are often excellent, but they suffer from two major drawbacks. It is very difficult to measure the sound pressure levels developed at the eardrum, which will be affected by the use of the circum-aural cushions (Stein and Zerlin 1963 and Tillman and Gish, 1964) and no audiometric standards relate to the use of domestic earphones.

The IEC artificial ear (IEC 318) allows the acoustic output of a range of supra-aural earphones to be measured but this is not suitable for the reliable measurement of circum-aural earphones even though a flat plate adapter is available for this purpose. Work is being persued on the development of adaptors for the measurment of specific circum-aural earphones, but currently no standardized reference threshold values exist.

There is no guarantee of consistency between different types of earphones which might be used in different clinics and since the comparability of results is one important aim of all audiometry, the argument must be to use audiometric earphones set in supra-aural cushions, choosing those models which have the flattest response over the speech frequencies until the work on circum-aural earphone measurement is sufficiently advanced.

The standard types of audiometric earphones have all been studied extensively and they have the advantage that their performance can be measured on an artificial ear or reference coupler. An artificial ear consists of a measurement microphone set inside an enclosure whose impedance characteristics approximate to those of the human ear. The frequency response of the earphones should be measured as part of the routine audiometric calibration procedure. For pure-tone audiometry, the frequencies between 125 Hz and 8 kHz are measured and, because the frequencies are tested singly, it is a relatively simple matter to make allowances for any small deviations of the earphone frequency response from the ideal. In speech audiometry the frequencies lying between 200 Hz and 4 kHz are particularly important and as all frequencies are present in the speech stimulus, it is very much more difficult to compensate for earphone frequency response. The audiologist has to rely, therefore, on the earphone response being as flat as possible over the important frequencies and should also select a pair of earphones which are as closely matched as possible from those available for use.

Two earphone types in particular, the Telephonics TDH-39 and TDH-49, are both widely used and are suitable for pure-tone audiometry. The TDH-39 however, shows a marked resonance at 6 kHz (Rudmose, 1964) and differences between metal and plastic cared versions (Sherwood, McNeil, Torr, 1995). This frequency is just above the main speech frequencies, but the TDH-49, which was designed to have more built-in damping and a flatter frequency response to higher frequencies, would probably be the preferable earphone type of these two for speech audiometry.

Loudspeakers

There is sometimes occasion to conduct speech audiometry as a free-field, or sound-field test, (the term free-field only strictly applies when there are true anechoic conditions) though speech material is more frequently used in this way in order to test patients using hearing aids. This latter form of testing is not strictly audiometry, but the test forms a useful part of the audiologist's repertoire and the considerations applying to the choice of equipment are the same in both cases.

In sound-field testing where the stimulus is presented to the patient via a loudspeaker, it is desirable that this should show low distortion and as flat a frequency response as possible over the speech frequencies. In addition it is necessary to ensure that the loudspeaker will generate sufficient levels for the loudest presentation which will be used. As with tape recorders, good domestic equipment will be perfectly adequate for speech testing. Many loudspeakers have excellent frequency responses up to and well beyond 6 kHz and a good power handling capacity, but the placing of the loudspeaker in the test room and the position occupied by the patient will interact to affect the received signal (Stream and Dirks, 1974). The measurement of the sound-field generated at the position of the patient's head needs some care.

The majority of audiometric test rooms, although acoustically treated, are not anechoic and for this reason problems arising from standing waves will occur if measurements of the loudspeaker output are made using pure tones. To avoid such difficulties, it is necessary to create a more uniform distribution of the sound in the room and this can be achieved with either bands of noise or warble tones — pure tones which are frequency modulated about a centre frequency. ISO 8253 Part 2 (1992) sets out the sound-field requirements for a free field, quasi-free field and diffuse field for pure-tone and narrow-band test signals for determining the threshold of hearing. Although this standard does not extend to speech audiometry it offers a measure for testing the suitability of a chamber and in addition it gives the requirements for the warble tones to be used. Using a measurement microphone placed at the position which will be occupied by the patient's head, the output of the loudspeaker can be measured using speech spectrum noise or white noise, whilst the relative frequency response of the loudspeaker in the room is measured with either warble tones or narrow bands of noise centred at 1/3 -octave intervals over the frequencies of interest. It should be remembered, however, that the presence of the patient in the room will affect the sound field slightly and that sound-field testing is not, generally, as well controlled and monitored as testing using earphones.

Values of threshold are now given in a revised version of ISO 226 which is now divided into two parts. Part 1 gives the reference threshold of hearing under free-field and diffuse-field listening conduction. Part 2, when produced, will give information on the revised equal loudness contours above threshold. Effectively Part 1 is a reworked version of the Minimum Audible Field (MAF) given in the previous composite ISO 226 standard and is now produced as ISO 389-7 (1996) reference threshold of hearing under free-field and diffused-field listening conditions.

A number of studies have been carried out to compare thresholds of hearing obtained under earphone and sound-field conditions. These have shown that the unaided sound-field thresholds are about 6 dB better than those measured using earphones, a difference that is probably accounted for by physiological noise (Anderson and Whittle, 1971). This difference in threshold should be remembered when interpreting the results of any sound-field measurements (Tillman et al., 1966).

Test rooms

All audiometry must be carried out in quiet conditions because of the masking effects of extraneous noise. The perception of the test signal is affected by noise which is within the same critical band as the stimulus and it is thus not sufficient to measure the overall noise level. The background noise in the test room must be measured in 1/3 - octave bands in order to ensure that it is not excessive at any frequency. The maximum permissible ambient noise levels for audiometry are referred to in section seven of ISO 8253-3. This indicates that the ambient noise level in a test room for speech audiometry are less stringent than for pure tone audiometry. The requirements stated in the right hand (RH) column of Table 4 of ISO 8253-1 (1989) for bone conduction audiometry are reproduced in Table 5.2. In practice these levels may be very difficult to achieve.

The background noise in the test room should be measured under normal working conditions, that is with test doors closed and with normal ventilation systems functioning. Intermittent sources of noise which might affect the test room, such as structure borne noise from other parts of a hospital, should also be taken into account as the figures in the table represent the maximum desirable levels when testing is taking place.

Table 5.2 Maximum background sound pressure levels for audiometry

1/3-octave band centre frequency (Hz)	Maximum SPL (dB re 20 μPa) ISO 8253-1 Table 4 RH column	1/3-octave band centre frequency (Hz)	Maximum SPL (dB re 20 μPa) ISO 8253-1 Table 4 RH column
31.5	63	630	8
40	56	800	7
50	49	1000	7
63	44	1250	7
80	39	1600	8
100	35	2000	8
125	28	2500	6
160	21	3150	4
200	15	4000	2
250	13	5000	4
315	11	6300	9
400	9	8000	15
500	8		

Effective masking level

When all of the equipment used for speech audiometry has been adjusted and objectively calibrated, two further subjective measures are necessary — the determination of the effective masking level of the audiometer's broad-band noise and the establishment of a normal response curve.

In speech audiometry, as in pure-tone audiometry, it is necessary to ensure that the non-test ear does not contribute significantly to the results. A signal applied to one ear will be transmitted to the other by bone conduction through the head with a loss of about 40 dB in level. If the pure-tone audiogram suggests that this bone-conducted signal will be heard, a masking noise must be applied to the non-test ear, using the wide-band noise facility of the audiometer (Liden, 1971).

Because of the existence of critical bands, the masking noise is most efficient when its energy is in the frequencies which are close to those being masked. The audiometer will probably provide either white or speech spectrum noise, neither of which is exactly matched to the spectrum of the particular voice used for the tests. It is therefore necessary to determine the effectiveness of the audiometer's masking noise for the test voice used (Coles and Priede, 1974).

Using a group of about 20 normal hearing adults, the audiometer is set at a level where at least 95% of the test lists are correctly heard. The masking noise is then added to the same ear as the speech and, using a different word list each time, the masking level is increased by 5 dB steps until the discrimination score just drops below 10%. The difference between the settings for the masking noise and for the speech is then equal to the effective masking level of the audiometer. If the effective masking level is +10 dB, this means that a masking noise set at 10 dB above the speech signal will just mask out the speech. It is good practice to balance the design of these measurements, using the lists in different orders and at different levels to eliminate any systematic effects. It is also important that the chosen subjects should have no familiarity with the test material.

Normal response curves

Differences in the test lists used, in the acoustical conditions of testing, in the accent of the local population and the instructions given to the patients, may all affect the results of the speech tests. For this reason it is necessary to establish a normal response curve with which the patients' results may be compared.

In order to do this, a group of normal hearing adults, who are representative of the population from which the patients will be drawn, are tested using equipment, test lists, pattern of presentation levels and instructions which will be used with the patients. Following the presentation of a number of word lists at different levels, the results are pooled to give an average response curve for normal hearing subjects.

Ideally the response curve should be established using a minimum of 20 people, but certainly no less than 10. In practice the normal listeners are often drawn from members of staff of the hospital concerned, but if this is the case, it is important that they are native to the local area and are not familiar with any of the test material. As when measuring the effective masking level, it is important to balance the order of presentation of the lists when establishing the normal response curve so that any slight differences do not distort the shape of the curve obtained.

Fuller and Moss (1985) noted that audiologists differ in the extent to which they elicit responses from patients when the stimulus is difficult to hear and the score is low. If different audiologists within the same clinic used markedly different instructions for speech audiometry, it would be advisable to establish a separate normal response curve for each audiologist, but if the instructions are fairly uniform this extra step is unlikely to be necessary.

Computer-controlled audiometry

Computerized applications of speech audiometry give the opportunity to examine other aspects of the patients' responses in addition to the rather crude right/wrong markings applied in the conventional test. In an early piece of research, Stevenson (1973, 1975) demonstrated some of the advantages of the sophisticated control and marking aspects of computerized systems. Using a tape recorder and a computer together as a hybrid system, he was able to examine the use of additional measures such as the recognition times and the particular confusions made at different levels of presentation.

Developments since Stevenson's work was carried out mean that it is now feasible to dispense with the tape recorder, storing the test words in digital form and using the computer to replay the stimuli, record the patients' responses and mark the test. These stimuli could be held on the computer's hard disk or on CD-ROM (using a sample frequency of 20 kHz the Boothroyd lists would take up approximately 15 Mb). Many of the improvements offered by such a system can readily be seen, although the possibilities need to be explored and evaluated carefully before they can be introduced into clinics for regular use — important preparatory work which is only just beginning.

The great advantage of a computer over tape recorder-based systems is flexibility. The speed at which a conventional test is performed is very largely determined by the timing of the words as they are recorded on the tape. This has to be chosen to be suitable for average patients and may be too fast for those who find the test difficult, or frustratingly slow for those who could cope with a faster pace. It is very simple to arrange for a computer to repeat words on demand, to present a test word only when a response has been made to the previous item and to adapt to the preferred pace of the patient. It is also possible to randomize the presentation of the stimuli to minimize any learning effect.

Multiple choice tests, giving the alternatives either in written form or as pictures, offer automatic marking of the tests and open up a further possibility of adaptive testing. In computer-controlled adaptive tests, the level of each stimulus or group of stimuli is determined by the patient's responses to the previous items — increasing the level if the previous items have been mis-heard and decreasing it if they have been correctly perceived. Items can also be selected to test more closely any particular discriminations which the patient finds difficult. In this way the speech reception threshold, optimum discrimination score and the presence of roll-over effects at high levels can all be explored without necessarily needing to use a whole word list at each level or to plot the whole of the discrimination curve. A shorter test conducted in this way would, of course, differ significantly from the current tests and the effects of both the multiple-choice items, the adaptive paradigms and the measurement of the levels of individual test items would have to be carefully studied and the results normalized before such testing could be introduced. James (1992) describes a new test of speech hearing acuity and existing speech and pure-tone tests which have been implemented on an integrated low cost computer-based system.

An alternative would be to use computer-synthesized speech, that is speech that is generated according to a series of rules. The quality of synthesised speech is rapidly reaching the high quality of digitally recorded material and this will mean that only the rules and not the speech are stored on computer, reducing the storage requirements and opening up possibilities of the use of regional dialects etc. The technology is improving quickly and computerized audiometry is becoming an economically viable alternative but it is important that normalizing studies are undertaken so that the full potential of computerized testing is exploited as the technology becomes available.

Chapter 6
Ensuring reliability and comparability of speech audiometry in Germany

KLAUS BRINKMANN and UTZ RICHTER

Speech audiometry is widely used in Germany, for example as a basis for the assessment of auditory handicaps and the selection of suitable hearing aids. It was recognized early on, however, that the results of speech audiometric tests carried out at different times, at different places and with different equipment were comparable to each other only if equivalent word lists, equivalent copies of the same recording of these word lists and speech audiometers with equivalent characteristics for the reproduction of the recorded speech were used.

A comprehensive concept of standardization in the field of speech audiometry has, therefore, been elaborated in Germany mainly in the decade from 1968 to 1977. More than 30 years later, the composition of these word lists may be completely representative of today's daily life language in Germany. Nevertheless, for the benefit of continuity it was decided not to modify the lists for the time being. Although many details have meanwhile been refined, the principles remain valid and have been adopted in recently developed international standards. This chapter describes the present state of the art in Germany.

Standardization of speech material for recognition tests

Lists of numerals and monosyllabic nouns

As early as 1961, as a first step, word lists for hearing tests using speech were laid down in the German Standard DIN 45621, based on the previous basic research work of Hahlbrock (1970). These lists comprise 10 groups, each containing 10 polysyllabic numerals and 20 phonetically balanced groups, each containing 20 monosyllabic nouns.

Examples of both tests are:

Numerals

Group 1: 98, 22, 54, 19, 86, 71, 35, 47, 80, 63

Monosyllabic nouns

Group 1: Ring Spott Farm Hang Geist Zahl Hund Bach Floh Lärm Durst
Teig Prinz Aas Schreck Nuß Wolf Braut Kern Stich

The numerals are pronounced evenly with uniform pitch, e.g. 'acht -
und - neun - zig', and are easy to understand if their level is high enough
to detect at least the vowels contained in them. The sound pressure level
corresponding to a 50% recognition score of numerals for otologically
normal subjects under monaural listening conditions is intended to form
the reference level for the hearing level scale for speech in Germany.

The monosyllabic nouns usually require a level which is about 10dB
to 20 dB higher than that of numerals to achieve the same recognition
score among subjects with normal hearing. Very often, subjects with
impaired hearing will not reach a recognition score of 100% even at very
high sound pressure levels. In Germany, the maximum speech recognition score in %, and the sound pressure level at which it occurs, i.e. the
so-called optimum speech level, are considered the most important
outcomes of hearing tests with monosyllables.

Lists of sentences

Besides the single polysyllabic and monosyllabic test words mentioned
before, a speech test consisting of short meaningful sentences developed by Niemeyer (1967) was standardized in Germany (DIN 45621-2).
This test comprises 10 phonetically balanced groups, each containing 10
sentences of four to six words. Each group thus consists of 50 words. An
example is as follows:

Group 1: 1. Geld allein macht nicht glücklich.
2. Böse Menschen verdienen ihre Strafe.
3. Mittwoch kommt uns Besuch passend.
4. Ich bin nicht naß geworden.
5. Uns're Eltern tanzen Wiener Walzer.
6. Lärmt nicht, Jungs, Vater schreibt.
7. Wer weiß dort genau Bescheid?
8. Er geht links, sie rechts.
9. Leider ist dies Haus teuer.
10. Dienstag wieder frisch gebrannte Mandeln.

The recognition score for these sentences is between that for numerals and that for monosyllabic nouns. The redundancy of information

inherent in sentences can be used to compensate for a discrimination loss that may occur with monosyllables if subjects with impaired hearing are tested or if hearing tests are performed in noisy environments. Speech audiometry with sentences, therefore, provides additional information on the ability of subjects to understand speech in daily life and has proved to be a useful tool especially for the selection of a suitable hearing aid.

Word lists for recognition tests in paediatric audiology

Special word lists, which are in use for testing the hearing of children, are standardized in the German Standard DIN 45621-3. Two alternative tests are specified: test A compiled by Biesalski et al. (1974) consists of three parts for (1) the age group below 4 years, (2) the group from 4 to 5 years and (3) the group from 6 to 8 years. Speech test B developed by Chilla et al. (1976) is intended for use with 3-to 6-year old children.

More recent research work carried out in Germany aims at the development of new speech tests such as closed set material, rhyme tests, a new sentence test and an improved speech test for children (Kollmeier, 1992).

Tests with different speech audiometers — basic ideas for standardization of test material recordings and speech audiometric equipment

In spite of the early standardization of word lists, the technical level of speech audiometry was still unsatisfactory in the late sixties as far as the comparability of the equipment used and the methods applied for calibration were concerned. At that time, German audiologists asked the German national institute for metrology, the Physikalisch-Technische Bundesanstalt (PTB), to evaluate the technical level of speech audiometry and to make suggestions for a new recording of the word lists, for an objective calibration procedure and for future standardization.

A series of investigations with different models of commercial speech audiometers was therefore started at the PTB, the results of which led to the following main conclusions.

Sound pressure level of speech

Various recordings of word lists according to DIN 45621 were in use at the time of the investigations above. According to the judgements of otologically normal test subjects, all of them showed large fluctuations in the loudness of the recorded words. A correlation analysis was performed in which the subjectively perceived loudness level of individual monosyllabic test words and their sound pressure level measured objectively using different devices such as a peak level indicator, a volume unit meter, a sound level meter with time weighting F ('fast'), and a sound level meter with time weighting I ('impulse') were compared (Brinkmann et al., 1969a).

The outcome of this investigation was that the indication of devices with a short integration time, such as the sound level meter with time weighting I, correlated best with the results of subjective loudness estimates. It was therefore decided to define the level of an individual word to be the sound pressure level (re 20 μPa) in dB as indicated by an impulse sound level meter according to DIN 45633-2[1] without any frequency weighting[2] but with an additional 'hold' circuit, and to use this well-specified instrument for the purpose of equalizing word levels in the course of the planned new recording of word lists (see below). Consequently, for the purpose of standardization in speech audiometry, the term 'sound pressure level of speech' was defined to be the mean impulse sound pressure level of all individual words of a test word group according to DIN 45621 and/or DIN 45621-2.

Recent developments in modern electronics allow alternative and more sophisticated methods of speech level measurement (Ludvigsen, 1992). No strong reasons are to be seen, however, to adopt these methods in Germany immediately, bearing in mind the enormous consequences such a step would have upon the continuity of speech audiometry and the comparability of test results. The recently issued International Standard ISO 8253-3 does not specify any preferred method, but leaves the question to national standardization.

The concept of free-field calibration of earphones

In Germany speech audiometry is performed equally in a sound field using loudspeakers as sound sources, and by means of earphones (and sometimes bone vibrators). To make test results comparable, a common basis must be established both for the determination of the sound pressure level of the transmitted speech and for equivalent specifications of frequency responses of the transmission system.

---

[1]The requirements of the former German standard DIN 45633-2 are almost identical to those of IEC standard 651 for type 1 instruments providing time weighting I.
[2]Fuller (1983) came to a similar conclusion regarding the suitable time weighting for measuring the level of single words. The apparent discrepancy between her results and those of the PTB with respect to frequency weighting (A vs. linear) can easily be explained by the fact that she used headphones for the reproduction of the test words, these having a real ear response with high pass filter characteristics due to leakage effects (see Figure 6.1), whilst the tests at the PTB were carried out via loudspeakers with an almost flat frequency response down to low frequencies.

Listening tests with loudspeakers are most frequently carried out under quasi free-field conditions with frontally incident sound waves. Reference to the sound pressure level in the undisturbed free sound field at a specified distance from the loudspeaker therefore seems quite logical. Sound pressure level measurements and frequency response specifications are then straightforward.

But how can the output of an earphone (or even a bone vibrator) be referred to free-field conditions? Acoustic or mechanical couplers, artificial ears or ear simulators usually applied in earphone and bone vibrator measurements are apparently unsuitable for this purpose. Acoustic couplers can only simulate the median acoustic impedance of the human ear (as claimed for artificial ears for supra-aural earphones according to IEC 318 and occluded ear simulators for insert earphones according to IEC 711) and can correctly measure the sound pressure level generated by the earphone at a well-defined point inside the human ear canal and under well-defined conditions (as an occluded ear simulator does with respect to the ear drum under no-leakage conditions of the earphone). However, they neither take into account leakage effects (which occur especially with supra-aural earphones on human ears) nor are they basically designed to represent sound diffraction effects caused by the head of a test subject under free-field listening conditions in a sound field.

Mechanical couplers can only simulate the mechanical impedance of the human head bone and can correctly measure the force exerted by a bone vibrator. However, they are not designed to include sound diffraction effects at the human head and the transfer function of the external and middle ear (Richter and Brinkmann, 1976).

The output of earphones (and bone vibrators) can, however, be referred to free-field conditions if instead of the coupler sensitivity level, the so-called free-field sensitivity level is determined. The free-field sensitivity level is 20 times the logarithm to the base 10 of the ratio of the free-field sensitivity to the reference sensitivity, 1 Pa/V. The free-field sensitivity at a given frequency and for a number of otologically normal test subjects is defined as the quotient of the sound pressure of a frontally incident plane progressive sound wave (0° sound incident) and of that voltage of equal frequency which must be applied to the terminals of the earphone (or bone vibrator) in order that the test subjects, on average, judge the sound wave and the sound produced by the earphone (or bone vibrator) as being equally loud, both sounds being received in the same ear (IEC 645-2).

Test methods for the determination of the free-field sensitivity level are described in textbooks (e.g. Zwicker and Feldtkeller, 1967; Brinkmann and Richter, 1989) and specified in IEC Standard 268-7 (in which the term is called a 'free-field comparison frequency response'). The method can be applied to all kinds of earphones (whether they are of the supra-aural, circum-aural or insert type) and even to bone vibrators (Richter and Brinkmann, 1976). Similar methods were used long ago when reference equivalent threshold sound pressure levels had to be established for new types of earphones (see ISO 389).

Once the free-field sensitivity level has been ascertained for a specified type of earphone, it can be determined in a simple manner for all other earphones of the same type without the necessity to always repeat the extensive loudness comparison measurements. For this purpose, any suitable coupler or artificial ear or ear simulator may be used. The coupler sensitivity at a given frequency is defined as the quotient of the sound pressure generated by the earphone in an acoustic coupler or ear simulator and the voltage applied to the terminals of the earphone (IEC 645-2) and can be determined without sophisticated measurement arrangements. For two earphones of identical design, the difference of their free-field sensitivity levels equals the difference of their coupler sensitivity levels. Consequently, if for a particular type of earphone and for each frequency, the difference between free-field sensitivity level and coupler sensitivity level is known, the free-field response can be determined for each earphone of this design by measuring the coupler sensitivity level.

Free-field and coupler sensitivity levels were determined for various types of earphones (Brinkmann and Richter, 1989) and bone vibrators (Richter and Brinkmann, 1976). A typical example is shown in Figure 6.1, which contains both the free-field sensitivity level and the coupler sensitivity of a (supra-aural) Telephonics TDH 39 earphone or a (circum-aural) Sennheiser HDA 200 earphone, respectively. In the case of the TDH 39 earphone, great differences between the two sensitivity levels can be seen both at low frequencies (mainly due to leakage effects at real ears) and at medium and high frequencies (due to insufficient acoustic impedance simulation and resonance effects in the coupler, and to sound diffraction effects inherent in free-field listening conditions). In the case of the HDA 200 earphone, the differences are far less severe at low frequencies, but still significantly high at frequencies around 5 kHz. For these and other types of audiometric earphone, the differences between the free-field and the coupler sensitivity levels as determined by the PTB are given in digital form in Table 6.1 (Richter, 1992). Some of these data are also contained in Annex A of IEC 645-2.

The concept of free-field calibration of earphones described earlier has been accepted for the purpose of standardization in speech audiometry in Germany at an early stage and has proved its utility in later investigations. It is now, as an option, also adopted in international standardization (IEC 645-2).

A survey of frequency responses of speech audiometers available at the time of testing showed typical deviations in the free-field responses of loudspeakers and earphones (Brinkmann et al., 1969b). Earphone

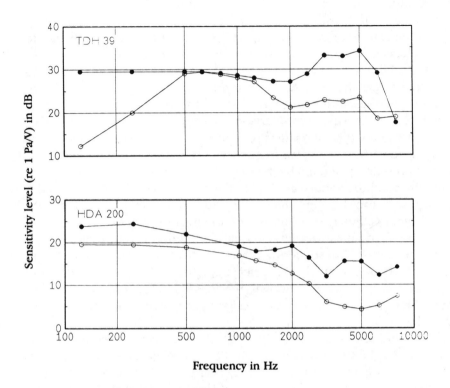

Figure 6.1 Free-field sensitivity level (∘—∘) and coupler sensitivity level (●—●) of a supra-aural Telephonics TDH 39 earphone (top) and a circum-aural Stennheiser HDA 200 earphone (bottom).

free-field responses are typically less flat than loudspeaker responses, especially in the frequency range from 2–6 kHz which is important for the correct discrimination of consonants. It could be proved by the listening tests described in the following paragraph that this fact must be given special attention in the standardization of speech audiometric equipment.

Outcome of early speech recognition tests

Speech recognition tests with a large group of otologically normal persons were carried out with five different types of speech audiometers both via loudspeakers in a free-sound field (binaural listening) and via earphones (monaural and binaural listening). The sound pressure level of the recorded speech material was directly measured in the field at the listener's position or referred to free-field conditions following the principles described in the preceding section. The results of these tests can be summarized as follows (Brinkmann and Diestel, 1970).

Table 6.1 Difference between the free-field sensitivity level G_F and the coupler frequency G_C for six types of earphone using an acoustic coupler according to IEC 303 or an ear simulator according to IEC 318, respectively, and 1/3 octave bands of noise as test signals (values rounded to the nearest half decibel)

Centre Frequency (Hz)	$G_F - G_C$ (dB)					
	Beyer DT 48 (i) (IEC 303)	Telephonics TDH 39 (i) (IEC 303)	Telephonics TDH 49 (i) (IEC 318)	Holmberg 95-01 (i) (IEC 318)	Optac Vario Cup/TDH 39 (ii) (IEC 303)	Sennheiser HDA 200 (iii) (iv) (IEC 318)
125	-16.5	-17.5	-19	-13	-18.5	-4
160	-15*	-14.5*	-17*	-11*	-15*	-4*
200	-13*	-12*	-14.5*	-9*	-12*	-4.5*
250	-11	-9.5	-12	-7	-9	-5
315	-9*	-6.5*	-9*	-5.5*	-8*	-4.5*
400	-7*	-3.5*	-5.5*	-3.5*	-6.5*	-4*
500	-5	-0.5	-2.5	-2.5	-5.5	-3
630	-3	0	-1	-3	-5.5*	-2.5*
800	-2	-0.5	-2	-2.5	-5	-2.5*
1000	-2.5	-0.5	-3	-0.5	-5	-2
1250	-1.5	-1	-2	-0.5	-5	-2.5
1600	-5.5	-4	-6.5	-5.5	-8	-3.5
2000	-7.5	-6	-9	-10	-9	-6.5
2500	-7.5	-7	-10.5	-13.5	-10.5	-6
3150	-6.5	-10.5	-12.5	-16	-14	-6
4000	-5	-10.5	-13	-17	-11	-10.5
5000	-1.5	-11	-8.5	-11.5	-17	-11
6300	-3.5	-10.5	-12	-8	-16	-7
8000	-2	+1.5	-7.5	+4	-7	-7

* Values derived by interpolation.
(i) Supra-aural earphone.
(ii) Supra-aural earphone in a sound attenuating enclosure.
(iii) Circum-aural earphone.
(iv) IEC 318 ear simulator fitted with a flat plate adapter.

On average, a 2.5 dB lower sound pressure level of speech was sufficient for binaural listening conditions to achieve the same recognition
score as for monaural hearing. The result was the same whether polysyllabic numerals or monosyllabic nouns were used as test material.

On average, identical free-field sound pressure levels were needed to
achieve a recognition score of 50% for numerals both in the case of
binaural earphone and binaural loudspeaker listening conditions which
shows that the concept of referring the sound pressure levels generated
by earphones to the free sound field as described before yields reliable
results.

However, on average, a 5 dB higher free-field sound pressure level
of monosyllabic test words was necessary to achieve the same recognition score under binaural listening conditions when the speech material was transmitted via earphones instead of loudspeakers. This result
seems to be in contradiction with the findings with numerals; however,
the reason for this discrepancy was easily found: the free-field
frequency responses of the earphones used with the audiometers
showed pronounced dips in the frequency range from 2–6 kHz. These
dips cause effects in the case of monosyllabic words (which contain
much information in consonants) while they do not influence the
recognition levels of numerals (which contain most of their information in their vowels). As mentioned in the previous paragraph, this fact
must be given due attention in the design of speech audiometric
equipment. At least with presently available audiometric earphones,
special equalizing networks will have to be introduced in speech
audiometers in order to obtain reliable results when performing
hearing tests with earphones.

With a sound pressure level sufficiently high to achieve a recognition
score of 100%, the responses of test subjects are quite rapid. If the
sound pressure level is, however, reduced, the answers are given with
noticeable hesitation. The testing time thus becomes longer the lower
the recognition level is. To obtain comparable results, the sequence of
words on a sound carrier must therefore also be given attention and it
must be standardized (Brinkmann et al., 1969a).

Recordings of word lists and sentence lists

Based upon the results of the investigations described above, the word
lists according to DIN 45621 and the sentence lists according to DIN
45621-2 were recorded and further improved in 1969 and 1973. Both
recordings were performed in a studio of the North German
Broadcasting Corporation by the same professional speaker.

In the case of the word lists, the levels of all individual test words, i.e.
100 polysyllabic numerals and 400 monosyllabic nouns were adjusted
to the same level by means of a sound level meter with time weighting

I. The pauses between the test words were adjusted in such a way that in the final version, the test words follow each other at regular intervals of 5 seconds (numerals) or 4 seconds (monosyllables).

In addition, a technical part was added consisting of three check tones of frequencies 125 Hz, 1 kHz and 8 kHz and a speech-simulating noise as previously recommended in G 227 (1964) of the Comité Consultatif International Télégraphique et Téléphonique (CCITT 1964). The spectrum level of this noise has its maximum at about 800 Hz and falls off at a rate of about 5 dB per octave at lower frequencies and of about 12 dB per octave at higher frequencies.

The tones may be used for a simple check of the frequency response of the speech audiometer in use. The noise signal is mainly intended for calibration purposes and is dealt with later in more detail. It may, however, also be used as an easy means of checking a given sound carrier with regard to the frequency spectrum characteristics.

This concept has now also been adopted in recent international standardization. ISO 8253-3 specifies that each copy shall, besides the speech test material, contain the following signals:

1. A signal for the calibration of the speech audiometer of a duration of not less than 60 seconds. The calibration signal shall be a weighted random noise, e.g. as specified in IEC 645-2, a band of noise centred at 1 kHz and having a bandwidth of 1/3 octave, or a frequency-modulated tone at 1 kHz having a bandwidth of at least 1/3 octave. The modulating signal shall be either sinusoidal or triangular with a repetition rate in the range 4–20 Hz.
2. Signals for testing the frequency response of the speech audiometer including the playback equipment and the recording. Such signals shall have a duration of not less than 15 seconds and consist of 1/3 octave bands of white noise centred at the preferred 1/3 octave frequencies according to ISO 266, in the frequency range 125 Hz–8 kHz.
3. Signals for testing the harmonic distortion of the speech audiometer. Pure tones of the frequencies 250 Hz, 500 Hz and 1 kHz shall be available with a duration of not less than 60 seconds each and a peak level corresponding to the highest peak level of the recorded speech test material.

The actual levels of test words and calibration signals were measured later on various commercial copies of the mother tape (Brinkmann, 1974a). A typical result is represented in Figure 6.2: the levels of all 500 test words are equal to within about ±1 dB. The average level of the speech-simulating noise deviates from the total mean level of the test words by not more than 0.1 dB. The noise level, however, shows fluctuations with time of about ±0.5 dB. The levels of the three check tones are 18.0 (±0.5) dB below the level of the noise.

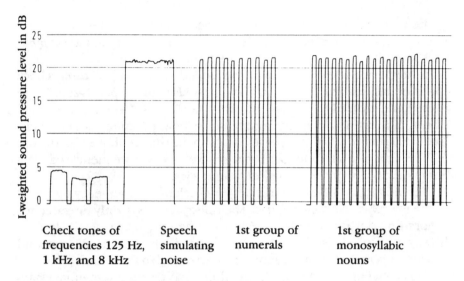

Figure 6.2 Levels of calibration signals and test words of the recording of word lists according to DIN 45621 (1969)

When recording sentence lists the speaker's voice level was monitored by means of a peak level indicator to obtain an optimum with respect to both a constant speech level and a natural melody of speech. In the final version, the standard deviation of the impulse sound pressure levels of all 500 words was only 2 dB, and the mean levels of the 10 groups did not differ by more than 1 dB from each other (Brinkmann, 1974b). It was therefore decided not to perform any further level adjustments. A speech simulating noise and three pure tones were added to the recording, which had identical level relations for the sound pressure level of speech, as for the recording of the word lists. Copies of both test recordings can therefore be used on a speech audiometer without any recalibration.

Speech recognition tests with otologically normal subjects

Extensive hearing tests were carried out with the two new recordings using large groups of otologically normal test subjects in order to determine the speech recognition reference curves and to evaluate the recognition score of individual test words and groups of words and sentences (Brinkmann, 1974a, b).

Equipment used

In the case of word lists, the tests were performed monaurally by means of laboratory speech audiometric equipment that included a high quality studio record player having a flat frequency response, a specially designed filter network with attenuation unit, a power amplifier and two supra-aural Beyer DT 48 earphones. The filter network was dimensioned so that the overall free-field sensitivity level of the earphones including the network had a value almost independent of frequency within the frequency range from 80 Hz – 12.5 kHz. This means that speech replayed via this equipment sounds as if it were replayed via a loudspeaker having a flat frequency response in an anechoic room.

The frequency response of the entire equipment referred to the free field was tested with a frequency measurement record. In the range between 100 Hz and 10 kHz it does not deviate by more than ±1.5 dB from the reference value at 1 kHz. Below 100 Hz and above 10 kHz, the sensitivity level decreases in a monotonous way, the –3 dB frequencies being 80 Hz and 12.5 kHz. Furthermore, the upper and lower frequency limit of the filter network could be altered in such a way that the sensitivity level of the equipment had already decreased by 3 dB at the frequencies 110 Hz and 7.5 kHz.

The individual frequency responses have been plotted in Figure 6.3: curve (a) represents the frequency response of the free-field sensitivity level of the earphone used (Beyer DT 48), curve (b) the free-field frequency response of the entire equipment without additional band limits.

In the case of sentence lists, monaural tests were carried out with similar equipment, but with a studio tape recorder instead of the studio record player. Additional hearing tests were performed binaurally using a high quality electrostatic loudspeaker in an anechoic room.

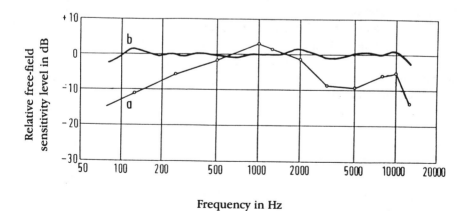

Frequency in Hz

Figure 6.3. Frequency response (referred to the free sound field) of the equipment used for the determination of the speech intelligibility reference curves. Curve (a) relative free-field sensitivity level of the Beyer DT 48 earphone used; curve (b) relative overall free-field sensitivity level of the speech audiometer

The overall frequency response of this equipment was frequency-independent within ±2 dB in the frequency range from about 80 Hz to about 15 kHz, except for two narrow dips near 120 Hz and 6 kHz.

Reference speech recognition curves

A group of 97 test subjects (157 ears) took part in the basic listening tests on numerals and monosyllabic words. They had fulfilled the criterion of having a hearing threshold level below 10 dB at each audiometric frequency up to 4 kHz; at either 6 kHz or 8 kHz a maximum hearing threshold level of 15 dB was allowed. The subjects were for the most part employees of the PTB (workshop and laboratory apprentices, as well as scientific, technical and administrative personnel). Apart from a few exceptions, the participants had no previous experience in the field of hearing tests.

All participants were tested at the same pre-set free-field sound pressure levels of speech using four out of 10 groups of numerals and four out of 20 groups of monosyllabic words chosen at random. In addition, a limited number of subjects (35 ears) were also tested in a corresponding manner with the audiometric equipment set at a limited bandwidth.

The arithmetic average values of recognition scores vs. free-field sound pressure level of speech together with the corresponding standard deviations are plotted in Figure 6.4 for the case of the broader bandwidth of the equipment. The curves are extrapolated beyond the range of the sound pressure levels tested and have the typical S-form. The sound pressure levels of speech corresponding to a 50% recognition score for numerals or monosyllabic nouns for monaural listening conditions are 18.4 dB and 29.3 dB, respectively. As might be expected, the slope of the curve for monosyllables is somewhat less steep than that for numerals.

The curves of the arithmetic average values in Figure 6.4 join almost asymptotically the 0% and 100% recognition score lines. In general the curves of individual listeners continue somewhat more steeply than the average value curves, not only in the range of the lower sound pressure levels but also in the range of the higher ones. For practical speech audiometry the curve of an 'average otologically normal subject' is therefore more relevant than the curve of the arithmetic average of a large group of subjects. For this reason, median instead of mean curves are given in DIN 45626 as reference speech recognition curves.

Parallel to the basic scale of 'free-field sound pressure level of speech (re 20 μPa) in dB', a second scale has been entered at the level of the 50% recognition score line referred to as 'Hearing level for numerals in dB', the origin of which is located at the sound pressure level of speech which otologically normal listeners need on average to recognize approximately 50% of the numerals, i.e. 18.4 dB.

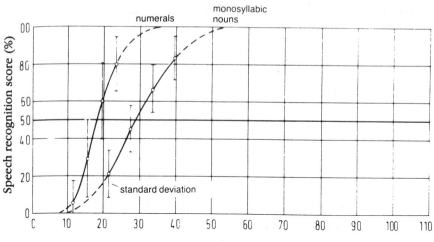

Figure 6.4 Recognition score of test words according to DIN 45621 as a function of the free-field sound pressure level of speech for monaural listening conditions (mean values and standard deviations of 157 otologically normal ears)

Due to the concept of earphone calibration in terms of free-field sensitivity levels, the reference curves are valid for monaural test word presentation both via any type of earphone or via any type of loudspeaker in a free sound field, on the premise of sufficiently flat free-field frequency responses. Additional listening tests (35 ears) showed that a slight limitation of the frequency range (lower cut-off frequency 110 Hz instead of 80 Hz, higher cut-off frequency 7.5 kHz instead of 12.5 kHz) has only a minor effect on the recognition curves. The curves valid for numerals are slightly shifted towards smaller sound pressure levels, presumably due to a reduction of the sound pressure levels of the test words at the same recognition level (influence of low-frequency cut-off). The shifting of the curve valid for monosyllables towards higher sound pressure levels is, on the other hand, probably a result of the high-frequency cut-off and the poorer discrimination accompanying it. Conclusions based on these results with respect to speech audiometer specification have been drawn.

The results for the sentence lists were derived in a similar way to those for the word lists and are presented in Figures 6.5 and 6.6. Figure 6.5 contains two curves: the right-hand curve represents the arithmetic mean recognition score vs. free-field sound pressure level based on tests with 59 subjects (91 ears) with normal hearing under monaural earphone listening conditions, the left-hand curve represents corresponding results based on tests with 15 subjects with normal hearing under binaural loudspeaker listening conditions in a free-sound field.

Both curves are almost parallel. The sound pressure levels of speech corresponding to a 50% recognition score are 21.0 dB (for monaural listening) and 18.6 dB (for binaural listening). This proves very clearly two facts: first, the speech volume increase with binaural hearing compared with monaural hearing is almost equal to 2.5 dB, a value formerly shown to be valid for speech with binaural earphone listening vs. monaural earphone listening. Second, and more importantly the calibration of speech audiometers based on free-field sound pressure level leads to correct and comparable results both for speech audiometry tests in a sound field and via earphones. It should be noted that this is valid only in the case of frontally incident sound waves in free-field audiometry. Any other angle of sound incidence would require different frequency response specifications and a different calibration of the equipment, due to the well-known sound diffraction effect of the human head as a function of the angle of sound incidence.

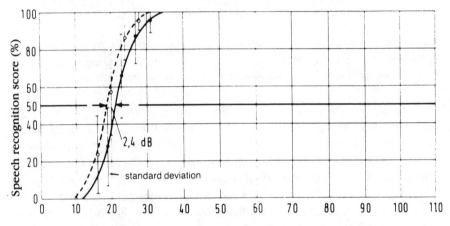

Free-field sound pressure level of speech (re 20 μPa) in dB

Figure 6.5 Recognition score of test sentences according to DIN 45621-2 as a function of the free-field sound pressure level of speech for different listening conditions. o— — —o, Monaural hearing via earphones (mean values of 91 otologically normal ears, 59 test subjects); •—•, Binaural hearing via loudspeaker in a free sound field (mean values of 15 otologically normal subjects)

The absolute response of the recognition curves for sentences is also reliable. This can be seen by a comparison with the equivalent curves previously obtained for numerals and monosyllabic words. In Figure 6.6, instead of mean values, the median curves are plotted in each case for the reasons given above. As could be expected, the sentence curve runs well between the two other curves. All three recognition curves have almost the same standard deviation with respect to the sound pressure level.

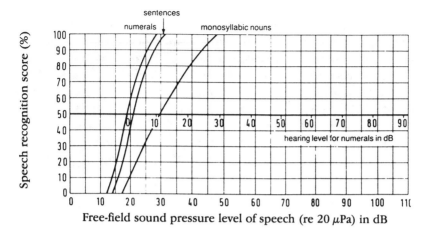

Figure 6.6 Reference speech recognition curves for different test materials and monaural listening conditions

In principle, the free-field sensitivity level of bone vibrators can be determined in a similar way to that of earphones as shown by Richter and Brinkmann (1976). Based on these measurements, speech audiometric equipment was set up using a Präcitronic KH-70 bone vibrator as a sound transducer. By means of an equalizing network, the frequency response of this equipment referred to the free sound field could be adjusted to be frequency-independent within ±3.5 dB in a range from 125 Hz to 8 kHz when the bone vibrator was applied to the test subjects' foreheads. Binaural listening tests using this equipment were initially carried out with a group of 12 otologically normal test subjects (Richter and Brinkmann, 1977) the number of which was later increased to 20. The same group was also tested binaurally by means of earphone equipment almost identical to that described above. In each case the same recording of monosyllabic words was used. The two resulting speech recognition curves are almost parallel and deviate by only 1.3 dB at a 50% recognition score (Figure 6.7). This shows that the concept of free-field calibration of speech audiometers is even applicable to bone vibrators.

In a later, more extensive study concerned with the bone conduction pure-tone threshold (Brinkmann and Richter, 1983) the remaining discrepancy between earphone and bone vibrator measurements could be explained to be most probably due to the influence of vibro-tactile sensation in the course of bone vibrator calibration

Recognition score of individual test words and groups of test words

The exact adjustment of the sound pressure level of individual test words to the same value does not necessarily result in all test words being equally understandable. On the contrary, considerable differences in speech recognition were found not only for monosyllabic words but also for the polysyllabic words when the results of the tests described previously in the chapter were evaluated. Some words were understood by almost all participants even at very low sound pressure levels while others were almost never repeated correctly even when presented at a level about 20 dB higher. This shows that not only the sound pressure level of a single word affects its recognition level but also other factors, such as the articulation by the speaker, the specific extent to which a word is known in each group of subjects or the possibility of confusing it with similar words.

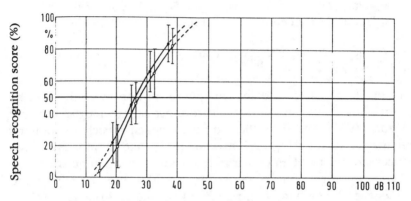

Free-field sound pressure level of speech (re 20 μPa) in dB

Figure 6.7 Recognition score of monosyllabic nouns according to DIN 45621 as a function of the free-field sound pressure level of speech for different listening conditions (means and standard deviations of 20 otologically normal subjects). ●—●, Binaural hearing via loudspeaker in a free sound field; ○—○, binaural hearing via a bone vibrator applied to the forehead

These large differences in recognition level within the standardized word lists are the main reason why the words have been adjusted to equal sound pressure level instead of equal recognition level. For equal recognition levels, the differences between the sound pressure levels would have been so great that the definition of an average speech level of the words in a group would have been very questionable.

Recent international standardization (ISO 8253-3) allows for both methods taking into account different audiometric traditions in various countries and the possible effect of different linguistic characteristics of various languages.

For practical use of the recorded test words it is of particular importance to know whether the individual test word groups can be interchanged, i.e. whether they can be understood equally well when being played back at the same level. The results of the hearing tests were therefore also evaluated in this light. The greatest recognition score difference between any two groups of numerals amounted to 10% (corresponding to one out of 10 words), while between any two groups of monosyllables differences of up to 15% may occur (corresponding to three out of 20 words). It may be concluded that the existing differences are not very severe and that the interchangeability of the groups can be guaranteed for tests with the usual accuracy.

Similar evaluations were carried out regarding the sentence tests. Maximum deviations in recognition scores were found to be about 10% between any two of the 10 sentence groups.

Standardization of the recordings of word lists and sentence lists

In order to ensure a wide acceptance of the recordings described above, and to provide suitable means for checking the electro-acoustical characteristics of a commercial copy, the technical specifications of sound carriers for hearing tests using these recordings have been laid down in the German Standards DIN 45626 (for the recording of word lists) and DIN 45626-2 (for the recording of sentence lists). Both standards contain the following basic information:

- The location of the mother tape of the recording.
- The frequencies and the levels of the pure tones at the nominal frequencies 125 Hz, 1 kHz and 8 kHz with tolerances.
- The frequency spectrum and the level of the speech simulating noise with tolerances.
- The levels of the test words (or sentences) with tolerances.
- The minimum signal-to-noise and cross talk ratio.
- The reference recognition score curves for the recordings as determined by the PTB (see Figure 6.6) for monaural hearing.

Together with the standards DIN 45621 and DIN 45621-2 containing the actual word and sentence lists, the two parts of DIN 45626 form the basis of a complete harmonization of speech audiometry in Germany. Sound carriers according to these standards are commercially available in the form of records, tapes, tape cassettes and compact discs (CDs). In practice, only CDs are used in recently type-approved speech audiometers.

Recordings of the word lists for speech recognition testing in paediatric audiology according to DIN 45621-3 are also on the market, however, their standardization is not yet being planned.

For the evaluation of hearing disability, special tables exist (Boeninghaus et al., 1973) which enable the audiologist to transfer the recognition score measured by means of a standardized recording into a single number describing the person's handicap.

Standardization of speech audiometer facilities

Parallel to the standardization of speech material recordings, specifications for speech audiometers have been evaluated and laid down in the German Standard DIN 45624. They are mainly based on the results of the investigations described in the preceding sections.

DIN 45624 was introduced to the IEC Working Group charged with the preparation of an international standard for speech audiometric equipment. The outcome of this work was recently published as IEC 645-2. Although not fully compatible with DIN 45624, IEC 645-2 contains the main elements of the former, and can be regarded as the best compromise to be reached on an international level. It is, therefore, intended to withdraw DIN 45624 as soon as the IEC standard is available in the German language as a DIN IEC standard.

Basically, IEC 645-2 deals only with instruments which use recordings of the test speech on a sound carrier for speech reproduction. Reproduction may be via earphones, loudspeakers or bone vibrators. Some requirements for the transmission of live voice are included in order to ensure the highest possible degree of reliability, recognizing that live voice speech audiometry is in many countries still widely practised, particularly with children.

Two methods of specification, calibration and testing are given for the output levels generated by earphones and bone vibrators, i.e. a free-field equivalent output level method or an uncorrected coupler output level method. When using the free-field equivalent output level method, all specifications are referred to the free sound field, independent of whether they concern frequency response, speech level accuracy or harmonic distortion, thus allowing quantitative comparisons of speech audiometric results obtained with different types of transducer.

Two types of speech audiometer, types A and B with respect to minimum facilities are specified. If reference is made to the free-field equivalent output level method, the type designation is A-E or B-E, respectively. German audiologists have expressed their intention to use only E-type audiometers.

The tolerances for the frequency response, for instance, are ±3 dB in the frequency range from 250 Hz to 4 kHz, 0 dB to -10 dB above 125 Hz and up to 250 Hz, and ±5 dB above 4 kHz and up to 6.3 kHz. This should be considered a compromise between the physically desirable tolerances (based on the information given above) and those technically feasible. With regard to audiometric earphones at present available, these specifications require special equalization networks. However, no alternative can be seen to achieve comparability of speech audiometric results with different sound transducers. Detailed information is given on how speech audiometers can be tested for compliance with these requirements.

The tolerance for calibration in terms of the sound pressure level of speech is ±2 dB. The calibration must be carried out using a calibration signal which is recorded on the sound carrier used and whose level in relation to the level of the test words is known. The use of speech simulating noise with the same level as the test words is used exclusively in Germany at present.

Harmonic distortion figures are also specified in terms of free-field related values which offers the possibility of comparing loudspeaker and earphone requirements (Richter, 1976). Again, test methods are described in detail.

Testing and calibration of speech audiometers

In the case of free-field speech audiometry via loudspeaker, testing and calibration are quite simple for the user. Testing mainly requires a sound level meter with known free-field sensitivity (together with some filter equipment if distortion measurements are to be included) and any suitable reference tape, record or CD. The calibration in terms of the sound pressure level of speech is carried out in two steps: first, the amplification of the speech audiometer is adjusted to achieve a specified reference level indication of the calibration signal recorded on the sound carrier used on the monitoring instrument incorporated in the audiometer. If this is done well, the audiometer is expected to produce the sound pressure level of speech indicated at the level control setting at a specified distance from the loudspeaker.

This can be checked easily by means of a sound level meter using the recorded calibration signal. The use of the speech simulating noise is clearly preferable for this purpose, mainly because calibration errors can be widely avoided in non-ideal anechoic rooms and due to loudspeaker sensitivity irregularities at single pure-tone frequencies. Moreover, because of its simple level relationship to speech, the reading of the sound level meter equals — for exact calibration — the setting of the audiometer level control when speech simulating noise is used.

Testing and calibration of speech audiometer earphones are as simple for the user as usual pure-tone audiometer testing and calibration. If it is borne in mind that the frequency-dependent difference between the free-field and the coupler sensitivity level of an earphone only depends on the type of earphone and not on the specific unit, all necessary measurements may be performed using a coupler (or artificial ear). The target values for coupler sound pressure levels both for testing the frequency response and for absolute calibration must be specified by the manufacturer of the audiometer (or the National Metrology Institute), who must determine the free-field sensitivity level of the earphone in question — the user is only concerned with simple coupler measurements (as in the case of pure tone audiometers). Again, the use of a speech simulating noise instead of a pure tone as a calibration signal is to be preferred. The method of determining the reference calibration levels for earphones used in type A-E or B-E speech audiometers and examples for common types of earphone are given below.

Recent experience with pattern evaluation of audiometers in Germany

In 1988, the German Verification Ordinance introduced a new and comprehensive test system for all pure-tone and speech audiometers used in medical applications (Richter, 1988). It provides, among other things, that prior to being marketed each new type of such audiometers must be subjected to an approval test by the PTB. The test is intended to verify that, within the test parameters, the design of the audiometer complies with the requirements of the relevant national and international standards regarding its measuring accuracy and the patient's safety, and that it is sufficiently reliable and correctly calibrated. If this is the case, the applicant is granted an approval mark, and an approval certificate is issued. The applicant is then entitled to certify single instruments of the respective audiometer type to be in conformity with the approved pattern and is authorized to sell them.

The approval certificate states constructional details of the audiometer submitted for the test. It indicates which tests must be carried out on each instrument prior to its being delivered to the user (conformity test) and which tests are to be conducted later by an accredited maintenance service at yearly intervals, and by the user at shorter intervals.

Most of the PTB requirements the audiometers have to meet during pattern evaluation, are based on international standards (IEC 645-1, IEC 645-2, OIML R 104) or German national standards (DIN 45624, DIN 45626).

In addition to meeting the requirements established in the standards, the audiometers must be designed such that they cannot impair the patient's hearing ability, and so that all metrological controls can be carried out (this concerns in particular, computer-controlled audiometers). Speech audiometers must be equipped with a digital speech reproduction unit (e.g. a CD player).

Between 1988 and 1992, 17 applicants submitted a total of 43 different models of audiometer to the PTB for pattern approval. Seventeen of these 43 instruments were pure-tone audiometers of types 3 to 5, and 26 were combined pure-tone and speech audiometers of types 2 and 3 (according to IEC 645 part 1). The following are the most important outcomes of the tests on these audiometers. None of the 43 different types of audiometer submitted passed at the first attempt. All instruments had to be returned to the manufacturers for modification, and some have not been re-submitted (Richter and Gössing, 1992).

The shortcomings found must be considered significant. Eight of the shortcomings encountered most frequently are listed, each requiring modification of audiometer design; these are listed in order of the frequency of their occurrence. The percentage shown in brackets indicates the frequency in relation to the number of possible cases. In almost all cases, two items from the list given below were concerned in each rejection.

- Electromagnetic compatibility (95%).
- Reference levels of pure tones transmitted via loudspeaker (80%).
- Frequency characteristics, bandwidth and centre-frequency of narrow-band masking noise (73%).
- Headband application force (72%).
- Minimum facilities required for a specific type of audiometer (42%).
- Tone switching (35%).
- Free-field frequency response of speech audiometer (35%).
- Unwanted sound radiated by the audiometer (20%).

In addition to the shortcomings listed above, which made modifications necessary, calibration errors had to be corrected in most of the instruments. In the case of pure-tone audiometers, these errors concerned mostly, the output levels of the bone vibrators (up to 13 dB) and those of the loudspeakers (up to 26 dB); in speech audiometers, the main concern was the sound pressure levels for speech transmitted via earphones (up to 9 dB).

These results unfortunately suggest another conclusion; as the great majority of the instruments submitted for testing were audiometers which had been on the market for some while, it must be assumed that almost all audiometers in use before 1989 are not in compliance with valid standards. This indicates that standardization alone does not ensure a sufficient degree of reliability while testing against the standards is not officially required by legislation.

Meanwhile, intervention by the German authorities has bought about a reorientation. Reliability and measuring accuracy have again come to the fore, and newly designed audiometers comply with the standards. The manufacturers have improved their measuring facilities, and their acoustic measurement standards are now traceable to the national standards maintained at the PTB. In addition, carefully measured reference threshold levels and free-field frequency responses are available for a great number of different sound transducers (circum-aural earphones, supra-aural earphones, with or without sound attenuating enclosures, insert earphones, bone vibrators and loudspeakers), (Richter, 1992).

Determination of the sound pressure level of speech provided by speech audiometers equipped with earphones

For the calibration of speech audiometers, a speech-simulating noise, for example according to DIN 45626 (or CCITT G 227 (1964)) may be used. As described above, such a signal is stored on magnetic tape or CD, together with German speech test material having the same impulsive sound pressure level as the test words. In Table 6.2, the relative 1/3 octave band levels $L_{f,i,rel.}$ of this noise are given (column 3), adjusted to result in a total level L_{total} of 0 dB when summed according to the rules of level addition, following the equation below.

$$L_{total} = 10 \lg \sum_{i=1}^{20} 10^{0.1 L_{f,i}} \, dB$$

Assuming transmission via speech audiometric equipment using earphones with ideally flat free-field frequency response, these electrical noise levels $L_{f,i,rel.}$ may be equally regarded as free-field sound pressure levels $L_{f,i,F}$ (re 20 μPa).

As described above in detail, the sound pressure levels produced by the same earphones in an acoustic coupler deviate from the free-field sound pressure levels by G_C–G_F, G_C, being the coupler sensitivity level, and G_F the free-field sensitivity level of the earphone in question. For earphones of the Beyer DT 48 type, G_C–G_F is given in column 4 of Table 6.2 The free-field sound pressure levels $L_{f,i,F}$ of the speech simulating noise given in column 3 will thus result in the coupler sound pressure levels $L_{f,i,C}$ as given in column 5. Level summation according to the equation above gives a total coupler sound pressure level of the noise of 5.8 dB.

A speech audiometer with an ideally flat free-field frequency response, with the speech sound pressure level control set, for instance, to 70 dB, and equipped with an earphone of type DT 48 must therefore be adjusted so that a total I-weighted sound pressure level of 75.8 dB re 20 μPa is measured in the coupler when the speech-simulating noise referred to above is used.

If the frequency response of the speech audiometer is not ideally flat, its real frequency response must also be taken into account in the calculation.

Table 6.2 Example for the determination of the speech sound pressure level provided by speech audiometers equipped with Beyer DT 48 earphones, assuming ideally flat free-field frequency response

Frequency Index i	f_i	$L_{f,i,rel.}$	C_C-G_F (DT48, IEC303)	$L_{f,i,C}$ (re 20 μPa)
	(Hz)	(dB)	(dB)	(dB)
1	100	−27.9	+18	−9.9
2	125	−24.4	+16.5	−7.9
3	160	−21.4	+15	−6.4
4	200	−18.4	+13	−5.4
5	250	−15.4	+11	−4.4
6	315	−13.4	+9	−4.4
7	400	−11.4	+7	−4.4
8	500	−9.9	+5	−4.9
9	630	−8.9	+3	−5.9
10	800	−8.4	+2	−6.4
11	1000	−7.9	+2.5	−5.4
12	1250	−8.9	+1.5	−7.4
13	1600	−10.9	+5.5	−5.4
14	2000	−13.4	+7.5	−5.9
15	2500	−16.4	+7.5	−8.9
16	3150	−20.4	+6.5	−13.9
17	4000	−24.4	+5	−19.4
18	5000	−28.9	+1.5	−27.4
19	6300	−32.9	+3.5	−29.4
20	8000	−37.4	+2	−35.4
		$L_{total} = 0$ dB		$L_{total} = 5.8$ dB

Final remarks

The concept of standardization in speech audiometry described above and realized up to now in Germany, guarantees reliable and comparable results if the various standards are complied with by the equipment actually used, if standardized speech audiometric test methods are used and if test rooms fulfil certain minimum requirements with respect to sound field conditions and background noise. The ongoing standardization in ISO in this field (ISO 8253-3) is in agreement with current practice in Germany, and will certainly be transferred into national standards. As described above, regular testing and calibration of speech audiometers together with pure-tone audiometers are covered by legal metrology, ensuring a high technical level of speech audiometric equipment in accordance with the most recent standards.

Chapter 7
Speech audiometry for differential diagnosis

PHILLIP EVANS

For over one hundred years (Wolf, 1874, cited in Lyregaard et al., 1976) speech has been used in a systematic way to assess hearing ability. Undoubtedly for very much longer than that, and to the present day, it has been the basis of informal tests for hearing impairment by parents, general practitioners, teachers and others.

Two factors predispose speech to this role. First is the common but arguable assumption that the primary function of human audition is that of communication with our fellows, that is the reception of speech. Thus, speech has face validity as a 'natural' and 'meaningful' stimulus for assessing auditory function. It is supposed that, if we can hear speech normally then our hearing is not significantly impaired. The second factor is the ready availability of speech as a stimulus, with no need for equipment to produce it.

These two factors combine to perpetuate the use of a technique that is unscientific in principle and unreliable in practice as a test of auditory sensitivity. Speech is a stimulus of high redundancy because the information in it is conveyed in several ways simultaneously. The complexity of the human neural system enables it to make optimum use of the information arriving at any time. The listener extracts the message by analysis of both acoustic and linguistic features, application of learned phonological and syntactic rules, interpretation of contextual clues (including, where available, non-auditory information) and prediction and deduction on the basis of semantic probabilities. It is likely that these mechanisms operate in parallel (Cutting and Pisoni, 1978). This makes the recognition of speech a rapid information processing procedure that is resistant to corrupting influences. Thus, the normal auditory system has little problem with moderately degraded speech material and an impaired system often copes well with good-quality speech in good listening conditions.

A hearing loss involving only part of the auditory frequency range may go undetected in an informal speech test which is not carefully controlled. Even a mild or moderate hearing loss of end-organ origin, involving the majority of the auditory range, may not cause noticeable difficulty with speech identification if the test is carried out at normal conversational levels in quiet, low-reverberent conditions (such as a doctor's surgery or a typical suburban living room). Yet, speech audiometry, properly carried out with calibrated equipment and standardized recorded speech material can be a useful tool for audiological diagnostic testing. It can give a reasonably accurate prediction of the best hearing threshold levels in the mid-frequency region of the auditory range. It may also provide useful 'site-of-lesion' information about an auditory impairment, to aid diagnosis.

Acoustically, speech is a complex auditory stimulus, the correct identification of which depends fundamentally (but not only) on satisfactory frequency resolution, frequency discrimination, intensity discrimination and temporal resolution. Psychoacoustic tests of such auditory analytical functions exist but they are time-consuming, difficult and tedious for both subject and tester. Tests using speech material are generally regarded as clinically more acceptable for identifying patients with poor auditory analytical capability and they have been found to be powerful tools for distinguishing patients with various types of auditory disorders.

Terminology

The clinical use of speech materials to aid diagnosis involves the testing of the patient's ability to accurately identify samples of speech or speech-like stimuli. The frequently used description 'speech discrimination testing' is usually not accurate as the patient is rarely asked to discriminate between two or more auditory stimuli or between a small number of possible responses. The current (1996) terminology specified in ISO 8253-3, is speech recognition rather than speech discrimination, speech intelligibility or speech identification and similar terms. The term 'speech intelligibility', arising from communications research, is more accurate but, in the clinical context, it needs to be carefully distinguished from the intelligibility of the subject's own speech to others. The same confusion can arise with 'speech testing', the common use of which is to be deprecated. The term 'speech audiometry' is, itself, rather unsatisfactory as the procedure does not measure auditory sensitivity (or any other fundamental psychoacoustical function) alone. The test result depends not only upon the condition of the peripheral auditory system and its primary central neural projections, but also substantially upon the nature of the speech material, the availability of visual cues, the extent of contextual information and the size of the response set (which is partly determined by the linguistic competence of the patient). Nevertheless, as the term 'speech audiometry' is so deeply entrenched in audiological terminology, it will be used here also, but with the foregoing reservations in mind.

Objectives

In the clinic, speech audiometry is most often used diagnostically to place the patient into one or more of a number of 'auditory function' categories, namely:

Normal auditory function.
Non-organic hearing loss.
Conductive hearing loss.
Sensory or end-organ disorder.
Peripheral-neural (NVIII) disorder.
Central auditory disorder.

Although a characteristic pattern of response (or rather a characteristic deviation from a normal response) may be found in conductive hearing loss (Figure 7.1) speech audiometry is rarely of value in such cases. Carefully masked air-conduction and bone-conduction pure-tone audiometry, combined with acoustic immittance and stapedial reflex measurements, is a more appropriate way of identifying and investigating middle-ear disorders. Speech audiometry cannot be relied upon to give an accurate prediction of everyday hearing ability following middle-ear surgery. However, it may be useful for identifying unusually poor speech identification capability in a patient in whom the conductive

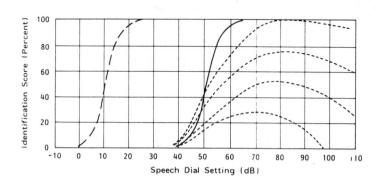

Figure 7.1 Typical speech identification functions for monosyllabic words in subjects with normal hearing (– –), conductive hearing loss (—) and sensorineural hearing losses (- - - -). In conductive hearing loss the effect is largely one of reduced sensitivity. In sensorineural disorders with similar pure-tone thresholds, the identification function tends to be flatter and the maximum score may be reduced, with greater reductions generally associated with NVIII lesions

component overlies a sensorineural hearing loss with considerable involvement of the acoustic nerve. The identification and differentiation of central neural disorders cannot readily be achieved with the use of conventional speech materials. The effects of central neural disorder on speech recognition are usually subtle and frequently different in kind from those of peripheral disorders. Several special techniques have been devised in an attempt to identify central auditory neural dysfunction and to distinguish cortical and brainstem disorders. They will be considered later in this chapter.

Materials and parameters

There are usually two measures sought in the use of speech audiometry for diagnostic purposes in the clinic. The first is a 'threshold' for the identification of the speech material to provide an estimate of auditory sensitivity, as measured by pure-tone audiometry. The second is the maximum speech recognition score achieved at supra-threshold intensities under optimum conditions.

In the United States, different speech materials are generally used to achieve each of these measurements with maximum accuracy. For measurements of maximum speech identification performance, lists of monosyllabic words are widely used. Initially, 'phonetically-balanced' (PB) word lists were developed at the Harvard Psychoacoustic Laboratory (Egan, 1948) for the testing of communications systems. They became popular for clinical audiological use, as the W-22 word lists (Hirsh, 1952), after modification at the Central Institute for the Deaf to restrict the vocabulary to commonly-used words. In addition to meeting the criterion of word-familiarity, the lists were constructed to be of equal difficulty and equal phonetic (actually phonemic) composition, approximately corresponding to that found in everyday speech.

More lists have subsequently been produced by other workers in the United States, but the W-22 lists have remained the most widely-used by clinical audiologists there. The maximum discrimination score achieved by a subject is generally referred to as 'PB_{max}' (Figure 7.2). Spondee word lists were developed (Hudgins et al., 1947; Hirsh et al., 1952) for speech threshold determination, as the identification functions are steeper than for monosyllabic words (Figure 7.2) due to the higher linguistic redundancy or predictability of spondees. On average, normally hearing listeners achieve 100% correct identification at an intensity 20–30 dB lower than for monosyllabic words (Rupp and Stockdell, 1980). The 'speech reception threshold' (SRT) is defined as the lowest intensity at which the listener correctly identifies 50% of spondee words. It is a reliable measure that correlates well with the pure-tone threshold average.

Jerger and Jerger (1976) pointed out several advantages of calculating a speech recognition 'threshold' using monosyllabic word lists,

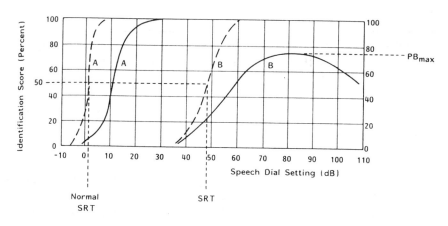

Figure 7.2 Typical speech recognition functions for spondees (– –) and monosyl-labic words (—). (A) Average functions for normal subjects; (B) functions for a patient with a sensorineural hearing loss. SRT = speech recognition threshold; PB$_{max}$ = maximum recognition score

though they found that the appropriate norm, with which to compare the patient's performance, depended upon the PB$_{max}$ achieved. Their results suggested that monosyllabic word lists are comparable with spondees in the accuracy with which they can be used to predict average pure-tone thresholds. Nevertheless, Rupp (1980) noted that the 'Guidelines for Determining the Threshold Level for Speech', published by the American Speech and Hearing Association in 1977, specify spondees as the standard test materials for speech threshold measurements.

In the UK, considerations of time availability in the clinic have led to monosyllabic word lists being used for both threshold estimation and measurement of identification ability. Only a few word lists have been published and used extensively in the UK. The MRC lists (1947), derived from the Harvard lists for the determination of an 'optimum' hearing aid frequency response, are generally thought to be too long and to contain too many uncommon words to be suitable for clinical diagnostic use. The Fry lists (Fry, 1961), with 35 words per list, are also often regarded as being too time consuming. The isophonemic word lists of Arthur Boothroyd (Boothroyd, 1968) have achieved widespread clinical use in the UK. Boothroyd published and recorded 15 lists, each comprising 10 consonant-vowel-consonant (CVC) monosyllables, with the same 30 phonemes appearing in each list in different combinations.

Phonemic balance, consistent with that in everyday spoken English, is precluded by the small number of phonemes in each list, but is not of great importance for diagnostic application (Lyregaard et al., 1976). The original recording by Boothroyd was felt by many to be unsuitable for use across the whole of the UK, because of his strong northern English accent. The lists were re-recorded in a 'standard' southern English accent on at least two occasions, at the Institute of Sound and Vibration Research (ISVR) in the University of Southampton and at the Royal National Institute for the Deaf, who inserted two non-scoring practice words at the beginning of each list. Original normative studies carried out at the ISVR, showed that the recognition (and hence the degree of difficulty) of three of the original 15 lists (nos. 9, 10 and 15) in the Southampton recording differed significantly from the remainder and they were therefore discarded.

Hood and Poole (1977) described a procedure for improving the reliability of the MRC word lists. A similar exercise was carried out at the ISVR on the re-recorded Boothroyd word lists. They have subsequently been used widely for clinical purposes in the UK and are generally referred to as the Arthur Boothroyd lists — Southampton recording: AB(S).

Markides (1978a) showed that the test/retest reliability of the AB(S) word lists is reasonably high, with correlation coefficients for identification scores ranging from 0.34 at near threshold levels to 0.79 at suprathreshold intensities. He presented normative data for children aged 6 - 11 years and for adults. As the words are less familiar to children than to adults, the slope of the identification function becomes shallower and the intensity for 50% recognition rises with decreasing age of the subject. However, the differences between adults and children are not great. Clinicians with extensive experience with the word lists know that they can be used even with subjects whose knowledge of English is minimal (Figure 7.3). In such cases the identification functions become still less steep, approximating those for nonsense words, where the linguistic redundancy of the material is minimal. The maximum identification score will, however, usually reach 100%.

Figure 7.4 shows the parameters of a speech recognition function obtained with monosyllabic word lists. The term 'optimal discrimination score' (ODS), proposed by Coles et al. (1973), is synonymous with PB_{max} but acknowledges that the maximum score is obtained or estimated at the optimum speech presentation level indicated by the identification function. It is also more appropriate in cases where the identification function rises throughout the measured intensity range and appears likely to reach a maximum score at an intensity above the maximum output of the equipment.

As the identification function of monosyllables has a considerably lower slope than that for spondees, particularly for patients with sensorineural hearing loss, the SRT (the level at which 50% correct identification is achieved) does not always agree as well with the pure-tone threshold average. Coles et al. (1973) proposed the use of the 'half-peak level' (HPL), which is the intensity (in arbitrary dial-level units) at which

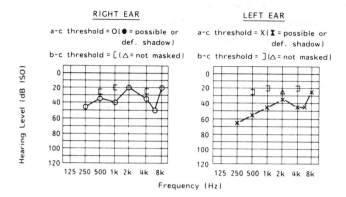

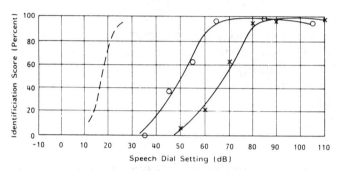

Figure 7.3 Pure-tone audiograms and speech audiograms of a 30-year-old woman from Bangladesh with no knowledge of English. Speech audiometry was carried out with AB(S) word lists, phoneme scoring (- - - , average normal curve for equipment used)

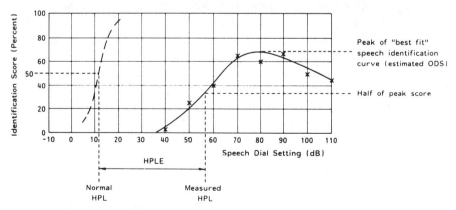

Figure 7.4 Speech recognition functions and measurement parameters for monosyllabic word lists; - - - , average normal curve; —, pathological curve, HPL, half-peak level; HPLE, half-peak level elevation; ODS, optimal discrimination score (the ODS should be measured at the optimum speech dial setting indicated by the 'best fit' identification curve)

the listener achieves 50% of their maximum score. The 'half-peak level elevation' (HPLE) is then the difference between the patient's HPL and the average normal HPL. The measure has the advantage that it can be applied to recognition functions in which 50% correct recognition is never achieved.

In determining the presentation level at which the maximum identification score of the patient is likely to occur, it is important that a full identification function is obtained by presenting word lists at various supra-threshold levels. Several authors (e.g. Coles, 1972; Rupp and Stockdell, 1980; Hood, 1981) note the error of attempting to measure the maximum score with a single presentation level. Boothroyd (1968) estimated that, for his 10-word lists, a single-list phoneme identification score of about 50% would have associated confidence limits of ±20%. Therefore a 'best-fit' curve should be determined by eye, according to the theoretical expectation of a sigmoid psychometric function, rather than joining up individual list scores, each with its associated measurement error. When measuring the maximum discrimination score at the peak of the identification function, it is important to present sufficient items to ensure adequate reliability of the score. For the Boothroyd lists, three lists are recommended for ODS measurement (Priede and Coles, 1976), giving 90 test items (phonemes).

Method

A suggested systematic procedure for obtaining a speech identification function using monosyllabic word lists, is outlined in Appendix I. For accurate and reliable results the word lists should be recorded and played back to the subject through earphones driven by an audiometer or an amplifier with variable attenuation. Live-voice presentation, even when monitored with a sound level meter, gives rise to unacceptable variability of intensity both within and between lists and to variations in pronunciations between different presentations of the same list (Brandy, 1966). Wide-band masking should be applied as necessary to the contralateral ear (Coles et al., 1973). The requirements for calibration of recorded material will be found elsewhere in this book (chapters 5 and 6) but it is important to realize that it is necessary for normal parameter values to be obtained or calculated for each set of play-back equipment used. Two items of calibration should be available for every combination of word-list recording and playback equipment:

1. The attenuator setting for the speech channel, which gives an average of 50% correct identification in a group of normally hearing subjects (the normal half-peak level or SRT).
2. The effective masking level of the equipment (i.e. the relationship between the dial levels for wide-band noise masking and the speech

material should be known, for a specified decrement in speech identification in normally hearing subjects, when ipsilateral masking is
introduced).

Each recording of the word lists will usually have a calibration tone
at the beginning, allowing the input level of the audiometer to be
adjusted to the same level on each occasion of use, thus ensuring that
the dial settings are consistent and that the normal parameter values
apply. It is important that the patient understands the requirement of
the test. The scoring of the word lists should be carried out on a
phoneme basis (Table 7.1) to improve the reliability of the test by
increasing the number of test items (Lyregaard et al., 1976). The patient
should be instructed to respond to any parts of the word he or she
hears. Suitable instructions are suggested in Appendix III. It is not
important that the exact wording be adhered to, as long as the main
points are covered.

Table 7.1 Examples of phoneme scoring (stimulus word: 'FISH')

Verbal Response	Marking	Scoring
'FISH'	FISH ✓	3
'FIT'	FI$\cancel{SH}$	2
'WISH'	$\cancel{F}$ISH	2
'FOSH'	F$\cancel{I}$SH	2
'FLIT'	FI$\cancel{SH}$	1
'FAT'	FI$\cancel{SH}$	1
'DASH'	$\cancel{F}$ISH	1
'FISHED'	FI$\cancel{SH}$	2
'DEBT'	$\cancel{FISH}$	0
(no response)	~~FISH~~	0

Clinical applications

Threshold estimation

Coles et al. (1973) compared speech HPLE values (for Fry's word lists)
with pure-tone thresholds in a large number of subjects with normal
hearing or acquired sensory hearing loss. They found that, with a high
degree of reliability, the HPLE lay within ±10 dB of the 'best-two-
average' (BTA) of pure-tone thresholds for 500 Hz, 1 kHz and 2 kHz,
with corrections for greater high-frequency and low-frequency threshold elevation as follows:

4 kHz threshold 11–20 dB poorer than BTA, add 1 dB to BTA.
4 kHz threshold 21–30 dB poorer than BTA, add 2 dB to BTA.

4 kHz threshold 31–40 dB poorer than BTA, add 3 dB to BTA.
4 kHz threshold over 40 dB poorer than BTA, add 4 dB to BTA.
500 Hz threshold 11–20 dB poorer than BTA, add 3 dB to BTA.
500 Hz threshold 21–30 dB poorer than BTA, add 10 dB to BTA.

The high correlation between HPLE and BTA (0.5 – 2 kHz), corrected for high-frequency losses, was similar to the relationship predicted by Fletcher (1950) for spondee SRT values. Priede and Coles (1976) showed that the relationship applied similarly to patients with hearing losses apparently of NVIII origin (Figure 7.5). Hood and Poole (1971) agreed with the general principle of a linear relationship between BTA and speech SRT for conductive hearing loss, but showed that it did not apply in patients diagnosed as having Ménière's disease. As Hood and

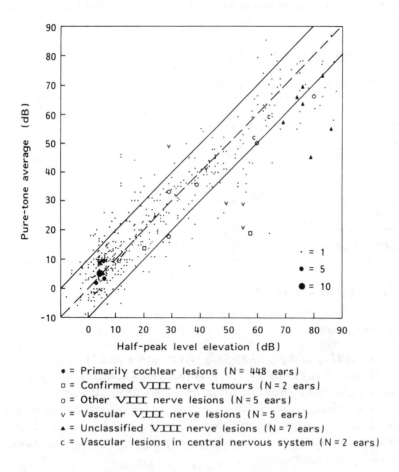

Figure 7.5 Relationship between pure-tone average threshold (see text) and speech identification half-peak level elevation in patients with cochlear and eighth nerve lesions. (From Priede and Coles, 1976, by permission)

Poole used monosyllabic word lists to test their subjects, their SRT measurements were not strictly comparable with spondee SRT values measured by Fletcher. Nevertheless, in such a restricted group of patients, which is characterized by variable, but often poor speech perception, it is likely that Hood and Poole would have obtained similar results with spondee word lists. However, Hood (1981) rightly noted the limitation of the SRT parameter in patients whose maximum speech recognition score is less than 50% and informal examination of Hood and Poole's (1971) group average data suggests that, if the HPLE value is taken as the speech recognition 'threshold' (rather than the SRT), a reasonably good agreement with the BTA would be obtained, as Coles et al. (1973) predicted.

Markides (1980), using Boothroyd's isophonemic word lists with hearing impaired children aged 9–14 years, calculated correlation coefficients between speech HPLE values and a variety of single-frequency and multi-frequency measures of pure-tone sensitivity. Of the two pure-tone threshold descriptors that gave the highest correlations with HPLE, the simplest formula was the best-two-average hearing level in the frequency range 250 Hz – 4 kHz, which estimated the speech HPLE within ±10 dB in every case. Markides pointed out the importance of low-frequency hearing levels in predicting the speech recognition threshold, but also warned that, for children with atypical audiometric configurations (e.g. predominantly low-frequency or U-shaped losses) the simple formula may not be reliable.

The speech HPLE for monosyllabic word lists is useful as a check on the reliability of pure-tone audiometric thresholds and has been shown to be a powerful measure for identifying non-organic hearing loss in clinical populations. Priede and Coles (1976) found that over 80% of patients with proven non-organic components in their hearing losses gave pure-tone average thresholds that were more than 10 dB greater than their speech half-peak level elevations (Figure 7.6).

Aplin and Kane (1985) found similar discrepancies between pure-tone average thresholds and half-peak level elevations in experimental subjects who were asked to simulate hearing loss. Sophisticated subjects (staff or post-graduate students of a university audiology department) were no more successful in matching their HPLE values to their average simulated pure-tone thresholds than were unsophisticated subjects. Like Priede and Coles (1976), Aplin and Kane found that their subjects frequently, but not always, gave consistent speech half-peak level elevations that suggested some degree of hearing loss, albeit considerably less than indicated by the simulated pure-tone audiograms. This conflicts with the widely held assumption that unsophisticated subjects (presumably including the majority of clinical non-organic cases) are unable to simulate a consistent hearing loss in speech audiometry, because the fluctuating nature of the speech signal makes it difficult for

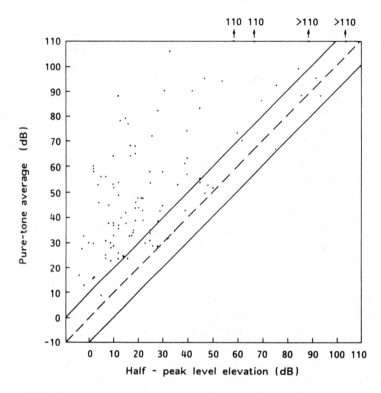

Figure 7.6 Relationship between pure-tone average threshold (see text) and speech recognition half-peak level elevation in patients with non-organic hearing loss. (From Priede and Coles, 1976, by permission)

the listener to maintain a chosen performance level reliably. Indeed, both Coles (1982) and Aplin and Kane (1985) identified anomalous patterns of responding in speech audiometry by non-organic cases, which enabled them to maintain artificially elevated half-peak level elevations. These include giving few partly correct responses ('all-or-none' responding) or making systematic errors such as responding only to every second or third test word or omitting the third phoneme in all or most of the test words. Priede and Coles (1976) described a procedure for speech audiometry, based on the loudness alteration technique advocated by Fournier in 1956, in cases of suspected non-organic hearing loss. By alternately lowering the intensity of the speech by 20 dB and raising it by 15 dB on successive lists, it is possible to confuse the patient and cause them to respond at progressively lower intensities, often to a level within normal limits.

Differentiation of sensory and peripheral neural disorders

Liden (1954) was one of the earliest authors to identify poor speech recognition as a characteristic of retrocochlear disorder. Prior to that time (e.g. Dix et al., 1949) and for several years afterwards (e.g. Hood and Poole, 1971), poor speech recognition was held to be a consequence of loudness recruitment, which was indicative of end-organ pathology, in contrast to the good recognition evident with high intensities in conductive lesions. Hood and Poole (1971) acknowledged that lesions of the acoustic nerve can cause recognition losses well in excess of those typically found in cochlear lesions with similar pure-tone thresholds, but pointed out that '. ... the speech audiogram can have little practical diagnostic value unless it can be interpreted within the content [sic] of the predictability of speech curves encountered in cochlear hearing loss'. Priede and Coles (1976) took a similar view in plotting optimum speech recognition scores against average pure-tone thresholds, corrected as recommended by Fletcher (1950), for cochlear and eighth nerve lesions. They found that the 90th percentile curve for cochlear ODS values approximated to the 10th percentile curve for neural cases. That is, the curve effectively separated 90% of the end-organ disorders from 90% of the eighth nerve lesions. The original data were obtained using Fry's word lists (Fry, 1961) but a 90th percentile curve was later calculated for the Boothroyd lists (Boothroyd, 1968) and both curves were published in notes accompanying recordings of the AB(S) word lists produced by the Institute of Sound and Vibration Research (Figure 7.7).

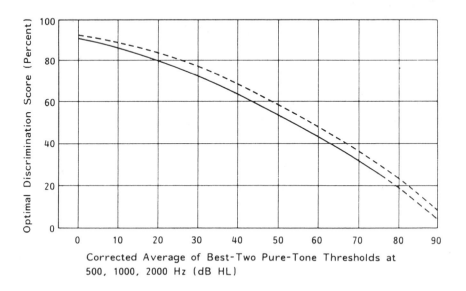

Figure 7.7 Criterion curves for distinguishing cochlear and eighth nerve lesions. When the non-test ear is properly masked, 90% of cochlear cases lie above the relevant criterion line and approximately 90% of neural cases fall below it. —, AB(S) word lists (three lists); – – – , Fry's lists (one list)

Priede and Coles (1976) suggested that the disproportionately greater speech 'discrimination loss' of neural lesions might be a result of temporal distortion of the neural signal arising from variable conduction velocities of the nerve fibres. This notion was supported by Borg (1982) who showed that speech recognition scores in patients with acoustic neuromata were well correlated with features of the auditory brainstem electric responses which are dependent upon temporal coding within the nerve. No such correlation was found in cochlear hearing loss. Hood (1981), while continuing to point to poor speech recognition in patients with Ménière's disorder, stated that 'Speech audiometry, however, can be of particular value in the differential diagnosis of cochlear and nerve fibre lesions since the latter *invariably* [my emphasis] exhibit poorer speech discrimination than the former.' Such is clearly not the case, as the data of Priede and Coles (1976) demonstrated, with evidence of wide variations and some overlap of the ODS values for cochlear and eighth nerve lesions with similar pure-tone audiograms. White (1980) cited several studies that also showed variability of speech discrimination scores in retrocochlear disorder. Jerger and Jerger (1971) found similar variations in PB_{max} scores obtained with PB-50 word lists in cochlear and retrocochlear cases, but noted a tendency in retrocochlear disorders (particularly eighth nerve lesions) for speech discrimination to deteriorate markedly at high speech stimulus intensities. They termed this phenomenon 'roll-over' and recommended the use of a 'roll-over index' of:

$$\frac{PB_{max} - PB_{min}}{PB_{max}}$$

where PB_{min} is the lowest recognition score recorded for stimulus intensities above that at which PB_{max} is obtained (up to a maximum of 110 dB SPL). Jerger and Jerger (1971) found that the roll-over index separated cochlear and eighth nerve cases without overlap. They acknowledged that many other investigators had not found the roll-over phenomenon to be diagnostically useful but noted the importance of recording a full speech identification function in order accurately to measure PB_{max} and PB_{min}.

Dirks et al. (1977) supported the use of the roll-over index, but emphasized the necessity of deriving a new diagnostic criterion value if speech materials other than the PAL PB-50 words (Egan, 1948) are used. In the UK, the roll-over index is not widely used, probably due largely to the influence of British authors (e.g. Hood and Poole, 1971; Priede and Coles, 1976; Hood, 1984) who have reported the occurrence of roll-over in certain cases of cochlear disorder, as well as eighth nerve lesions. Nevertheless, in the United States, the roll-over index continues to be advocated (White, 1980) as a means of increasing the sensitivity of speech audiometry to retrocochlear disorders.

Evaluation of central auditory nervous system disorders

The reported effects of central auditory nervous system (CANS) lesions upon auditory perception are highly variable. With bilateral lesions of the auditory cortex (e.g. Jerger et al., 1969) it is possible for the patient to experience severe auditory impairment, particularly with respect to the discrimination of speech. Such cases are rare, however, and most central neural lesions appear to give rise to varying but often relatively subtle perceptual disabilities (compared with lesions of the cochlea or acoustic nerve). Standard monosyllabic word recognition tests are generally insensitive to cortical disorders and Hurley (1980) summarized results from the literature showing that brainstem lesions give inconsistent results with such tests.

A large number of special test procedures have been suggested for the investigation of CANS disorders, using speech or non-speech stimuli. Although non-auditory variables, such as intelligence and linguistic competence of the subject can substantially affect the results of speech-based tests (Davis et al., 1976) the familiarity of speech encourages patients into more consistent and reliable performance than is usually observed with non-speech stimuli.

Brainstem lesions

Speech-based tests of brainstem function generally investigate aspects of binaural interaction which arise from the binaural representation of auditory information through crossing neural pathways at various levels. They include the binaural fusion of speech presented dichotically with the test material split either spectrally (e.g. Matzker, 1959), or temporally as in the RASP test (discussed by Lynn and Gilroy, 1977). In brainstem disorders, identification of the dichotic signal is often not significantly better than that achieved with monaural presentation of each part of the divided speech material. The phenomenon of binaural release from masking, or masking level difference (MLD), giving improved signal detection and recognition when either the signal or the masking noise (but not both) is made anti-phasic between the two ears, has been widely used as a test of brainstem function. A similar improvement in recognition is observed with masked speech stimuli (Olsen et al., 1976). The MLD effect is disrupted by brainstem disorder, but also unfortunately by cochlear or eighth nerve impairment, so that its reliable application may be limited to patients with normal auditory sensitivity.

Cortical disorder

Owing to the complexity of the CANS, a limited impairment of cortical function may have little effect upon the perception of good quality speech, analysed by an intact peripheral auditory system. Most tests of cortical dysfunction therefore rely upon a reduction in the redundancy of the speech material to improve their sensitivity. This may be achieved by degrading the acoustic signal conveying the speech information, in terms of spectral content or temporal structure (see Hurley, 1980 for a review of these procedures). Speaks and Jerger (1965) aimed to reduce the redundancy of speech material linguistically as well as acoustically. They developed third-order synthetic sentences which give an advantage over monosyllabic words in having temporal variations in frequency and intensity that approximate 'real' sentences, while conveying minimal contextual and syntactic clues.

For assessment of CANS dysfunction, competing running speech is presented simultaneously with the synthetic sentences, to either the ipsilateral or contralateral ear. Keith (1977) reviewed results showing the synthetic sentence identification (SSI) test to be effective in differentiating acoustic nerve, brainstem and cortical disorders and in identifying the site of the lesion, though he emphasized the need to consider SSI results in conjunction with those of other auditory tests. Hurley (1980) however, reported that the test was not in wide use in the United States.

Probably the best standardized and most evaluated test of CANS function is the staggered spondaic word (SSW) test (Katz, 1962). Katz, (1977) and Brunt, (1978) described the application of the test and reviewed a sizeable body of data available. Although the test uses dichotic binaural presentation of partially overlapping spondées, it appears to be most sensitive to cortical disorder.

Although tests of CANS dysfunction continue to be used and further developed in other countries, they have generally fallen out of favour in the UK. This is largely because of lack of confidence in the specificity and reliability of such tests, coupled with the rising popularity of auditory brainstem response measurements. Undoubtedly, much of the early published research data on CANS behavioural tests were of doubtful value because of the poor anatomical and patho-physiological specification of the central lesions being studied. Certainly, also, the tests are highly susceptible to the effects of concomitant peripheral auditory disorder. With regard to central speech tests in particular, it is not clear whether the decrement in performance observed with increasing age of the subject (Bosatra and Russolo, 1982) is due to speech-specific central neural dysfunction or to deterioration of peripheral auditory coding that is known to occur with advancing age (e.g. Patterson et al., 1982). Nevertheless, similar criticisms can be levelled at electrophysiological tests of central auditory neural function that have enjoyed a rapid and not wholly justifiable ascendancy in the audiological armamentarium over the last two decades.

Future developments

Lyregaard et al. (1976) concluded, for both theoretical and practical reasons, that the efficient diagnostic application of speech audiometry is limited to CANS disorders, requiring reduced-redundancy test materials.

However, with the considerable advances that have been made in auditory physiology and psychoacoustics over the last 20 years, the opportunity now exists for the development of a more analytical and functional approach to diagnostic assessment; investigating basic auditory processing.

Psychoacoustic tests are now clinically more acceptable with the use of adaptive procedures, but speech-based tests such as the four-alternative-auditory-feature (FAAF) procedure (Foster and Haggard, 1979) offer the additional advantage of stimulus familiarity. Synthesized speech features (Fourcin, 1979) allow precise control of parameters of the speech signal and investigation of specific aspects of auditory processing. Dramatic improvements in neuro-radiological procedures should help to overcome some of the specificity problems involved in the assessment of central auditory nervous system disorders.

Appendix I

Method of performing speech audiometry with monosyllabic word lists

(a) The first word list should be presented at a level which is comfortable to the patient and is likely to give rise to a high recognition score. Estimate the level at which the patient is likely to score 50% correct (the half-peak level or HPL). This can be calculated by adding the HPL for normals to the average of the patient's best two pure-tone thresholds for the test ear (over the frequency range 250 Hz – 4 kHz). The presentation level of the first word list should be at the estimated HPL + 10 dB.
(b) Calculate the contralateral masking level required for the first speech level, using the formula in Appendix II.
(c) Test at estimated HPL + 10 dB, estimated HPL + 0 dB, estimated HPL – 10 dB and at 10 dB lower levels until the recognition score drops below 10%. The contralateral masking level should be adjusted in line with the speech presentation level.
(d) Test at HPL + 30 dB and in increasing 20 dB steps to complete the speech audiogram curve (up to the maximum output of the audiometer or the loudness discomfort level of the patient).

(e) Sketch by eye the 'best fit' sigmoid speech identification function, as judged from the recognition scores plotted on the chart.

(f) Except where the identification score, averaged over three adjacent test levels, is 95% or more measure this maximum or optimum recognition score separately. To do this, present three word lists at the level which is judged by eye to be most likely to give the maximum speech recognition score.

Appendix II

Masking for speech audiometry

For accuracy of masking, the effective masking level of the audiometer should be known (see chapter 5, this volume). Coles and Priede (1975) published formulae for the masking of the non-test ear in speech audiometry and their derivation is outlined in Coles and Priede (1974). The formula to determine the masking noise dial setting when the effective masking level is known is:

$$D_m = D_s + E_m + maxABG_{nt} - 40$$

where: D_m = masking noise dial setting; D_s = speech dial setting; E_m = effective masking level; and $maxABG_{nt}$ = maximum difference between air-conduction and bone-conduction pure-tone thresholds in the non-test ear for any frequency in the range 250 Hz – 4 kHz.

Where the effective masking level is not known, the formula derived by Coles and Priede is:

$$D_m = M_w + D_s - C_s - BBC_{nt}$$

where: D_m = masking noise dial setting; M_w = the threshold in the non-test ear for the wide-band masking noise; D_s = speech dial setting; C_s = speech dial setting at which an average of 50% speech recognition is obtained by a group of normally-hearing listeners (i.e. the normal half-peak level); and BBC_{nt} = best bone-conduction threshold in the non-test ear in the range 250 Hz – 4 kHz.

Appendix III

Instructing the patient

The following instructions are suggested for use in speech audiometry using monosyllabic word lists with phoneme scoring. It is not important that the exact wording be adhered to, as long as the main points are covered:

'You are going to hear someone speaking single words through the earphones, one ear at a time. The words are spoken slowly like this . . . BUS . . . FUN . . . SHOP . . . TOY. . . At the beginning the words will be at a comfortable level but they will gradually become quieter and then later they will be much louder. Please listen carefully and repeat after each word whatever you think you heard. Even if you hear only part of the word or a word that does not seem to make sense, or even a single sound like /a/, /o/ or /ch/, please repeat it because it adds to your score. From time to time you may hear a rushing noise in the opposite ear to the speech. Ignore the noise and concentrate on repeating the words that you hear. It is important to go to quite loud levels, but if the words or the rushing noise get uncomfortably loud, let me know. Do you have any questions?'.

Chapter 8
The uses and misuses of speech audiometry in rehabilitation

ROGER GREEN

Rehabilitation is a wide area of audiology, and speech audiometry has been used extensively within it. However its uses can be summarized into two main categories. First, it is used to measure a patient's ability to understand speech and so to predict the degree of handicap they are likely to suffer. Second, it is used to evaluate treatments, such as the fitting of a hearing aid or the introduction of an auditory training programme.

Other chapters in this book describe the practical details of tests appropriate to each of various roles, and the procedures which would yield the best results with these tests. However, speech audiometry has still not reached the degree of precision that will enable it to do all that we would wish. There are many reasons for this, not least of which is the nature of the medium itself, as we shall see. Its predictions are muddy rather than clear. Furthermore it has considerable potential for abuse. The role of this chapter is in a sense then to play devil's advocate, in an attempt to make the reader aware of the limitations of speech audiometry's as well as its strengths

This chapter will begin by looking at the meaning of the term rehabilitation. It will go on to discuss how speech audiometry has been used to measure disability and evaluate treatments. It will focus in particular on hearing aid intervention as this is both a common treatment and one with which speech audiometry is often linked. The use that has been made of speech audiometry in making inferences both about handicap and treatment benefit will be discussed. It will be necessary to look at some theoretical issues (in particular test sensitivity and reliability) in order to achieve a clearer understanding of the need for choosing appropriate test conditions and of the importance of making critical interpretations of the test results. Finally some practical suggestions will be made though these will refer more to the qualitative than the quantitative uses of speech audiometry.

Auditory rehabilitation

The aim of auditory rehabilitation will vary from clinic to clinic. In some institutions it is considered sufficient simply to fit a hearing aid on the assumption that self-induced rehabilitation will automatically follow. At the other extreme, considerable effort may be expended in quantifying the extent of the patient's auditory disability, and then fitting aids and conducting auditory training programmes which focus on bringing about as much reduction in that disability as possible, in order to alleviate the resulting handicap. A clear, if modest, definition of the aim of auditory rehabilitation is necessary if the place of speech audiometry within a rehabilitation programme is to be understood. A possible definition of rehabilitation then is as follows:

> Rehabilitation is the process by which patients are enabled to come to terms with the disabilities which result from their hearing impairment, and to reduce as far as possible the impact of those disabilities on their daily life.

It is also worthwhile, in the context of this definition, to differentiate between the terms impairment, disability and handicap. Hearing *impairment* describes the extent of the underlying dysfunction of the patient's auditory system. This impairment is commonly (though not exclusively or exhaustively) 'measured' by the pure-tone audiogram. A hearing impairment will in turn give rise to *disabilities* in performing various more complex processing tasks such as discriminating speech. The relationship between such disabilities and the underlying impairment that gives rise to them is not straightforward. For example, two patients with the same pure-tone audiogram may not have the same ability to discriminate speech. Finally the patient's degree of *handicap* will be governed by the extent to which their disabilities interfere with their way of life. Thus a mild high frequency hearing loss may provide a serious handicap to a young teacher coping with speech at different distances and in a sometimes noisy classroom. The same loss may go almost unnoticed in a retired person whose life is mainly centred around the home.

Disability measurement

It is often thought useful to measure the effect of the patient's hearing loss on their ability to discriminate speech. There is as expected some relationship between the speech discrimination scores and the pure-tone audiogram, with typically correlations of around 0.6 – 0.7 being found between the pure-tone average and the maximum speech discrimination score (see Figure 8.1). The degree of correspondence of this relationship suggests that some idea of a patient's difficulties in coping with speech discrimination can be obtained from the pure-tone audiogram alone. Poorer audiometric thresholds are associated with poorer speech discrimination. However it seems to be also true, for reasons discussed elsewhere in this book, that the pure-tone audiogram does not tell the whole story. Patients with identical audiograms will not always give similar speech discrimination scores. Most clinicians will be familiar with the patient who seems to be having a lot more difficulty coping than their pure-tone audiogram would have lead them to expect, or the patient who appears to be doing surprisingly well despite their impairment.

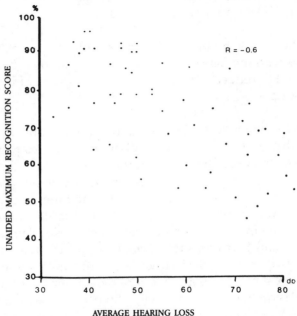

Figure 8.1 Relationship between hearing loss (averaged across frequency), and unaided maximum recognition score (FAAF Test)

If measures of speech recognition are to be useful in rehabilitation then they must tell us something about the patient's ability to cope in the world outside the audiology clinic. In other words we should be able to make predictions about the degree of handicap from such disability measures. Unfortunately a close relationship between disability and handicap does not exist though it is often assumed, with the result that many unfounded inferences are made from one or two brief speech recognition measures. This practice underlies the all too familiar situation in which the general medical practitioner conducts his own version of speech audiometry (by interview in a one-to-one situation in a quiet consulting room) and makes unjustified predictions based on the 'test result' ('I had no trouble making myself understood, therefore you do not have a hearing handicap in any situation').

In the audiology clinic more precise, quantitative measures of speech recognition are possible, such as maximum recognition score, speech reception threshold and so on. However such increase in precision is in a sense only useful if it allows us to predict the extent of the patient's handicap. If a patient has a maximum recognition score of 82% what can we say about their ability to cope as a secretary in a noisy open plan office, or as a nurse needing to understand patients on an intermittently noisy ward? Some light is shed on this issue by examining studies in which Hearing Handicap Questionnaire scores have been compared with speech discrimination scores in order to see how closely related they turn out to be.

Several such questionnaires have been developed (High et al., 1964; Noble and Atherley, 1970; Berkowitz and Hochberg, 1971; Ewertsen et al., 1973). Usually they contain questions relating to typical real life situations and require the patient to circle the category of answer that best fits their experience. Extracts from the Hearing Measurement Scale are shown in Table 8.1.

Table 8.1 Extract from the Hearing Measurement Scale (Noble and Atherley, 1970)

Against each relevant question put a circle round the short form of the phrase that most closely describes your experience.

---

1. Do you have difficulty hearing in a conversation with one other person when you're at home?

    | All | Mo | Half | Occ | Ne |

2. Do you have difficulty hearing in group conversation at home?

    | All | Mo | Half | Occ | Ne |

3. Do you have difficulty hearing in a conversation when you're with one other person outside? (by 'outside' is meant some place outside the house where you would be talking to others)

    | All | Mo | Half | Occ | Ne |

4. Do you have difficulty hearing in group conversation outside?

    | All | Mo | Half | Occ | Ne |

All = all the time, Mo = most of the time, Half = about half the time, Occ = occasionally, Ne = never

---

Several studies have compared such measures and some of these are summarized in Table 8.2. Thus Jupiter (1982) showed a correlation of

0.57 between speech recognition measured under headphones and handicap. (A higher correlation was found between the handicap score and free-field speech measures, implying perhaps that more 'realism' in the clinic does enable better prediction of real-life handicap, at least for some tests and conditions.)

Table 8.2 Correlations between speech recognition ability and self-assessed hearing handicap

Study	Speech Recognition (40 dB SL)	Sound-field Speech Recognition (50 dB HL)
Jupiter (1982)	−0.57	−0.74
Bernstein (1981)	−0.63	−0.65
Weinstein and Ventry (1983)	−0.50	−0.54
Berstein (1981a)	−0.50	−0.74

Findings such as these seem to emphasize three points. First, there is some relationship between discrimination scores and handicap. Second, the relationship depends on the test conditions under which speech discrimination was carried out. In the Jupiter study, for example, free-field test scores using voice levels typical of normal speech intensities were more closely related to handicap than scores measured under head- phones and at higher signal levels than are typical in everyday life. It seems then that more 'realism' in the clinic may enable better prediction of real life handicap. Third, the relationship between the two measures is at best only loose, which implies, hardly surprisingly, that there is more to handicap than can be encompassed in a single measure of disability.

Handicap is a multi-dimensional entity, reflected in all the different situations that a person comes across in their daily life. For example, Gatehouse (1990, 1994) showed that some 50% of the variance in self-report handicap questionnaire scores is explained by age, IQ and personality differences. In order to tighten up the relationship between what goes on in the clinic and in real life it would be necessary to measure speech discrimination in a variety of situations similar to those encountered by the patient. Thus it would be necessary to measure speech in quiet and in a variety of different background noises, in condi- tions with various degrees of reverberation, using a variety of different voices, both live and amplified, with and without lip reading. Clearly this is not a practical proposition in most clinics.

It seems that we do not have a disability measure which easily and accurately predicts handicap. However it is worth considering just how close we can make the relationship. In other words which test or clinically feasible combination of tests best allows us to predict hearing handicap? This is currently a question to which research has not supplied a complete answer, but some insight is obtained from studies in which the correlation between handicap and both disability (e.g. speech recognition) and impairment (e.g. pure-tone average) measures have been compared. Table 8.3 shows the results of a number of studies in which handicap scores were related to both speech discrimination scores and the pure-tone average (the former correlations are negative because as speech discrimination scores get smaller, i.e. worse, handicap scores get larger). The correlations are better for the pure-tone results than for the speech results.

Table 8.3 Correlations among pure-tone sensitivity supra-threshold speech recognition ability and hearing handicap in selected studies

Study	Sample Age	Sample X PTA	Sample Scale	Pure-tone Average Loss and Hearing Handicap	Speech Discrimination Score and Hearing Handicap
High et al. (1964)	21–73	38dBHL	HHS	0.65	–0.46
Berkowitz and Hochberg (1971)	60–87	36dBHL	HHS	0.57	–0.30
Noble and Atherley (1970)	35–65	37dBHL	HMS	0.60	–0.58
Rosen (1978)	16–65	?	SHHI	0.58	–0.33
Weinstein and Ventry (1983b) (from Weinstein, 1984)	65–92	37dBHL	HHIE	0.62	–0.42

HHS = Hearing Handicap Scale; HMS = Hearing Measurement Scale; SHHI = Social Hearing Handicap Index; HHIE = Hearing Handicap Inventory for the Elderly.

These studies suggest that handicap is in fact better predicted from the pure-tone audiogram than from speech measures. The fact that speech audiometry is a relative rarity in rehabilitation may then be due to more than just lack of equipment or time. It may also be that pure-tone audiometry gives in practice a better 'feel' for the degree of handicap than speech discrimination measures even though the latter seem at first sight more valid.

We have discussed so far the possibility of predicting a patient's handicap from speech discrimination scores. We have seen that the relationship appears to be only a loose one. Therefore if we are to use speech tests what use can such scores be put to in helping each individual? What can we say to them as a result of their discrimination scores? Perhaps the most useful concept we can get across is that of 'distortion'. It is important for patients to understand that there is more to their hearing impairment than simply a loss of sensitivity, that the 'distortion' introduced by their damaged ear can make it difficult to unscramble even loud speech.

The extent of this difficulty is well demonstrated by measures of maximum recognition. The fact that many will score less than 100% at any level provides a good starting point for discussing the difference between clarity and loudness that puzzles so many patients. It also provides a starting point for discussing the likely benefit that a hearing aid will provide, as the degree of cochlear distortion which underlies less than perfect recognition scores must limit the potential success of an aid. However this takes us into a further area of rehabilitative speech audiometry.

Treatment evaluation

Rehabilitation involves more than simply predicting and assessing handicap. Indeed its primary function is to provide treatment aimed at alleviating that handicap as much as possible. Various forms of rehabilitative intervention exist, for example the fitting of a hearing aid, or the use of an auditory training programme. The success of such a treatment is sometimes monitored with the help of speech audiometry. Thus a patient may be given speech discrimination tests before and after undertaking an auditory training programme and the difference between scores used as a measure of the effect of the programme. Comparison of aided and unaided speech scores is a frequently suggested method for measuring the effect of a hearing aid. Indeed the latter idea is so common that even if many clinics do not use aided/unaided comparisons, such procedures probably linger close to the top of many a list of priorities intended for implementation just as soon as time and finances permit. It is therefore worthwhile focusing on the potential of speech discrimination as a means of hearing aid evaluation.

In practice recognition scores are obtained with and without a hearing aid. Let us for example take a situation in which a patient's recognition score unaided is 70% and aided is 90%, with a fixed input level typical of normal conversational speech. Is such information useful? What can we do with it? Firstly it may seem to indicate that the aid is definitely helping. However most hearing aids, unless grossly misfitted, will provide some benefit. In that sense we have achieved a result which is so highly predictable anyway as to not really warrant the time taken to do the test.

A more useful comparison may be between the unaided maximum recognition score (rather than the score at normal speech levels) and the aided maximum recognition score. Suppose we do this and find that the patient's unaided maximum score is 80% and the aided score 90%.

This result suggests that the aid is indeed doing more than simply making speech louder. It is also clarifying it to some extent, as the maximum recognition score has improved by some 10%.

Such a comparison suggests that the hearing aid is providing some benefit (though we will have cause to question this inference shortly). However a further question arises here. Is the aid fitted the best possible aid for that patient, or would a different aid demonstrate an even greater improvement? This question takes us into the area of predicting optimum benefit, in which an attempt is made to predict the best possible improvement in speech recognition score we can expect, given certain background information about the patient. If such a prediction can be made with any certainty then it should be possible to compare the predicted recognition score with the measured recognition score and so decide whether a particular hearing aid is providing optimum benefit. As an illustration of the problem, Figure 8.2 shows the relationship between the unaided maximum recognition score and the 'benefit' provided by a hearing aid (difference between aided and unaided score). The relationship between the two is approximately defined by the following equation:

PREDICTED AIDED SCORE = (UNAIDED SCORE)/2 + 50

Thus if the unaided score was 80%, the predicted aided score would be 90%. In this study (Green and Bamford, 1986), aids were carefully fitted according to the configuration of the individual audiograms. However it is still not possible to state with certainty that each represents the best aid for each patient (indeed strictly speaking we can never be sure we have the best of all possible aids). Furthermore there is still a considerable 'spread' of scores, so that it is difficult to predict with any certainty the aided score for each patient. The correlation between the aided and unaided scores is not high (r = 0.5). A patient with an unaided score of 80% could have an aided score anywhere between 85% and 100%.

It is possible to predict aided scores with more certainty if we take into account more background information about the patient. Thus in the same study a closer relationship (r = 0.9) was obtained when a different speech test was used and certain other background information was taken into account, such as the patient's age, audiometric configuration and unaided most comfortable level (MCL).

The interesting thing about this result is that it was obtained by choosing from a considerable amount of background information (such as age, degree, slope and configuration of hearing loss, measures of cochlear distortion, hearing aid frequency response slope) those features of the situation which contributed most to predicting the aided score. Thus prediction of the 'benefit' provided by a hearing aid was

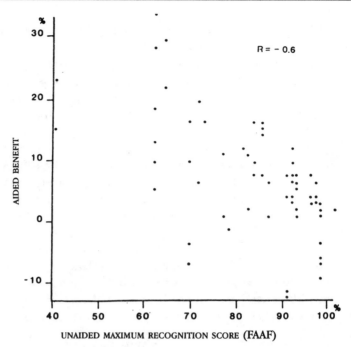

Figure 8.2 Relationship between unaided maximum recognition score and aided benefit. The relationship demonstrates the extent to which benefit (aided-unaided score) experienced by patients is predictable from their unaided recognition score. Patients with lower unaided scores tend to show more measurable benefit than patients with higher unaided scores

possible to some extent from the patient's unaided score for the same test. Prediction was considerably improved by allowing for the age of the patient, the unaided MCL and the configuration of the audiogram. However one feature included which made very little difference to prediction of the aided score was the slope of the hearing aid frequency response. Changing the slope does not appear to significantly influence the aided score. Thus we can to some extent predict this score, we can measure it, but in many cases we can do very little to influence it. Again this calls into question the usefulness of performing speech audiometry as a means of measuring the success of a hearing aid fitting other than for detecting an aid which is grossly misfitted.

Treatment comparisons

Speech testing has also been used as a tool for differentiating between treatments. For example we may wish to compare the benefit provided by several different hearing aids, in order that the most successful can be selected for the patient. Various procedures for performing such a comparison have been suggested. The most straightforward is simply to compare the aided recognition scores for the various hearing aids under identical conditions. This form of speech testing formed part of a procedure for comparative evaluation of hearing aids first described by Carhart (1946a,b). Because of its face validity and subsequent influence on comparative evaluation, it is worth describing the Carhart procedures in some detail. Carhart's original procedure consisted essentially of five steps:

STEP 1   Measure the subject's unaided sound-field speech recognition threshold, threshold of discomfort and recognition score at a fixed sensation level (25 dB SL).

STEP 2   Fit the first hearing aid for evaluation. Set the gain so that the subject reports a speech signal 40 dB above normal speech threshold as being comfortably loud. Measure the aided speech recognition threshold and threshold of discomfort.

STEP 3   Set the aid on maximum gain and repeat the aided speech recognition threshold and threshold of discomfort.

STEP 4   Set the gain so that the subject reports a speech signal 50 dB above normal speech detection threshold as being comfortably loud. Measure the speech recognition threshold in noise (Carhart advocated two types of noise, white noise and saw tooth noise).

STEP 5   Reset the aid as in STEP 2 and remeasure the aided speech recognition threshold (as a check for reliability). Measure the speech recognition score at a 25 dB sensation level.

Steps 2 to 5 were repeated for each hearing aid to be evaluated. The method enables a number of dimensions of hearing aid performance to be examined, in particular the recognition in quiet and background noise, and the aided dynamic range.

Experience with the procedure has led to a number of modifications. For example the full procedure proved time consuming and so not practical for comparing more than a few hearing aids. The signal and noise levels, as well as types of noise have also been varied to suit the tastes of the clinician performing the procedure. However, in its modified form the Carhart method still finds favour.

The status of hearing aid selection and evaluation has changed substantially since Carhart's day as a result of thorough and critical examination of the issues. The background to this area is well covered in many audiology texts (Ross 1978; Schmitz 1980; Byrne 1983) and it is not the author's intention to review that material in any detail here. Briefly the usefulness of comparative evaluation was brought into question following a number of studies which seemed to show that differences between hearing aids were simply not detectable (e.g. Shore et al., 1960; Resnick et al., 1963) unless aid parameters were manipulated so as to be grossly inappropriate (e.g. Jerger et al., 1966). It was not clear whether this failure to differentiate between aids was due to the fact that the aids used really were equivalent or simply because the speech tests used were just not sensitive enough to reveal any differences.

Interest in comparative evaluation continues. There are two main reasons for this. Firstly, with the developments in microelectronics and consequent versatility in hearing aid design, the debate about individual selection has reopened, particularly in the form of a plethora of hearing aid selection procedures (e.g. Shapiro, 1976; Berger et al., 1977; Seewald and Pascoe, 1978; Byrne and Dillon, 1986: Seeward and Ross, 1988). Often the claims of such procedures are backed by their apparent success as measured by speech recognition scores. Secondly, speech tests themselves have developed to the point where they are now more likely to be sensitive to differences between hearing aids.

Quality judgement

One development in this area is in the introduction of more qualitative comparisons between hearing aids. In this type of test patients may be asked to listen to speech through each of a number of different instruments and to decide on the basis of this listening test which aid they prefer. Various versions of this test occur. For example one rather elaborate procedure has been developed by Studebaker et al. (1982). In their procedure speech signals from a large number of aids are pre-recorded on two channels of a tape recorder. Each possible pairing of the hearing aids is recorded and comparison between pairs is performed by the patient switching between channels on the tape recorder. In Studebaker's method the pairs 'compete' against each other rather like soccer teams aiming for a place in the World Cup. This method enables a fast switching between pairs so that subtle differences between aids can be more readily identified than may be the case in more conventional speech audiometry. It also enables each patient to sample in one session all the aids held in a clinic's stock, or at least all those recorded. However the difficulties associated with making such recordings make it clinically rather a formidable undertaking.

In its simplest form, quality judgement is probably the method used most often to differentiate between aids. It is common practice for the patient to try a number of aids in the clinician's office and each time to be asked 'How does that one sound?'. Indeed this situation is so common that a note of caution must be introduced concerning the validity of its underlying assumption. This assumption is that when a patient makes a judgement about a particular aid this judgement says something meaningful about that aid. In other words if the patient states that they prefer aid A to aid B, there is some essential difference between aids A and B that is causing them to say this. In a study by Green, Day and Bamford, (1986) different hearing aids were compared using this quality judgement type of task. Each time a patient, listening to speech in various types of background noise, was asked which of two hearing aids they preferred.

The results showed a marked order effect, suggesting that regardless of the type of aid fitted, the more frequently preferred aid was the one fitted second. This preference for the second aid persisted even when the 'two' aids tried were (unbeknown to the patient) actually the same aid. In a similar study, McClymont et al (1991) also showed that patients can express a strong preference between two aids which are actually the same (although they did not find an order effect). The implication here is that a patient's quality judgements, or more casual comments, about different hearing aids do not necessarily reflect important differences between aids. It may have more to do simply with the patient adapting to the environment (acoustic and otherwise) in which the aid is being fitted.

Speech recognition and benefit

In an earlier section we examined the relationship between speech recognition measures of disability and a patient's degree of handicap. It was demonstrated there that the two measures are only loosely related. Inferences about handicap are also implicit in taking speech recognition measures of the effect of a hearing aid.

Such tests are performed partly on the assumption that differences between unaided and aided scores will reflect the degree of benefit, or reduction in handicap, experienced by the patient in real life. Furthermore differences between hearing aids measured in the clinic are assumed to reveal which hearing aid is most likely to provide the greatest benefit for the patient outside the clinic. Does this prove to be the case? Benefit is a difficult thing to measure. Like handicap it comprises many dimensions, such as how well the patient copes with the aid in quiet conditions, noisy conditions, at home, at work and so on. Often benefit is encapsulated in overall measures such as patient satisfaction or hours for which the hearing aid is worn. Table 8.4 is taken from a study (Gerber and Fisher, 1979) in which different test conditions were used to measure recognition scores and these differences were then correlated with the patient's average use (hours per day) of their hearing aid. As much as 50% of variability in the patient's aid use was predictable from their recognition scores, though this depended on the particular test and conditions used.

Table 8.4 Rank order for predicting the subject's use of a hearing aid

	Signal-to-noise Ratio	Correlation (r)² Between Test Score and Aid Use
Carhart	−10 dB MCR	(50.8%)
SSI	−10 dB MCR	(48.1%)
SSI	−20 dB MCR	(47.8%)
SSI	0 dB MCR	(41.6%)
Carhart	−20 dB MCR	(36.1%)
Carhart	0 dB MCR	(34.6%)
Carhart	+20 dB MCR	(13.8%)
Carhart	+10 dB MCR	(11.8%)
SSI	+10 dB MCR	(8.4%)
SSI	+20 dB MCR	(0.4%)

The figures show the correlation between aid use and scores from the Synthetic Sentence Identification Test (SSI) and W-22 word lists (Carhart) with various levels of competing signal. MCR = Message to Competition Ratio.

In particular the study reveals that a test becomes most sensitive as a predictor of hours of use in a restricted range of signal-to-noise ratios. Discrimination scores in quiet seem to bear little relationship to hours of use. Discrimination scores in high levels of background noise are also poor predictors. However across a range of intermediate conditions some relationship does exist between speech discrimination and hours of use. This relationship is apparently tightened up considerably if further background information is also taken into account.

Foster et al. (1981) looked at how well the amount of use of a hearing aid (hours per day) could be predicted, and found that if allowance was made for the patient's recognition score, tolerance thresholds, age and some other easily obtained background information, almost 80% of the variability in use time could be accounted for.

The relationship between speech recognition and patient satisfaction is more complex. It might be expected for example that if patients do show better speech recognition with one hearing aid rather than another, then they would also tend to prefer it. A number of studies have given results that suggest that this is not in fact the case. Thompson and Lassman (1969) for example showed that although a frequency response which provided more high frequency emphasis gave better speech recognition scores, patients tended to prefer aids with less high frequency emphasis. Haggard et al. (1981) found a slight tendency for more favourable responses about the benefit of a hearing aid from subjects whose speech results show less rather than more improvement. The reasons for this somewhat paradoxical finding must presumably lie in the overriding importance of the 'tone colour' of a hearing aid. Punch (1980) for example has shown that the amount of low frequency in a hearing aid strongly influences patient judgement about it. The more low frequency, the more they like it. Whatever the reasons, it puts the clinician in something of a spot. Speech audiometry is performed as a means of evaluating hearing aids. Common sense suggests that the aid with the best recognition score is best for the patient. Unfortunately it is also more likely to be received by the patient with less than optimal enthusiasm. The way out of this impasse is not clear. However it seems likely that any relationship between speech recognition and satisfaction is likely to change over time. Indeed such an influence presumably is implied in the often heard comment that 'I didn't like the aid at first but now that I am used to it I think it is much better'.

Treatment evaluation over time

If treatment evaluation by using speech recognition is to be useful in rehabilitating patients then it must, as has already been stated, tell us something useful about the patient. In the light of the discussion of the previous section what it actually tells us is in some sense paradoxical, in that the aid the patient performs best with will not necessarily be the aid they prefer. However rehabilitation is not instantaneous and very little work has been done on the way changes occur over time in measures such as speech recognition, patient satisfaction, hours of use and so on. It may well be that patients will grow to like the aid which gives them better recognition, once they have had time to adjust to it. Alternatively it may be (though intuitively this is less likely) that an aid which initially demonstrates poorer recognition, shows a marked improvement as the patient becomes accustomed to it. The point is that we do not really know yet what kind of predictions we can make about the long term rehabilitative prospects of a particular aid, simply based on speech recognition scores, which again throws their quantitative application into doubt.

So far in this chapter we have concerned ourselves with looking at the rehabilitative uses to which speech audiometry has been put. We have stressed the need for looking not simply at the test scores but further at what those scores tell us about a patient's handicap and likely benefit from a hearing aid. Indeed such considerations suggest that speech audiometry has a rather limited potential in one particular but common area of rehabilitation, namely the fitting of hearing aids. However, given that limitation it is necessary to look at some important underlying concepts that will enable us to be more effective in selecting tests and conditions which are most likely to be of use.

Sensitivity

Much misuse of speech audiometry results from a lack of understanding of how speech tests work. In particular tests are often used in situations and under conditions which render them insensitive to the process under examination, or in which they become so unreliable that the scores derived from them are meaningless. Thus a clinician trying to assess a patient's speech recognition using live voice in free field may well obtain different scores in different conditions simply because of uncontrolled changes in the level of the clinician's voice. We have already seen the effect of background noise on the sensitivity of speech tests as predictors of aid use.

If we wish to differentiate between two hearing aids we need a speech test that is sensitive to differences between hearing aids. For example if two aids differ in terms of their frequency response a speech test will only successfully differentiate between them if it contains items which are made easier with one frequency response than with the other. This may appear obvious but tests are frequently employed in the hope that they will be sensitive to these differences, rather than because such sensitivity has been proven. This practice has largely stemmed from the idea that because speech can partly be defined in terms of frequency, changes in frequency response will therefore elicit changes in the ability to perform tests containing speech items. Although this has a grain of truth it misses two important points. First speech is very redundant, so that changes in frequency/gain characteristic of the hearing aid or impaired ear or both, through which the speech is being perceived need to be rather extreme if differences are to be detectable. Second the time domain is also important in defining the speech signal. Indeed the transient quality of many speech sounds suggests that it is likely to be at least as important as the frequency domain.

Clinicians theoretically have some control over test sensitivity by choosing a test that is known to be sensitive to differences they wish to examine. Unfortunately the day is not yet with us when they can decide what they wish to use speech audiometry for and then consult a 'catalogue' of tests and procedures in order to find a test known to be particularly effective for that use.

Some progress has been made in specifying target sensitivity. There now exist tests specifically for hearing impaired children and comprising items taken from the language typical of such a population such as BKB sentences (Bench and Bamford, 1979), or modelled after tests for adults but incorporating items suitable for children (Jerger and Jerger, 1982). The FAAF test (Foster and Haggard, 1979) claims sensitivity to high frequencies and should therefore be useful for both hearing aid work and assessing disability in milder high frequency impairments.

Further control can be exercised by selection of the conditions under which the test is performed. If for example two hearing aids are to be compared on a patient with a mild hearing loss there may be little point in measuring maximum discrimination in quiet, as scores are likely to be close to 100% with both hearing aids. Alternatively if the test is performed using a considerable amount of background noise the patient may score 0% with both aids. In neither of these conditions is the test proving 'sensitive' to hearing aid differences. Somewhere between these two extremes the test is likely to reach its greatest sensitivity (assuming, as we have already discussed, that it has any sensitivity at all to differences between aids).

Unfortunately this point of maximum sensitivity is seldom known. It is likely to depend on the test itself, the nature of the background noise and the type and degree of hearing loss of the patient being tested. However experience suggests that tests are likely to be most sensitive when the patient is scoring in the region of 50–90% and Dillon (1982) has shown that theoretically at least the best point to aim at is a score between 70% and 90%.

Reliability

Perhaps the greatest misuse of speech tests arises from a poor understanding of the idea of test reliability. Scores on an ideal speech test will be exactly repeatable. However in practice if a patient performs a speech test and scores say 70% it would be unrealistic to hope that every time they performed the test under those conditions they scored exactly 70%. If this were the case and if with another aid they scored 72%, we could be confident in asserting that this difference represented a small but significant improvement for the second aid. In practice the test score will show some random variation from test to test. Furthermore this variability will depend on the test itself and on the conditions under which it was performed.

There is in fact a trade off to be made between the sensitivity of a test and its reliability. It is possible to make a test perfectly reliable. To do this it is simply necessary to make the test very easy, so that the patient always scores 100%, or very difficult so that they always score 0%. Unfortunately at these points we have a test which is perfectly reliable but, as discussed above, completely insensitive. As the level of difficulty increases and the patient's score falls below 100%, so the sensitivity is likely to increase and the reliability decrease. Technically the rate at which they change is not quite the same for sensitivity as reliability. Thus sensitivity is greatest between 50% and 100%, and variability at 50%. The region of test difficulty which maximizes this sensitivity/reliability trade-off is the region of maximum efficiency.

Minimal differences

A critical concept is that of minimal differences. We have stated that if the test is not ridiculously easy or hopelessly difficult then the test score will have associated with it a degree of variability. Given a test score of 70% on one occasion, repeating that test on a separate occasion will give a score which is not necessarily or even probably the same. The problem arises when the two scores are obtained from two different treatments, for example two hearing aids. How large a difference would there need to be between scores before we could say with any certainty that the difference really was due to a difference between hearing aids and not simply due to the expected variability associated with the test.

It turns out that we can calculate the variability associated with a particular speech test. This variability depends almost entirely on the number of items in the test and the test score itself. Figure 8.3 represents the 95% confidence limits for establishing significant difference between two test scores for a typical speech test containing 30 items, such as the AB word lists (Boothroyd, 1968) when scored phonemically, i.e. 10 words in each list with three phonemes per word making 30 phonemes per test. The area bounded by the curves represents the amount of uncertainty associated with any particular test score. If we use the horizontal axis to represent patient test scores for a particular condition, we can determine for any score how much smaller or greater a second score (e.g. with a different hearing aid) needs to be before we can say with any certainty that the difference between scores really is due to a difference between hearing aids. Assume that a patient scores 70% with hearing aid A and 85% with hearing aid B. Follow the 70% grid from the horizontal axis to the points where it is crossed by the curves. Reading these points off the vertical axis establishes that the second aid must score 47% to be regarded as significantly worse than the first aid and 90% to be regarded as significantly better.

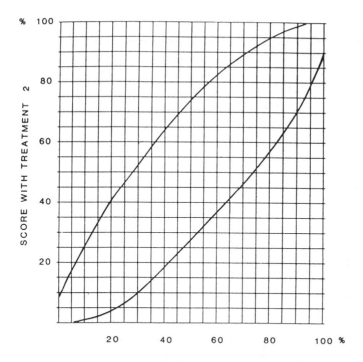

Figure 8.3 Minimal differences between treatment scores for significance (95% confidence limits). If the score for treatment 2 falls within the boundary of the curves at the points of intersection with the score for treatment 1, then the difference between scores cannot be attributed with any certainty to a difference between treatments

The striking point here is that the differences do need to be quite large before any importance can be attached to them. It would have been tempting to see the second aid as being better than the first as the difference in discrimination score was 15%. Examination of the 95% confidence limits shows that the size of this difference could simply be due to chance. Note also that the size of difference which can be regarded as significant depends on the scores themselves. For scores in the 50% region, differences need to be larger than for scores close to either extreme (100% or 0%) before significance can be attached to them. The only steps that can be taken to improve the reliability of the test scores without sacrificing sensitivity involve increasing the number of items on a test. This can be done by repeating the test more than once for each condition or by using a test which intrinsically contains more items. Figure 8.4 shows reliability plots for a number of typical test situations, and in the Appendix the same data are presented in tabular form. From these figures a number of comparisons can be made. For example if in the above situation the test had been performed twice for each hearing aid and scores obtained were those averaged over two lists, then we could regard the test scores as suggesting a significant difference between aids. Given a score of 70% the second score need only be 83% to be regarded as significantly better. If the scores had been obtained with the FAAF test where the minimal score is also 83% significance could again be accredited to the differences.

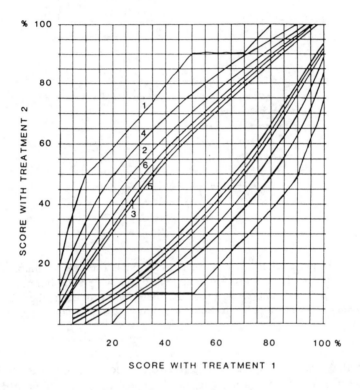

Figure 8.4 Minimal differences (95% confidence limits) for: 1. AB Words (% of Words Correct; 1 List); 2. AB Words (% Phonemes Correct; 1 List); 3. AB Words (% Phonemes Correct; 2 Lists); 4. FAAF (% Correct; 1 Page); 5. FAAF (% Correct; 1 Complete List); 6. BKB Sentences (% Correct; 1 List).

These concepts should be valid whatever rehabilitative situations are being compared, whether it is aided vs. unaided scores, comparison between aids, comparison of auditory training programmes or discrimination in quiet at different distances from the speaker. They serve again to emphasize the limitations of current speech audiometry in individual rehabilitation. Speech tests are useful in research as they can be performed a lot of times on different subjects. However speech audiometry is not a very precise instrument for use with individual patients, and its quantitative uses in that role are not therefore particularly great when only one or two test scores are considered.

It is possible with shorter speech tests to take several measurements of recognition at different levels and so plot aided recognition functions. This has the advantages of testing across a range of performance levels for the subject (and so including regions of greater sensitivity) and comparing the plotted performance/intensity curves. The variability associated with such curves will be less than that associated with a single test score. Figure 8.5 demonstrates the use of this procedure in comparing performance at different signal-to-noise ratios using monaural and binaural combinations of different aids (Jerger and Jerger, 1985).

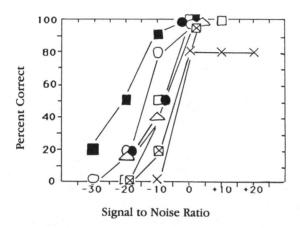

Figure 8.5 Unaided and aided paediatric speech recognition scores as a function of the message-to-competition ratio (MCR). The Sound Pressure Level (SPL) of the test sentences was 50 dB. The SPL of the competing sentence messages was varied to produce MCRs from +20 to –30 dB. Test conditions are listed in the order of administration. × = unaided, pretest; □ = Aid A, binaural; ■ = Aid B, binaural; ○ = Aid B, left ear; ● = Aid B, right ear; △, Aid C, binaural; ⊠, unaided, post test

Test types

If speech audiometry is to be performed in a rehabilitative setting then the test chosen should be governed by the use to which it is intended to be put. Much previous discussion has centred around work with hearing aids, but speech audiometry does have its wider uses. For example Watts and Pegg (1977) used speech recognition scores to assess the effects of an auditory training regime. By comparing a group of subjects who were given lip reading and auditory training with a group of subjects who were given only lip reading, they were able to show that discrimination scores did indeed improve with auditory training.

A useful test to incorporate into an auditory training programme would be the FAAF test. Although it requires a computer for scoring to obtain a full feature analysis, the resulting breakdown of scores into particular feature errors should enable those areas of difficulty to be targeted and monitored with serial repetitions of the test. An audio visual-version of the test, FADAST (Summerfield and Foster, 1983), is also available so that lip reading skills can be explored.

The problem with longer tests such as the FAAF test (which takes about 7 minutes to run) is that for optimal sensitivity some idea of response rate is necessary so that conditions can be suitably adjusted (either by increasing the noise level or decreasing the speech level). A test procedure currently under development is an 'adaptive procedure' in which, rather than running the test in fixed conditions, test.conditions are continually adjusted until a target rate of response is achieved. Such a procedure has the advantage that the scoring region likely to be most sensitive can be selected. However in practice the procedure is not straightforward (again being best handled by on line computing techniques) and in the case of FAAF will not produce feature error scores. The time taken to perform FAAF (other than as an adaptive procedure) tends to prohibit its use for plotting recognition functions and test lists such as the AB word lists or Jerger's paediatric speech intelligibility test (Jerger and Jerger, 1982) would be more useful here. Many tests even in the most favourable conditions are not easy enough for the profoundly deaf and tests such as the connected discourse tracking test (De Filippo and Scott, 1978) may provide help here. This test is run by a patient trying to follow and repeat continuous discourse, either with or without lip reading. The number of words correctly repeated per minute can be used as the score. Such a test has been used for example in monitoring the effectiveness of cochlear implants. It does however require good language skills on the part of the patient.

Test conditions

The conditions under which the test is performed can be manipulated to be more or less representative of 'real life'. Thus speech testing has been performed with a variety of different background noises. Continuous white, pink or speech-like noise are typical. If more 'realistic' noises are introduced such as canteen noise, traffic noise or whatever then the reliability of the test score tends to deteriorate owing to the intermittent nature of such noise.

Another approach to realism has been through using different amounts of reverberation on the assumption that many important living environments will be considerably more reverberant than the clinic in which tests are usually performed. The range of reverberation times commonly encountered is considerable. Results from a study by Wills (1985) for example suggested that a hearing impaired child moving between a normal classroom and a partial hearing unit classroom, could experience reverberation times varying between 0.36 and 1.42 seconds, depending both on the classroom itself and the number of people in the room at any one time. Moncur and Dirks (1967) were able to show that speech discrimination deteriorated in reverberant conditions when background noise was present.

Directional effects can also be explored. Directional microphones are a feature of some hearing aids, and studies using directional vs. non-directional microphones have demonstrated their effectiveness. However placement of speakers in a test room can be critically important in such studies, both for the speech signal and the background noise. Owing to head shadow effects signals tend to be louder to each ear from its respective side and softest from the rear. Using rear speakers for the noise and optimally placed speakers for the speech does tend to produce scores favouring directional microphones. However it is likely that factors such as the amount of reverberation present in a room will have some influence on directional advantage, and it is unclear to what extent laboratory demonstrations of such advantage carry over into the patient's normal environment.

The problem with any manipulation of test conditions is the same problem we have come across repeatedly in this chapter. We can perform tests and obtain scores under more or less any condition we choose. However inferences from such scores about individual rehabilitation cannot be more than very general. Furthermore equally valid inferences can often be made with information already obtained. We have seen for example that handicap is better predicted from pure tone thresholds than from speech discrimination scores, and that only gross differences between hearing aids will be apparent unless considerable time and effort are devoted to obtaining scores in a variety of conditions.

Qualitative uses of speech audiometry

If the reader detects a note of scepticism concerning the strictly quantitative uses of speech audiometry in rehabilitation with individual patients, let me redress that somewhat by pointing to its qualitative value.

Patients are often impressed by the improvement which an aid can provide in their discrimination score if both are performed with stimulus levels appropriate for normal speech. It is not difficult in this situation to get a significant improvement and this improvement can be a powerful tool for 'selling' the idea of a hearing aid. AB word lists are useful here due to their speed of administration and provision of a number of equivalent lists. Speech tests performed with and without lip reading give a sometimes dramatic demonstration of the extent to which a patient relies on lip reading skills. This can be done live voice (with care) using AB words or BKB sentences, or by using lip reading tests such as FADAST or the audiovisual version of BKB (Rosen and Corcoran, 1982).

A speech test such as FAAF serves to focus a patient's attention on particular areas of difficulty and as such serves as a useful catalyst to patient counselling and as a guide to auditory training needs.

With children it is very often useful to 'score' tests not so much by the number right or wrong as by the way in which their behaviour changes as they go from certain to uncertain responses. It is an attribute of tests such as BKB that their steep performance/intensity functions can cause rapid changes in behaviour from confidence to hesitation and faltering with small changes in intensity. Again this can be a telling demonstration to parents of both the extent of a child's loss and, if aided tests are also performed, the benefit provided by the hearing aid.

Even here a word of caution is appropriate with regard to mild and difficult-to-fit losses, such as steeply sloping high frequency losses. Occasionally in these situations, patients may score as well without the aid as with, in the quiet confines of the clinic using normal levels of voice, and attempts to demonstrate aided benefit may end up doing the reverse, so undermining efforts to encourage the use of the aid. Testing with these patients needs to be approached carefully, with greater emphasis placed on the quality of the sound and the relative effort which they have to put in when listening unaided, rather than aided.

In summary, if time and effort are to be expended in performing speech audiometry on individuals as an aid to rehabilitation, its limitations must be understood. Only a loose relationship between speech scores and handicap exists. Current speech tests are not particularly sensitive to differences between hearing aids. Furthermore speech test scores show considerable variability. On the positive side rehabilitation will be helped if patients and their families understand what is happening to them. Speech recognition scores often provide a meaningful demonstration of the patient's difficulties, and so can be used to lead them to a better understanding of the nature of the problems for which they have sought our help.

Appendix

Critical differences

These tables show the lower and upper limits beyond which two treatments can be said to be significantly different at the 95% level of confidence.

For example, assume that a patient performs one AB word list with hearing aid A (scored as phonemes correct) and scores 60%. For hearing aid B to be significantly better, they would need to score 80% with it (37% for it to be significantly worse).

A — Critical differences for FAAF

	% Correct 1 Page			% Correct 1 Complete List	
Score	Lower	Upper	Score	Lower	Upper
0	0	10	25	14	39
5	0	25	26	15	40
10	0	35	28	15	41
20	5	50	30	18	45
25	5	55	31	19	46
30	10	60	33	20	48
35	10	65	34	20	49
40	15	70	35	21	50
45	20	75	36	23	51
50	20	80	38	24	52
55	25	80	39	25	54
60	30	85	40	26	55
65	35	90	41	28	56
70	40	90	43	29	58
75	45	95	44	30	59
80	50	95	45	30	60
85	60	95	46	31	61
90	65	100	48	33	63
95	75	100	49	34	64
100	90	100	50	35	65
			51	36	66
			52	38	68
			54	39	69
			55	40	70

B — Critical differences for AB Words

	% Words Correct 1 List	
Score	Lower	Upper
0	0	20
10	0	50
20	0	60
30	10	70
40	10	80
50	10	90
60	20	90
70	30	90
80	40	100
90	50	100
100	80	100

Critical differences for AB Words (continued)

	1 List		% Phonemes Correct 2 Lists			2 Lists (continued)		
Score	Lower	Upper	Score	Lower	Upper	Score	Lower	Upper
0	0	7	0	0	5	52	35	68
3	0	17	2	0	10	53	37	70
7	0	23	3	0	12	55	38	72
10	3	30	5	0	15	57	40	73
13	3	33	7	2	18	58	42	75
17	3	37	8	2	20	60	43	77
20	7	43	10	2	23	62	45	77
23	7	47	12	3	25	63	47	78
27	10	50	13	5	27	65	48	80
30	10	53	15	5	28	67	50	82
33	13	57	17	7	32	68	52	83
37	17	60	18	7	33	70	53	83
40	20	63	20	8	35	72	55	85
43	20	67	22	10	37	73	57	87
47	23	70	23	10	40	75	58	88
50	27	73	25	12	42	77	60	90
53	30	77	27	13	43	78	63	90
57	33	80	28	15	45	80	65	92
60	37	80	30	17	47	82	67	93
63	40	83	32	17	48	83	68	93
67	43	87	33	18	50	85	72	95
70	47	90	35	20	52	87	73	95
73	50	90	37	22	53	88	75	97
77	53	93	38	23	55	90	77	98
80	57	93	40	23	57	92	80	98
83	63	97	42	25	58	93	82	98
87	67	97	43	27	60	95	85	100
90	70	97	45	28	62	97	88	100
93	77	100	47	30	63	98	90	100
97	83	100	48	32	65	100	95	100
100	93	100	50	33	67			

C — Critical differences for BKB Sentences

% Correct

	1 List			2 Lists	
Score	Lower	Upper	Score	Lower	Upper
0	0	4	56	41	70
2	0	10	58	43	71
4	0	14	59	44	73
6	2	18	60	45	74
8	2	22	61	46	75

C — Critical differences for BKB Sentences (continued)

% Correct

	1 List			2 Lists	
Score	Lower	Upper	Score	Lower	Upper
10	2	24	63	48	76
12	4	26	64	49	78
14	4	30	65	50	79
16	6	32	66	51	80
18	6	34	68	52	80
20	8	36	69	54	81
22	8	40	70	55	83
24	10	42	71	58	84
26	12	44	73	59	85
28	14	46	74	60	85
30	14	48	75	61	86
32	16	50	76	63	88
34	18	52	78	64	89
36	20	54	79	65	90
38	22	56	80	66	90
40	22	58	81	69	91
42	24	60	83	70	93
44	26	62	84	71	93
46	28	64	85	73	94
48	30	66	86	75	95
50	32	68	88	76	95
52	34	70	89	78	96
54	36	72	90	79	96
56	38	74	91	81	98
58	40	76	93	83	99
60	42	78	94	85	99
62	44	78	95	86	99
64	46	80	96	89	100
66	48	82	98	91	100
68	50	84	99	93	100
70	52	86	100	96	100
72	54	86			
74	56	88			
76	58	90			
78	60	92			
82	66	94			
84	68	94			
86	70	96			
88	74	96			
90	76	98			
92	78	98			
94	82	98			
96	86	100			
98	90	100			
100	96	100			

Chapter 9
Speech tests of hearing for children

ANDREAS MARKIDES

All tests of hearing using speech as stimulus are conveniently grouped under the heading of speech audiometry. Such tests are used for a multiplicity of purposes. In addition to their function as valuable checks on pure tone audiometry, they also contribute in differentiating between sensory and neural dysfunctions, in evaluating a patient's every day difficulties in hearing, in assessing the practical significance of therapeutic, educational, rehabilitative and compensatory procedures and in studying various factors affecting speech perception.

The main concern here is with those speech tests of hearing, specially designed for English speaking children, that evaluate a child's ability to make correct phonemic classification mainly on the basis of acoustical information. Such tests are commonly referred to as speech articulation, speech intelligibility, speech discrimination or speech recognition tests. In this chapter the latter term will be adopted and used throughout mainly because it describes more accurately the process involved (Olsen and Matkin, 1979).

This chapter begins with a brief description of the historical developments of speech audiometry and it goes on to consider the wide variety of speech materials used in the construction of speech recognition tests. The major criteria for the construction of speech tests of hearing for children are then presented and discussed. This is followed by a description of the main speech tests of hearing for children in current use in the United States of America and in the United Kingdom, with the latter ones being discussed in more detail. The chapter concludes with two major recommendations for developments in this area. The main speech recognition tests for children currently used in the UK are given in the Appendix.

Historical developments

Specially designed speech recognition tests have been in regular use for just over 40 years. It is of interest to note, however, that speech was

used as test material for hearing assessment as far back as two
ago when Ernaud and Pereire in the middle of the eighteenth ce..
and Itard at the beginning of the nineteenth century used speech to
evaluate the effects of auditory training on their patients' speech perceptual abilities (Urbantschitsch, 1895).

It is true that these early attempts in the measurement of hearing for
speech have very little in common with what we now refer to as speech
tests of hearing. They did, however, stimulate discussion especially
among otologists towards the end of the nineteenth century (Gruber,
1891). This debate was also facilitated by a series of timely scientific
inventions that had a considerable influence on the development of
speech audiometry. In 1876 Alexander Graham Bell invented a transducer that converted sound energy to electrical energy and vice versa.
In 1887 Thomas Edison patented the phonograph, which was later
suggested for use in the measurement of hearing for speech (Bryant,
1904).

At the beginning of this century these and other inventions brought
about rapid developments in electro acoustic communication systems.
These systems called for precise and quantifiable measurement of their
speech reproducing capabilities and the first person to respond to this
need was Campbell in 1910. Campbell was involved with telephone
transmitting equipment at the Bell Telephone Laboratories in the USA.
His evaluative method, referred to as 'articulation testing', involved a
speaker reading out a list of nonsense syllables at one end of the telephone and a listener trying to identify these syllables at the other end.
The percentage of correctly identified syllables was taken as a measure
of relative intelligibility (Levitt and Resnick, 1978). Many of the materials and methods used by Campbell were later found to be relevant for
evaluating hearing (Fletcher and Steinberg, 1929).

The major development in this direction came from the Psycho
Acoustic Laboratory of Harvard University and from the Central Institute
for the Deaf (CID), in the USA. It was just after the Second World War
that Egan (1948) developed the now well known PAL 20 PB-50 Lists. It
soon became evident, however, that many patients had difficulties with
the vocabulary used in these lists as they contained a number of generally unfamiliar words. In 1952 Hirsh and his associates at the CID
devised a modification of Egan's word lists referred to as the CID W-22.
According to Martin and Pennington (1971), and Martin and Forbis
(1978), this is the most extensively used monosyllabic (open set
response) test in the United States.

These tests and subsequent ones were comprehensively dealt with by
a number of authors especially Davis and Silverman (1978) and Bess
(1982). In view of this, and the contents of chapter 12, it is not intended
to repeat the same information here. Only a selection of the most widely
used tests will be mentioned in a historical context.

Over the last 20 years a large number of speech tests of hearing using a variety of speech materials have been developed in the United States. Using nonsense syllables Resnick and his associates (Levitt and Resnick, 1978; Resnick et al., 1976) developed the well known nonsense syllable test (NST). Using monosyllabic words (open set response) Tillman, Carhart and Wilber (1963) developed a new test of the consonant-vowel-consonant (CVC) variety based on the criteria of phonemic balancing.

Similar tests using monosyllabic words but of a closed set response type (multiple choice) were also developed, the most popular being the modified rhyme hearing test (MRHT) by Kruel and his associates (Kruel et al.,1968). Using sentences as stimulus materials Silverman and Hirsh (1955) introduced their everyday speech sentence test, which was developed and recorded at CID. The most commonly used sentence test in the USA at present, according to Bess (1983) is the synthetic sentence identification (SSI) test which was developed by Speaks and Jerger in 1965. Similar developments were also evident in the UK. Lists of words were constructed by Fry and Kerridge (1939) as part of a study sponsored by the Medical Research Council which led to the development of the MedResCo hearing aid used in the UK National Health Service. A later study, Fry (1961) at University College, London, developed phonetically balanced word lists for use with adults. The same author also designed a speech test of hearing based on sentences again with deafened adults in mind. There were also developments in speech audiometry for children which will be dealt with later in this chapter.

Speech materials

Since the early report of Fletcher and Steinberg (1929), a wide variety of speech materials have been employed in the construction of speech recognition tests. They have included individual sounds, nonsense syllables, PB monosyllabic words, disyllabic words, sentences and continuous discourse. Darbyshire (1970) and Ling (1978) for example recommended the use of isolated sounds as stimulus material for evaluating the hearing potential of very deaf children. In 1929 Fletcher and Steinberg devised several lists of nonsense syllables. It has been claimed on numerous occasions that speech tests of hearing consisting of nonsense syllables have certain advantages (Edgerton and Danhauer, 1979). It is true that they lack meaning and therefore their auditory recognition is not dependent on the vocabulary of the listener.

It must not be forgotten, however, that this lack of meaning in turn can also be a disadvantage since the listener does not commonly need to identify meaningless speech material. Also the composition of such syllables by definition does not follow the normally allowed sequence of the language and thus the combination of the sounds uttered are not necessarily the appropriate representations of the phonemic sequence in the language. Moreover, nonsense syllables are so abstract that they baffle many listeners and their auditory recognition is also greatly affected by previous experience (Berger, 1971). It was mainly because of these reasons that Fletcher (1929) recommended the use of monosyllabic words for speech tests of hearing.

The use of monosyllabic word lists in speech recognition tests has been widely accepted. This is mainly due to the fact that such tests must consist of relatively non-redundant items, otherwise the multiplicity of clues available to the listener can obscure some of the inability to differentiate speech sounds by their acoustical properties. Such tests, however, do not eliminate contextual clues and it is not always clear to what extent they are true measures of the ability of the listener to make phonemic classifications based solely on auditory clues (Hirsh, 1964).

In principle, tests using sentences are preferable because they are nearer to the speech material that the listener is exposed to in everyday life. It is well known, however, that the meaning of a sentence and word sequence can easily be conveyed by one or two key words and therefore, speech recognition scores derived from sentences are highly influenced by guessing. It is mainly because of this factor that the same hearing ability under similar listening conditions gives a higher score for sentences than for isolated words. As it has been repeatedly shown that there is a close correlation between the results of sentence and word recognition tests the use of the latter can be justified in view of the great saving of time that they afford. Sentence tests have a useful role to play, especially when used with people who are so deaf that they cannot understand amplified speech without having a great deal of help from context.

In view of the linguistic redundancy inherent in sentences and also the fact that it is exceedingly difficult to construct equivalent sets of 'real' sentences in terms of vocabulary, word familiarity, word length, sentence length and syntactic structure, Fry (1964) departing from traditional procedures suggested the use of 'artificial' sentences based on the probabilities of word sequence. This suggestion was immediately taken up by Speaks and Jerger for experimentation and in 1965 they reported in favour of the test, but cautioned on the high learning effect associated with such material.

The most logical speech message to use for speech recognition testing is continuous discourse (Hirsh, 1952). One major deterrent to the use of such materials is the difficulty of quantification. Ulrich (1957) devised such a test based on a 15 minute lecture on 'The Food Resources of Africa' which can be administered to a group of listeners and scored in terms of information retained. Its use has been very limited indeed.

In all routine uses of speech recognition tests the responses of the listener must be recognized and quantified by the tester. The tester is therefore placed in a listener's position, thus creating an unwanted variable. Moreover, many subjects, especially children, have accompanying defects of speech so that scoring can become extremely difficult and prone to errors since the examiner tends to be uncertain as to whether the imperfect spoken response is due to faulty hearing or faulty speech or both. To remove, or at least to lessen, the examiner's involvement in the recognition score, tests of multiple choice (Watson, 1957) or of the word completion type (House et al., 1963, 1965) have been compiled.

This approach has three important advantages over classical speech recognition techniques. First, the message set is always closed and of controllable size. Second the testing procedures can be easily automated thus minimizing experimental error and finally, the learning or practice effect can be determined with relative ease. Such tests have serious drawbacks in that the final score is contaminated by a chance factor and when word completion is involved by the spelling, handwriting legibility and reading ability of the subject. It must be remembered that speech tests of hearing should investigate the listeners' hearing function not their speech production or their mental, physical, linguistic or educational abilities.

Speech tests of hearing specially designed for children

Before presenting and discussing the various speech tests of hearing which have been specially developed for hearing impaired children in the UK it seems appropriate to consider the major criteria upon which such tests are based. When using speech tests of hearing with children our primary concern is threefold. First, we would wish to establish the intensity level at which the child can just detect the presence of speech — the speech detection threshold (SDT). Second, we want to establish the intensity level above which the child is not prepared to tolerate speech — the uncomfortable loudness level (ULL) and third, we want to find out how well the child recognizes speech at several supra-threshold levels with a view to maximizing residual hearing. Tests and procedures for the first two items are simple and have been presented and discussed by Markides (1980). Tests of speech recognition, our present concern, are more complicated.

Major criteria

According to Watson (1957) the major criteria for valid speech recognition tests for children are the following:

1. They should be constructed of monosyllables.
2. The words should be within the vocabulary range of the child.
3. The lists should be phonetically balanced.
4. The lists should be equal in difficulty.
5. The responses required must not involve a skill which will cause the subject any difficulty or the tester any uncertainty.

The use of monosyllabic words, preferably of the CVC type, is recommended because contextual clues are relatively absent with such materials. It is true that the same can be said for nonsense syllables. Watson (1957) however found that nonsense syllables make too difficult a test for children. He observed that the tendency among children when presented with nonsense materials was to try and perceive them as real monosyllables.

The monosyllabic words used must be within the vocabulary of the children for which the test is intended. If they are not the most likely happening is for the children either to make no response at all or to respond with the nearest known word in their vocabulary. In speech recognition tests the listener is comparing the words heard with a large portion of the vocabulary contained in their memory. Therefore, word familiarity (Broadbent, 1967) together with the number of alternatives with which each word may be confused (Miller et al., 1951; Rosenzweig and Postman, 1958) have been found to influence speech recognition scores. Ideally the monosyllabic word lists developed for speech recognition testing should be phonemically balanced. In other words the frequency of occurrence of the phonemes in each word list should reflect the frequency of the occurrence of the phonemes as found in the English language. According to Egan (1948) the minimum number of monosyllabic words required in each list to achieve such a phonemic balance is 50.

Since it is necessary to assess speech recognition ability at several supra-threshold levels or in a variety of acoustic conditions it is essential to have a number of word lists. These word lists should be of equal difficulty (not more than 8% variability) so that the differences in scores obtained reflect the relative ability of the listener to recognize speech and are not due to inequalities in difficulty between lists.

Finally, the type of response required must reflect the child's ability to hear and this must not be contaminated by any other factors. For example, an oral response is inappropriate for those children with severe articulatory problems because the tester cannot be sure whether such a response is due to faulty hearing or faulty articulation, or both. Similarly, it is inappropriate to accept a written response because this may reflect the child's ability to write correctly rather than their ability to hear. In this context it also needs to be mentioned that the tester's hearing should be near normal otherwise difficulty will obviously occur in assessing the oral responses of the child.

Tests

This section will be divided into two parts. The first part will present in summary the most commonly used speech recognition tests for children used in the USA. The second part will present and discuss in more detail the speech recognition tests for children in current use in the UK. This emphasis is deliberate. The former tests have been well documented by previous writers (Bess, 1983) whilst the latter have been existing in relative obscurity.

United States of America

One of the first workers to design and develop a speech recognition test for children was Hudgins. He introduced his test, consisting of four monosyllabic word lists based on familiar words in 1944 and referred to it as the phonetically balanced familiar (PBF) lists. A similar test was also developed by Haskins in 1949. It consisted of four lists, 50 words in each list, and was called the phonetically balanced kindergarten 50s (PBK-50s) test.

These two tests were based on an open response design and as such they proved rather difficult for young children below the age of 6 years. This difficulty led to the development of speech recognition tests based on the closed set or multiple choice format (Sortini and Flake, 1953; Pronovost and Dumbleton, 1954; Myatt and Landes, 1963). The test devised by the latter authors was later on revised and improved by Ross and Lerman (1970) and it soon became known as the word intelligibility by picture identification (WIPI) test. It is suitable for 3- to 6-year-olds and consists of four lists of monosyllabic words arranged into 25 plates with each plate having a six-picture matrix.

A similar test was also developed by Katz and Elliott in 1978. Their test referred to as the Northwestern University — children's perception of speech (NU-CHIPS) test, was specially designed for very young (3-year-old) inner-city children. It consists of four monosyllabic word lists with 50 items in each list. Erber (1974, 1977, 1980) developed a series of tests, the most widely known being the last one. This is a simple test specially designed for children with severe to profound hearing loss and who, owing to severe linguistic retardation are unable to respond to traditional word recognition tests. This test is known as the auditory numbers test (ANT). It requires that the child can count from 1 to 5 and it is suitable for children in the age range of 3 to 8 years.

In 1976 Weber and Redell were of the opinion that tests for children based on single words underestimate the speech recognition abilities of hearing-impaired children. Because of this, they constructed sentences using the stimulus words of the WIPI test developed by Ross and Lerman (1970). This test, referred to as the WIPI sentences, consists of four 25-sentence lists. The child's task is to identify and point to the picture on the WIPI six-picture matrix plate that best represents the spoken sentence.

Bess (1983) reported that a number of authors were in favour of using adult monosyllabic material of the open set response type with young children. It may be that certain adult lists can be used effectively with some children, but the consensus of opinion on this matter is that the selection of speech materials for children should be within the children's speech and language competence. There is no doubt that some hearing impaired children, mainly because of severe linguistic retardation, are unable to take part in conventional speech recognition tests. In order to assess the speech perceptual abilities of such children, Ling (1978) put forward a rather simple speech recognition test referred to as the five sound test using three vowels /u/, /a/ and /i/ and two consonants /ʃ/ and /s/. According to Ling, these sounds cover the frequency range of all phonemes and the vowels contain sufficient harmonics to convey suprasegmental information.

Another test in this category which deserves special mention is that developed by Finitzo-Hieber and his associates (1980). They developed a non-linguistic test for very young children around 3 years old. Their test is based on 30 environmental sounds (plus one practice item) and is referred to as the sound effects recognition test (SERT). The 30 environmental sounds are divided into three lists with each list consisting of 10 items represented on four-picture matrix plates.

United Kingdom

According to Watson (1957), one of the first workers to develop a speech recognition test specially designed for children in the UK was Kendall (1953, 1954) working in the University of Manchester under Professor Ewing.

THE KENDALL TOY TEST (KT TEST)

The KT test was intended for very young children (3 to 5 years old) who had developed a moderate vocabulary. It consists of three lists, each list containing 10 monosyllabic words which are represented by small toy replicas. Each word list contains a range of the most common vowels, diphthongs and consonants. The test is administered in a free-field situation using live voice which is monitored with a sound level meter situated close to the child's ear.

First of all the child is presented with each toy replica and is encouraged to name it. This procedure is followed in order to make sure that the objects in the test are within the known vocabulary of the child being tested. All 10 toy replicas are then presented and arranged on the table in front of the child. The child is then required to point to the appropriate toy when they hear the instruction 'Show me the . . .'. In order to lessen the possibility of a chance response and also to give some practice before beginning the test, an additional five toys are placed with the 10 test items.

This is a useful little test and provided the tester takes special care in monitoring the loudness of their speech, quite a lot of information can be gained not only regarding the speech detection level but also of the child's speech recognition abilities at several supra-threshold levels. Since this test can only be administered in a free-field situation (and masking is not practical for very young children) both the SDT measurement and the speech recognition scores obtained relate only to bilateral hearing. This test is widely used in paediatric audiology clinics throughout the country.

The Manchester tests

In order to meet the special needs of school aged hearing-impaired children, Watson (1957) working at Manchester University developed a series of speech tests comprising the Manchester Junior (MJ) lists, the Manchester picture vocabulary test (MP) and the Manchester sentence (MS) lists.

The Manchester junior (MJ) lists
This test was specially designed for hearing-impaired children from about the age of 6 and upwards. It consists of four word lists with 25 monosyllables in each list. Each list is scrambled once thus giving a total of eight 25-word lists. Although a serious attempt was made to achieve phonemic balance, this, owing to the small number of words in each list and also to the restricted vocabulary used, proved very difficult to meet. The end result however reflects a reasonable compromise. The test was tape recorded and standardized on normal hearing children. The eight-word lists proved to be equal in difficulty giving a normal speech recognition curve based on whole word scoring which rises by 5% per dB. This test has proved to be satisfactory for children with minor linguistic retardation. It presents, however, difficulties to children with severe linguistic retardation and associated speech problems.

The Manchester picture (MP) vocabulary test
This multiple choice test was developed for hearing impaired children of 6 years and over who because of their handicap are unable to take part in an open set type of speech recognition task. It consists of six lists of 20 monosyllables each. The vocabulary used is simple. An attempt

was made to secure homogeneity and equality of difficulty between word lists but experience has shown that there exist significant differences in difficulty between the lists. The lists are not phonemically balanced but the words in each list are carefully chosen to give as wide a selection as possible of the phonemes from the English language.

The test is configured in the form of three sets of 20 cards each. At the initial stages of the development of this test each card contained six pictures. Later on the number of pictures drawn on each card was limited to four. One of the pictures on each card illustrates the stimulus word whilst the other three relate to words containing the same vowels or the same consonants as the stimulus word.

The administration and scoring of this test is carried out as follows: The child is presented with the practice card and is asked to name the pictures on the card. The tester then asks the child to 'show me the . . . .' When the child shows that they understand the procedure then the tester (or preferably a helper) introduces the other cards one by one giving the child sufficient time between each stimulus word to respond. Only one stimulus word is given for each card. If the child is uncertain or mistaken in their choice the word given must not be repeated — the tester should proceed to the next item.

This test is usually administered in a free-field situation using monitored live voice. With cooperative children it can also be administered through a closed circuit system comprising of a tape recorder, speech audiometer attachment and earphones. The responses of the children are scored on the number of words correctly identified, expressed as a percentage of the total number of words in each list. The test was standardized with normal hearing children listening through a closed circuit arrangement. The normal speech recognition curve obtained showed a slight curvilinear rise of 4% per dB covering the 10% to 90% recognition function. It must not be forgotten that this is a multiple choice type of test and as such chance cannot be entirely ruled out and guessing is certainly taking place. Watson (1957) suggested that when the highest score obtained by a subject at any level is less than 20% this should be ignored as it might have come about as result of chance.

The test was revised and updated by Hickson in 1987. The revised version, referred to as the Manchester Picture Test (1984), is based on the same format as the original test. It consists of eight lists of matrices with 10 matrices in each list. Each matrix contains four pictures — one test item and three distractors. Hickson accepts that the word lists in the revised version are not phonemically balanced, but she is of the opinion that the phonemes contained in the test as a whole have a frequency of occurrence representative of that found in connected spoken English.

THE MANCHESTER SENTENCE (MS) TEST

This test was developed to ascertain the speech recognition abilities of hearing impaired children when presented with connected speech. It consists of five lists of 10 sentences each. The sentences consist of familiar statements, commands and questions and they reflect a linguistic level within the abilities of hearing impaired children of 10 years and over. The test was standardized with normal hearing pupils in the 7 to 9 year age range. The normal speech recognition curve obtained has a gradient at its linearly rising section of 5% per dB.

THE AB ISOPHONEMIC WORD LISTS

At present the most widely used speech recognition test for children in the UK is the one developed by Arthur Boothroyd in 1968. This test is commonly referred to as the AB isophonemic word lists and consists of 15 10-word lists with each list containing the same 30 phonemes, 10 vowels and 20 consonants. The monosyllabic words used in constructing the test were of the consonant-nucleus-consonant (CNC) type and were selected from the author's vocabulary — first names and obscenities excluded. This test has several major advantages over the other tests so far mentioned in this section.

1. It consists of short word lists thus allowing the exploration of a large number of listening conditions within a relatively short period of time (this factor is very important in busy audiology clinics).
2. The considerable number of word lists employed (N=15) reduces the possibility of repeating various word lists within a session thus diminishing the effects of learning factors.
3. The recognition score is based on the number of phonemes correctly repeated and thus, according to Boothroyd, produces a high interlist equivalence and good reliability.

The test also has several shortcomings. A considerable number of the words used are not within the vocabularies of junior children and some of these words are emotionally biased. Boothroyd was of the opinion that the phonemic scoring employed in the test diminished the influences of linguistic factors but this is an opinion which is strongly contested. Furthermore the word lists because of their short nature, do not reflect the phonemic balance of the English language.

Three versions of this test were produced on tape. The first version reflected a strong northern English accent whilst the second version recorded at the Institute of Sound and Vibration Research, University of Southampton, reflected a 'standard' BBC type of English accent. Using the first version, Boothroyd (1968) reported a maximum gradient of speech recognition of 4% per dB for children in the age group 5–9 years. Using the second version Markides (1978a) reported varying gradients of speech recognition depending on the age of the normal hearing children. For 6 year olds, he reported a 4.2% rise per dB from 10 – 90% recognition score. For 7 and 8 year olds, this rise was 4.8% per dB and for 9, 10 and 11 year olds it was 5% per dB. A third version of the lists was produced by the Royal National Institute for the Deaf and is commercially available. This version contains all the lists and has two practice words at the beginning of each list.

THE McCORMICK TOY DISCRIMINATION TEST
This test has great similarity to the Kendall toy test. It was developed by McCormick in 1977 and was intended for very young children (2 to 5 years old).

The test is used to estimate a child's word discrimination threshold for words spoken in quiet. It consists of 14 toys, arranged to form seven near-minimal pairs with similar sounding names (e.g. spoon/shoe, horse/fork). Care was taken to select items which were known to normal children with a mental age of 2 years.

The test is administered in a free-field situation using live voice which is monitored using a sound level meter. Real examples of the toys known to the child are placed on the table, and the child is required to point to or touch the appropriate toy when he or she hears the instruction 'show me the ....'. The tester varies the voice level used, in order to estimate the minimum level at which the child can correctly identify the toy requested, on approximately four out of five occasions. For clinical purposes, the child 'passes' if the minimum level is below 40 dB. A semi-automatic version of this test is available (Ousey, Sheppard, Twomey and Palmer, 1989).

THE E2L TOY TEST
This test was developed by Bellman and Marcuson (1991) to evaluate the hearing status of children 3 to 5 years old, with English as a second language.

The test consists of one list of 12 English words which was compiled using words previously shown to be among the early English words learned by children from the Indian sub-continent. These 12 words have been arranged into six pairs with matched vowels. Initial results have been encouraging. This test has recently been validated (Bellman et al. 1996).

THE BKB SENTENCE LISTS
A speech recognition test for children using sentences, produced in the UK is the BKB sentence lists (Bench, Koval and Bamford, 1979). This is an open set response test and according to the authors it better reflects the natural language usage of hearing impaired children. The construction of this test was based on the responses of hearing impaired children in the age range 8 – 15 years when asked to describe familiar pictures depicting everyday activities from home and play situations. It consists of 21 lists of 16 sentences (not more than seven syllables in each sentence). Each list contains 50 stimulus words. The scoring is achieved

by calculating the percentage of key words repeated correctly. A simplified version of this test referred to as the picture-related BKB sentence lists for children (BKB-PR) was also developed. This simplified version consists of 11 lists of 16 sentences with 50 stimulus words in each list. This test has potential but has not yet been widely accepted or used in the UK.

REED SCREENING HEARING TEST

The Reed hearing test (Reed, 1959) consists of a set of cards, each one containing four pictures. The pictures each depict a single object which on one card have a common vowel, e.g. mouse, house, owl, cow, but with differing consonants. There are eight cards in all. The child is required to point to the picture that is named, e.g. 'show me the cow'. After a practice with the tester in front of the child to ensure that the correct names are associated with the pictures and that the child understands the test, the test is repeated with the tester 2m behind the child and speaking in a normal conversational voice. Three or four cards are used and if the child fails to select the correct picture more than once or twice they should be referred for a full audiometric examination. If the child is successful the test should be repeated with a whispered voice and the child should be referred if they fail on more than one or two pictures.

Reed revised the test and it was published by the Royal National Institute for the Deaf in 1970 as the RNID Hearing Test Cards. The pictures were revised by the RNID in 1987.

OTHER TESTS

Several other attempts (Dodds, 1972; McCormick, 1977; Holsgrove and Halden, 1984) have been made in producing speech tests of hearing suitable for children in the UK. The tests developed have not been widely accepted.

Conclusion

Most of the speech recognition tests for children currently used in the UK were designed and developed more than 30 years ago. They are in need of updating and there is also an urgent need to construct and develop new tests for children of all ages especially for those children below the age of 5 years. The restricted use of speech audiometry in the UK National Health Service (Fuller and Moss, 1985) has not increased, partly due to the lack of use for diagnostic purposes. However the introduction of standards for speech audiometric equipment (IEC 645-2, 1993) and for procedures (ISO 8253-3, 1996) should improve the quality of speech audiometry undertaken.

Appendix

Main speech tests of hearing for children in the United Kingdom

The Kendal Toy Test (K.T.test)

Preliminary Practice List	*KT/1*	*KT/2*	*KT/3*
chair	knife	fork	house
church	bath	cat	spoon
nail	soap	tree	fish
ring	car	watch	duck
plane	bus	match	cow
	tin	dog	gate
	boat	horse	brick
	pig	bed	shoe
	brush	key	cup
	pipe	egg	plate

The following distractors should be used:

pin	ball	mouse
duck	sheep	book
jar	hen	string
comb	mat	glove
wheel	doll	plane

The Toy Discrimination Test

cup/duck
spoon/shoe
man/lamb
plate/plane
horse/fork

The E2L Toy Test Word lists

bus/brush
sweet/key
egg/bed
car/bath
plate/plane

The Manchester Junior (MJ) Lists

MJ/1	*MJ/2*	*MJ/3*	*MJ/4*
farm	bad	ship	book
bird	dish	home	kind
school	keep	cup	train
but	milk	made	last
play	boy	egg	three
duck	some	day	pot
them	fall	fish	does
soon	house	took	field
pig	put	park	had
doll	time	shoe	poor
for	know	horse	give
shop	bed	night	ball
hand	five	just	mouse
have	with	seat	hair
from	yes	man	big
cat	sheep	hat	room
green	her	bus	saw
door	down	long	can
white	good	chair	stick
nice	car	boat	good
that	take	seen	when
come	red	black	wash
brown	dog	road	floor
get	has	girl	one
could	gun	cow	said

MJH/5	*MJ/6*	*MJ/7*	*MJ/8*
hand	with	took	good
white	put	seat	room
but	milk	chair	last
then	car	road	one
doll	down	egg	ball
farm	bad	ship	pot
nice	fall	horse	kind
from	dog	bus	big
door	know	seen	train
soon	keep	cow	wash
for	time	cup	had
bird	sheep	long	mouse
that	red	day	said
shop	food	girl	hair
play	gun	night	book
come	bed	hat	give
cat	some	home	can
school	yes	boat	when
get	has	fish	field
green	boy	shoe	stock
pig	five	black	poor
could	house	man	does
have	her	park	three
duck	take	made	saw
brown	dish	just	floor

The Manchester Picture (MP) Vocabulary Test (Modified Version)

List 1	List 2	List 3	List 4
pin	ship	pig	sea
well	leg	fire	tie
boot	bus	cup	duck
coat	dog	saw	cake
star	cat	house	bird
dish	drum	bed	doll
tie	three	cake	plate
stair	fish	sock	spoon
fly	three	chair	ring
man	wall	mouse	light

List 5	List 6	List 7	List 8
key	hill	brick	sheep
bell	pen	pipe	kite
moon	book	sun	foot
boat	shop	wall	spade
car	cap	cow	man
ball	gate	dog	bat
tap	teeth	car	cup
house	star	bus	feet
snake	foot	seat	brush
bun	mat	leg	moon

The Manchester Sentence (MS) Test

List A
1. The *girls mother* has a *new red hat*.
2. *Some people send cards* at easter.
3. The *tits built* a *nest* in the *apple tree*.
4. *Mother* will *bake* a *cake* for *my birthday*.
5. *Indians make birch bark canoes*.
6. *Some countries have summer* in *December*.
7. *Is* a *twopenny stamp blue* or *brown*.
8. *Leave* the *door* key *under* the *mat*.
9. *Put,* a *tight bandage round* his *thumb*.
10. *Very early houses* had *roofs* of *straw*.

List B
1. My *friends father drives a blue car*.
2. *Would you like some water* with your *meal?*
3. *Swallows sometimes fly near* the *ground*.
4. *People squeeze lemons* to *get the juice*.
5. The *brown deer licked* its *baby fawn*.
6. *Stars seem brighter* on a *dark night*.
7. *Open* your *sun book* at *page fifty-two*.
8. *School ends* at *ten past four*.
9. *Put clean paper on top* of the *table*.
10. The *name of some towns end* in *-ham*.

List C
1. You *can't buy fish* in a *bakers shop*.
2. *New shoes* are *often tiring* to *wear*
3. *Most mice* have *long thin tails*
4. The *shops don't open before eight*.
5. *People sometimes cross* a *fence* by a *stile*.
6. *Many plants begin* to *flower* in *may*
7. The *American flag* has *red* and *white stripes*.
8. *Buy some toothpaste* in the *chemist's shop*.
9. *Most car engines* are *cooled* by *water*.
10. *Tigers* and *leopards* are *members* of the *cat family*.

List D
1. *Father comes home* from *work* at *six*.
2. *Please sew a button on* the *vest*.
3. The *man* had *cheese* and *dry buscuits* for *supper*.
4. *Fresh water fish are caught* with *flies*.
5. We *do not often have snow* in *September*.
6. *Many women use gas* for *cooking*.
7. *Bears often sleep* on the *branch* of a *tree*.
8. *Fetch some sticks* to *lay* the *fire*.
9. The *box* of *nails weighs half* a *pound*.
10. *Men used* to *hunt animals* with a *spear*.

List E
1. We *read a fairy story after tea*.
2. *Father carried* his *white shirt upstairs*.
3. *Frogs come out* of the *water* to *breath*.
4. The *boy likes bread* and *jam* for *tea*.
5. *Trees* do *not grow* on *high mountains*.
6. *Farmers usually cut* their *hay* in *June*.
7. *Put* the *glass jar under* the *water*.
8. *Don't come home without* your *cap*.
9. *Six o'clock is too late* to *start*.
10. The *first wheels* were *made* from *slices* of *log*.

AB isophonemic short word lists

No. 1	*No. 2*	*No. 3*	*No. 4*	*No. 5*
ship	fish	thud	fun	fib
rug	duck	witch	will	thatch
fan	gap	wrap	vat	sum
cheek	cheese	jail	shape	heel
haze	rail	keys	wreath	wide
dice	hive	vice	hide	rake
both	bone	get	guess	goes
well	wedge	shown	comb	shop
jot	moss	hoof	choose	vet
move	tooth	bomb	job	June

No. 6	*No. 7*	*No. 8*	*No. 9*	*No. 10*
fill	badge	bath	hush	jug
catch	hutch	hum	gas	match
thumb	kill	dip	thin	whip
heap	thighs	five	fake	faith
wise	wave	ways	chime	sign
rave	reap	reach	weave	bees
goat	foam	joke	jet	hell
shone	goose	noose	rob	rod
bed	not	got	dope	vote
juice	shed	shell	lose	shook

No. 11	*No. 12*	*No. 13*	*No. 14*	*No. 15*
man	have	kiss	wish	hug
hip	whizz	buzz	dutch	dish
thug	buff	hash	jam	ban
ride	mice	thieve	heath	rage
siege	teeth	gate	laze	chief
veil	gauge	wife	bike	pies
chose	poach	pole	rove	wet
shoot	rule	wretch	pet	cove
web	den	dodge	fog	loose
cough	cosh	moon	soon	moth

RNID hearing test cards

1.	EGG	PEG	HEN	BED
2.	CUP	DUCK	JUG	BUS
3.	SHIP	DISH	PIG	FISH
4.	KNIFE	PIPE	PIE	KITE
5.	KEY	SHEEP	FEET	TREE
6.	HAT	CAT	LAMB	FAN
7.	DOG	COT	DOLL	SOCK
8.	OWL	HOUSE	MOUSE	COW

Chapter 10
Speech perception tests for profoundly deaf listeners

VALERIE HAZAN

Introduction

Normally hearing listeners are aided in their communication by the fact that there is a great deal of redundancy of information in speech. Within the acoustic signal itself, speech contrasts are marked by a multiplicity of acoustic cues. In addition, listeners glean further information from visual cues and from the meaning and structure of the sentence. Thanks to this multiplicity of information, normally hearing listeners can perceive speech relatively well even in poor listening conditions, such as in the presence of noise, where some speech cues are masked or absent.

Profoundly deaf listeners are at a disadvantage as most of this redundancy is lost, due to a reduced audible frequency range, poor frequency selectivity and high susceptibility to masking. Even with powerful hearing aids, profoundly deaf listeners may only receive a very small amount of the auditory information contained in the speech signal. Studies on the perception of speech by profoundly deaf listeners have shown that they usually show some ability to discriminate vowels, which are marked by low-frequency acoustic cues, and that some listeners may be able to discriminate consonants differing in voicing (e.g. /b/ vs. /p/) but that profoundly deaf listeners show a poor ability to use the acoustic cues to place of articulation (e.g. to distinguish between /b/ and /d/) and some cues to manner of articulation (e.g. to distinguish between /s/ and /t/). They may therefore have to rely to a great extent on visual and contextual information for speech communication.

Standard speech audiometry tests, which present single words or sentence material at different intensity levels, may be much too complex for this listener population, and produce a 'floor' effect, with scores near zero. This is frustrating for the listeners, and yields very little useful information as to their perceptual abilities. There is therefore a need for a different set of speech audiometry tests for profoundly deaf listeners, which take full account of the fact that the visual channel (i.e. lip reading) is crucial for this listener population, and which will aim to quantify how well the listener is able to make use of visual cues to speech. There is also a need for finely grained tests, which, rather than looking at the perception of words or sentences, assess the listener's ability to make use of specific acoustic cues, which are the 'building blocks' of speech. These tests might indicate, for example, that a profoundly deaf listener may well be able to tell whether a speech sound is voiced or unvoiced, even though more subtle distinctions, such as the ability to hear the difference between the sounds /b/ and /d/, are impossible. An ability to perceive individual patterns, even if the whole of the speech signal is not accessible to the listener, is beneficial as it will enable the listener to perceive a specific speech feature, such as voicing, manner or place of articulation, which combined with other features obtained through the visual channel, can lead to an accurate perception of the sound produced.

In addition to acoustic and visual information, a third crucial source of information in decoding speech is the contextual information that is present at lexical, syntactic and semantic levels. This contextual information limits the choice of possible words given the preceding information perceived and is a major contributor to perception, especially in situations where the auditory signal is of poor quality. Tests which aim to assess the effect of contextual information on perception are useful as listeners show individual differences in the ability to make use of this information (e.g. Kalikow, Stevens and Elliott, 1977).

The need for a quantitative assessment of a listener's ability to make use of speech pattern and lip reading information is especially important given recent developments in hearing aid design aimed at profoundly deaf listeners who do not gain any benefit from conventional hearing aids. One approach is to simplify the sounds presented to the profoundly deaf listener by extracting and presenting specific speech patterns rather than the complete speech signal.

An example of speech pattern processing aids of this type is the SiVo aid (Faulkner et al., 1992), designed as an aid to lip reading, which extracts voice pitch and voiceless frication information from speech and presents them in the form of highly simplified patterns. Speech pattern information may also be presented via a tactile aid or via a cochlear implant. In order to evaluate a patient's suitability for such aids, it is imperative to have a proper assessment of the use this patient is able to make of the acoustic patterns contained in the speech signal. As many of these aids are aids to lip reading, focusing on speech features which are not cued visually, it is essential to have, for listeners being assessed for such aids, an analytic assessment of both lip reading ability and speech processing ability.

Finally, as in all speech audiometric testing, it is crucial, in test development and selection, to consider what source of information is being evaluated in any one test. In order to obtain specific information on the use made of acoustic or visual information, the information provided by context, which is difficult to quantify, needs to be kept at a minimum, for example by presenting consonants in nonsense words. While analytic tests of this kind provide very useful specific information about speech pattern perception, they are poor predictors of a person's overall communicative ability, as important sources of information are removed.

For such an assessment, sentence- or paragraph-level material is required. There is therefore a need, ideally, for a battery of tests, each evaluating a different level of speech perception, from the most analytic speech pattern processing level to the most global sentence processing level reflecting the combined use of acoustic, visual and contextual information. Some examples of tests at these different levels are presented here. A more detailed account of factors to be considered in the development of speech audiometry tests for profoundly deaf listeners can be found in Dillon and Ching (1995).

Although there is a wide range of test material available, the reality is that speech perception tests are little used in audiology clinics, due to time and financial pressures. However, many of the tests described here are routinely used by teams involved in the design and development of cochlear implants, tactile aids and speech pattern hearing aids, and in the evaluation and rehabilitation of profoundly deaf listeners being fitted with such aids. Most of the tests described here were used in a multi-site evaluation of cochlear implantation by the Department of Health and protocols for their use in this study were defined in a document produced by the Institute of Hearing Research (IHR) (1991).

Audio-visual speech perception tests

Lipreading cues, which profoundly deaf listeners have to rely on heavily for speech communication, provide a lot of information about the place of articulation of consonants, especially for sounds such as /p/, /b/, /f/, /v/, which involve highly visible articulators. However, they provide little information about the manner of articulation of the consonant (i.e. whether a plosive, fricative, nasal or approximant). Also, as voicing is a result of vocal fold vibration which is not visible, no visual information is given about features which are linked to the presence or absence of voicing. This includes events such as the timing of voicing onset which will mark whether a consonant is perceived as being voiced (e.g. /b/) or unvoiced (e.g. /p/), but also, at the suprasegmental level, information about the prosody (or intonation) of a word or sentence. Prosodic information can indicate the difference between a question or a statement, where the stress falls in a sentence and the way in which a sentence is segmented into its components. Summerfield (1983) defines four groups of consonants (/p b m/, /w/, /f v/ and /θ ð r t d n l s z ʃ ʒ t ʃ dʒ j k g ŋ h/) that lip readers can distinguish quite easily. Using visual cues alone, distinctions between consonants belonging to the same category are much more difficult to make. Vowels differ primarily in terms of their duration, and in the amount of lip rounding and opening present. Although vowels can quite easily be identified when presented in clearly articulated, isolated words, much of the distinctiveness between vowels appears to be lost in running speech (e.g. Summerfield, 1983).

Thankfully, there appears to be some complementarity between auditory and visual cues so that features such as voicing, which are poorly cued visually, are quite robustly cued via the auditory channel, even in situations when the auditory signal is highly degraded or when the listener has a very limited range of residual hearing. Providing voicing information in addition to lip reading, such as is done in certain speech pattern extraction aids, can improve consonant identification by around 30% (Faulkner et al., 1992). Certain distinctions between manners of articulation (such as nasals vs. fricatives) are also quite robustly transmitted via the auditory channel and can therefore disambiguate information presented visually.

The aim of audio-visual speech perception tests is to evaluate a listener's ability to make use of cues provided visually, either alone or supplemented by acoustic information. Two types of tests can be used. Analytic tests aim to abstract from contextual information, in order to get an evaluation of the ability to perceive cues to specific phonemes. They might therefore present nonsense words with a fixed phonemic structure (e.g. vowel-consonant-vowel). It is recommended to present these tests in video-taped form, in order to avoid any bias that might result from the variation in test condition and individual differences in cues provided via live presentation. More global tests, using sentence- or paragraph-length material, are used to model conditions which are closer to a normal listening situation.

Analytic tests

The intervocalic consonant (VCV) test (Rosen et al., 1979) is a good example of a test which has a simple structure and is easy to run, yet can be quite powerful in terms of the information it yields about a profoundly deaf listener's use of acoustic patterns and visual cues.

The VCV test investigates the perception of intervocalic consonants in nonsense words. Most commonly, a video-taped test with four repetitions of each of 12 consonants (/p b t d k g f v s z m n/) in a /a-a/ vowel environment is used. Each nonsense word is spoken with a falling intonation, with a stress on the second syllable. The listener is required to write down the consonant perceived, choosing from the consonants listed on the answer sheet. This is therefore a closed set test, as the listener is given a fixed number of alternative responses. The test is usually presented in a 'lip reading-alone' condition, in order to get a baseline evaluation of the use of visual cues, and in other conditions, in which the visual information is supplemented with various kinds of auditory input. These might include for example a lip reading + speech condition, in which condition the full speech signal is presented, and a lip reading + pitch information, in which the visual channel is supplemented by a single acoustic pattern representing voice pitch.

The data obtained are presented in the form of a general confusion matrix with stimulus plotted against response. Statistics are also provided in the form of both raw percentages and percentages of 'information transferred' (which are adjusted for chance level) for features such as voicing, and place and manner of articulation. It is important to use percentages which have been corrected for chance, as the chance level is different for voicing scores (two alternatives: voiced or unvoiced) than for place (four alternatives: labial, labio-dental, alveolar, velar) or manner scores (three alternatives: plosive, fricative, nasal). Figure 10.1 shows the patterns of confusions obtained with lip reading alone, lip reading with a conventional hearing aid, and lip reading with a speech pattern aid (SiVo) for a profoundly deaf listener (identified as Subject 1 in Faulkner et al., 1992). The patterns of confusions obtained in these tests give information on the kind of acoustic and visual cues that the listener is using in the test. For example, with lip reading alone, only three groups of consonants are distinguished: /m b p/, /f, v/, /n z d t s g k/. The client makes fewer confusions with a conventional hearing aid than in the unaided condition, but is still making many confusions in terms of voicing and manner of articulation (e.g. /m/ consistently perceived as /b/, /b/ perceived as /p/). However, when pitch information alone is added as an aid to lip reading, confusions are further reduced, and, for example, /m/ is almost always correctly perceived as it is the only labial consonant to be continuously voiced. Overall, the ability to decode a sound in terms of its voicing and manner of articulation improves significantly for this listener. It can be seen that the VCV test is sufficiently sensitive to show differences in a listener's perception using two types of hearing aid, and can be used to highlight specific areas of difficulty in speech pattern perception. It is very important to analyse patterns of confusion, rather than merely look at percentages of correct responses, as these patterns of confusions give clues as to the cause of the confusion, and as to the type of training that might be needed with this client.

Another word-level audiovisual test is the FADAST (four-alternative-auditory-disability) test (Summerfield and Foster, 1983) which is an audiovisual version of the FAAF test (Foster and Haggard, 1979). The FADAST uses audiovisual presentation of a set of monosyllabic English words. Each word presented is accompanied by a subtitled group of

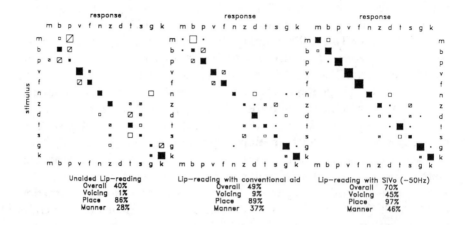

Figure 10.1 Confusion matrices for VCV test presented in three conditions. The size of the square is proportional to the number of responses. ■, Correct responses; ▨, errors in terms of voicing. □, errors in manner of articulation.

four possible responses involving one vowel contrast and one conso-nant contrast (e.g. 'bull', 'wool', 'bell', 'well'). The whole test has a balanced distribution of contrasts that are relatively easy, and contrasts which are relatively difficult to discriminate by vision alone. As this test has a closed set response protocol with a very limited set of real-word alternatives, the pattern of confusions obtained is not as indicative of a person's processing difficulty as those obtained from the VCV test.

Sentence-level tests

Sentence-level tests aim to provide a more global assessment of the combined use of visual, acoustic and contextual information provided within the sentence. These tests present a situation which is much closer to normal communication, but no longer enable much prediction as to the specific information being used by the listener, as so many sources of information are involved.

The BKB sentences (Bench and Bamford, 1979) are an example of material which aims to look at the accuracy with which words can be identified in simple sentences. These sentences were initially developed for audiometric use, but video-recorded versions of the test have also been produced (Rosen and Corcoran, 1982; EPI Group, 1986). All sentences are meaningful and there is no attempt to quantify the effect of contextual information. As these lists were initially intended for use with partially hearing children, the sentences, which were taken from natural language samples from this same population, are short, with simple syntactic structures and relatively common words. They are therefore highly suitable for use with listeners with very limited residual hearing and low vocabulary knowledge. Another advantage of this material is that it is extensive, consisting of 21 standardized lists of 16 sentences containing 50 key words. It is therefore particularly suitable for rehabilitative work or hearing aid fitting where a number of testing sessions may be required. Studies have shown that not all lists are of equal difficulty and that learning effects are obtained with this material, especially for good lip readers, although scores appear to stabilize after the first three lists (Rosen and Corcoran, 1982). However, Foster et al. (1993) have provided correction factors for the video-recordings of this test which are most commonly in use (EPI Group, 1986) so that results from different lists can be compared; they also provide a set of recommendations for the use of these audiovisual tests.

The SPIN (speech in noise) sentence tests (Kalikow, Stevens and Elliott, 1977) have been designed to quantify the relative use being made of acoustic and contextual information. This test is usually presented with background noise (e.g. speech babble) and can be presented in audio-alone or audio-visual conditions. Each sentence list consists of 50 sentences. The only word being scored is the final word of the sentence, which is always a noun. Sentence lists are twinned, both lists containing the same 50 key words. In one list, a key word is presented in a high predictability context (e.g. 'For your birthday, I baked a *cake*') whilst in the other list, it is presented in a low predictability context (e.g. 'We were discussing the *cake*'). The difference between the high predictability and low predictability scores for the two lists gives a measure of the use made of contextual information.

One potential problem with this material is that it is rather time-consuming to administer as two lists of 50 sentences are needed for a proper evaluation to be made. Also, it only tests the perception of a single word category (i.e. monosyllabic nouns).

A simple yet highly effective test which aims to get even closer to a normal communicative situation is the connected discourse tracking test (CDT) (De Filippo and Scott, 1978). The test material is extracted from books suitable for readers with a low vocabulary knowledge. These books contain sentences with simple syntax and easy vocabulary. The tester reads a passage from the book, sentence by sentence, and the task of the client is to repeat the passage verbatim. The tester can repeat the text as often as is necessary or use any (verbal) strategy in order to get the message across. The score is simply the number of words communicated per minute. This test can be run in lip reading alone vs. lip reading with different types of auditory input, to evaluate the improvement in communication seen with the addition of, for example, pitch information. Although listener performance can be affected by a number of factors, such as text complexity, talker strategies and learning of the task (e.g. Hochberg, Rosen and Ball, 1989), which may affect the cross-comparison between different test conditions, the test is popular due to its simplicity, relative closeness to a natural communicative situation, and because it is not reliant on finite lists of fixed material. The effect on scores of the use of different talker strategies in cases of 'blockages' for example, when a receiver is incapable of recognizing a given word after several attempts, is a cause of concern, and, recently, there have been attempts to standardize methods for administering and scoring CDT tests (e.g. Spens, 1995).

At present, the tests described are typically recorded on high-quality video-cassettes. The advantage of video-recorder-based presentation is that the equipment required is relatively cheap and easily available. However, in recent years, many computer-based systems have been developed which allow much greater flexibility in the use of the material, and which also allow for the automatic scoring and storage of results. Many systems developed in the last ten years have made use of laser-disc technology (for a review, see Sims and Gottermeier, 1995). The recently-released IHR computer-based test battery for predicting and measuring outcomes from cochlear implantation in adults (POCIA) (Summerfield, Haggard and Foster, 1996) contains a complete set of word- and sentence-level tests, together with questionnaires and non-speech tests included in the IHR recommendations for the evaluation of clients with cochlear implants. The quality of video playback on multi-media computers is now high enough to allow for the presentation of audiovisual tests stored on hard disk, and computer-based training and evaluation systems which make full use of this latest technology are beginning to appear.

Psychoacoustic tests

In order to perceive even the simplified speech signal presented through certain speech pattern hearing aids, a listener needs to have a sufficiently unimpaired cochlea to make some basic temporal and spectral distinctions. Tests are therefore necessary which evaluate these very basic abilities. For example, if it is found that a client's cochlea is so damaged that voiced sounds cannot even be distinguished from unvoiced sounds, it will be of no use to fit this client with an aid which contrasts pitch information (for voiced sounds) with noise information (for unvoiced sounds). The use of simple psychoacoustic tests may also save from unnecessary testing, as it would be of no use to present complex speech audiometry tests to a listener who has extremely poor temporal and spectral processing.

The following psychoacoustic tests are included in the IHR recommendations for test protocols for the evaluation of cochlear implant patients published in 1991, but are no longer included in the more recent recommendations which are about to be implemented. At present, these tests are typically presented in tape-recorded form, but there is a distinct advantage in using a computer-based testing procedure, as adaptive test procedures, which adjust the length and complexity of the test to the subject's ongoing performance, can then be run. This reduces the time needed to reach a threshold level in performance. PC-based packages are beginning to be commercially available.

The Gap Detection test measures the minimal duration of a silent interval that can be detected in the middle of a burst of noise. This ability is important for the perception of fluctuations in amplitude, which gives important information about the spectral envelope of the speech signal. Normal listeners can detect gaps as short as 5 millisecinds (e.g. Rosen, Faulkner and Smith, 1990). If the minimal detectable gap is greater than 40 to 50 milliseconds, poor results are expected on tests of speech perception.

The 'scratch–buzz' test is a test of periodicity–aperiodicity discrimination that measures the minimum duration of a signal needed to classify a sound as a 'buzz' (train of pulses) or a 'scratch' (band of noise). Again, a minimum duration of 50 milliseconds or above gives a prediction of poor performance on tests of speech perception.

Speech pattern tests

In the last 50 years, speech researchers have aimed at gaining a better understanding of which speech pattern cues are the most important for perception by normally hearing listeners. The main speech pattern cues marking contrasts in voicing, and manner and place of articulation have been defined (for a review, see Pickett, 1980). There is more recent evidence that the relative perceptual importance given to cues to a contrast may vary according to the context in which the sound appears and also vary across individual listeners (e.g. Hazan and Rosen, 1991).

Speech pattern perception research has mainly been based on the use of identification tests. These tests involve high-quality computer-generated (synthesized) pairs of words that differ in only one sound (e.g. 'goat' vs. 'coat'). The reason for using synthesized speech in identification tests of this kind is that natural speech is too complex and uncontrolled for the investigation of speech pattern use. For example, natural tokens of the pair 'coat' – 'goat', which could be used to investigate the perception of voicing in initial plosives, would differ in aspects unconnected with the initial plosive, such as overall intensity, duration and quality of the vowel. When testing the perception of these tokens, it would be impossible to determine what information the listener was making use of in discriminating between the two sounds. The problem is remedied by the use of high-quality copy-syntheses, which sound highly natural, yet give the experimenter total control over the speech patterns presented to the listener. In this way, 'irrelevant' differences between the two sounds will be neutralized and only one or two specific speech pattern cues marking the contrast under investigation are altered.

The potential of these tests as speech audiometry material, used to evaluate individual listeners' use of speech pattern information, has been recognized (Fourcin, 1976), and they have been piloted with a variety of listener populations, including hearing impaired children (e.g. Hazan et al., 1991) and adults with central disorders (Fourcin et al., 1985). Following these pilot studies, a new PC-based system, the 'speech pattern audiometer', is being developed commercially for clinical use (Hazan et al., 1995).

Speech pattern tests, which form the basis for speech pattern audiometry, thus provide the intermediate step between psychoacoustic tests, which investigate basic temporal and spectral processing abilities, and natural speech. As stated earlier, an acoustic-feature based approach to speech testing, in which one is aiming to assess which speech pattern cues are being used by a listener, is of particular relevance given that many new aids to lip reading for this population of listeners are also speech pattern-based. An assessment of which speech pattern cues are being used by a profoundly deaf listener is needed so that the most appropriate hearing aid is fitted, one which makes the maximal use of the listener's residual hearing.

Speech pattern tests can also be used for assessing the effect of specific speech training, or for longer-term assessment with deaf children, in order to monitor their development of speech perception abilities. The minimal pairs included in the test battery are chosen on the basis of knowledge of speech perception development, which is marked by an ability to perceive increasingly complex speech pattern combinations. By testing listeners on word pairs graded in terms of speech pattern complexity, it is possible to assess the stage of speech perceptual development achieved. Since the speech pattern elements in the words can be individually manipulated, an assessment can be made of the relative perceptual weighting given by the listener to each of the cues marking the contrast. In Figure 10.2, examples of stylized speech patterns for two contrasts are presented. The vowel contrast ([ɜ]-[a]) assesses the use of simple, steady patterns (first and second formants). This test could be run in a condition in which both formants are present and in a 'first formant alone' condition, in which the second formant has been removed. A comparison of a listener's performance on these two conditions could indicate whether the listener seems to be making the distinction using first formant information alone or whether both formants are being used. The voicing contrast (/g/–/k/ as in GOAT– COAT) is a more complex contrast which assesses the use of two

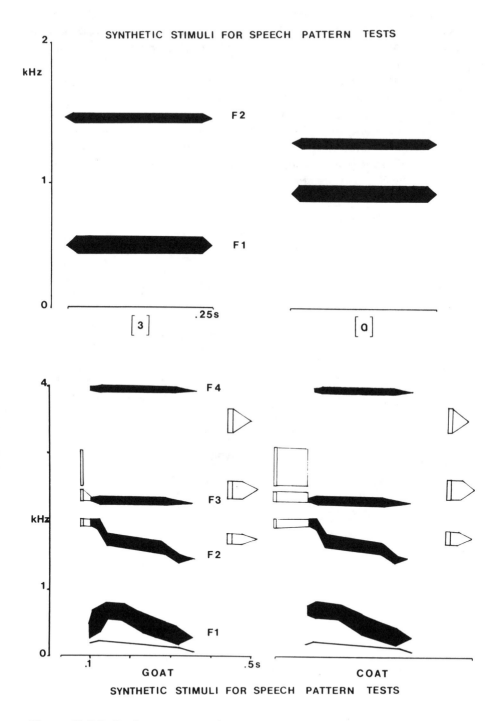

Figure 10.2 Stylized spectrograms showing the endpoints of the vowel ([ɜ]-[a]) and voicing (Goat–Coat) contrasts

important cues: voice onset time, i.e. the duration between the plosive burst and vowel onset, and first formant onset. Again, the relative use made of both these cues can be evaluated via manipulation of the speech patterns.

From each minimal pair, a series of speech sounds (a 'continuum') is produced in which one or several of the acoustic cues are varied in equal steps. This use of a continuum of stimuli mirrors, in a controlled way, the variability seen in natural speech patterns due to intra- and inter-speaker differences in production. A listener's ability to group slightly different productions of a sound into a single phonemic category ('categorical perception') is an essential skill for speech percep-

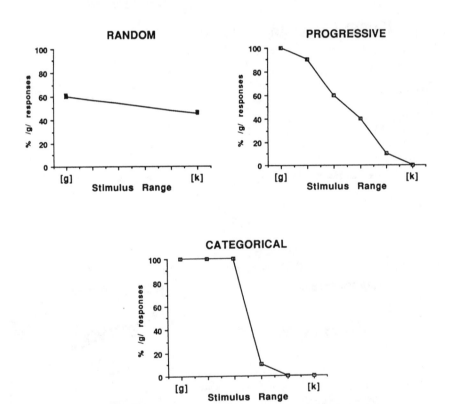

Figure 10.3 Three types of identification function configurations. When a listener is unable to consistently identify even clear exemplars of 'goat' and 'coat', a 'random' configuration is obtained. At a second stage, a listener might be able to consistently identify the 'coat'–' goat' endpoints, but be less consistent in the labelling of other stimuli along the continuum. A 'progressive' configuration is then obtained. 'Categorical labelling' is obtained when the listener can consistently classify stimuli into two clear categories. A categorical function is characterized by a sharp gradient

tion. The test is presented in the form of an adaptive forced-choice labelling test, where each of these sounds is presented to the listener a number of times. The listener's task is to decide whether the sound perceived was, say, 'coat' or 'goat'. The output of each test is an identification function, which plots the percentage of 'goat' responses against the stimulus continuum (which gradually goes from a clear 'goat' to a clear 'coat'). Different stages in the development of the ability to label the stimuli are reflected by different configurations of the identification function (from random to categorical) (see Figure 10.3). Statistical methods can be used to evaluate the significance of any change in identification function configuration between two test conditions (for further details, see Hazan and Rosen, 1991). Speech pattern tests can be run on a PC, using an adaptive testing procedure so that the duration and difficulty of the test are dependent on the listener's responses.

As these tests are not dependent on a client vocabulary knowledge, they are repeatable, with no significant learning effects. They are also analytic, quick to run and provide results which can be generalized to other speech sounds as they assess the ability to use subcomponents of speech. This makes them eminently suitable for example, for comparing the usefulness of different hearing aids for a given listener, or for evaluating long-term development in speech perception ability or the effect of some specific speech training.

Conclusion

In conclusion, a large range of speech material covering all levels of assessment is available for use with profoundly deaf listeners. The VCV intervocalic consonant test, the BKB sentences and connected discourse tracking, which represent three levels of audio-visual assessment, from the most analytic to the closest to natural communication, are included in the IHR recommendations for reception assessment. It is hoped that in the next few years, these and the speech pattern tests, which represent the link between natural speech tests and psychoacoustic tests, will also become more widely used, not only by cochlear implant and other research teams, but by the wider community of audiologists, speech and language therapists and hearing therapists.

Chapter 11
Testing visual and auditory-visual speech perception

GEOFF PLANT

Introduction

Tests of a hearing impaired person's speech reception skills have traditionally concentrated on the assessment of the subject's ability to understand speech via listening alone. The materials used for testing usually consist of lists of monosyllabic words (Egan, 1948; Hirsh et al., 1952; Fry, 1961; Clark, 1981). Tests using nonsense syllables (Levitt and Resnick, 1978; Edgerton and Danahauer, 1979), and sentence (Davis and Silverman, 1970; Bench and Bamford, 1979; Kallikow, et al, 1977) materials have also been developed, but they have not won widespread acceptance in audiological practice.

Auditory alone testing using monosyllabic words can provide very useful information on a person's speech perception skills. This is especially true if a detailed analysis is made of a subject's error responses (Stevenson, 1975; Robertson and Plant, 1983). Such an approach, however, cannot adequately assess an individual subject's everyday communication skills. Typically, with the obvious exception of telephone calls, most conversations are conducted face-to-face. In face-to-face conversations the receiver has access not only to the acoustic signal, but also to the visible movements of speech.

The importance of these visible movements to the hearing impaired receiver should not be underestimated. Lip reading — 'the correct identification of thoughts transmitted via the visual components of oral discourse' (O'Neill and Oyer, 1981) — represents the primary mode of speech reception for many profoundly and severely hearing impaired people. There are many instances where people with less severe losses also need to use lip reading to supplement the auditory signal. Speech perception via audition alone may be impossible for many hearing impaired people in noisy and/or reverberant conditions. Even in quiet listening conditions many moderately hearing impaired people report

208

that they understand speech more easily if they can both hear and see the speaker. Comments such as 'I can hear much better with my glasses on' and 'I don't hear so well in the dark' are familiar to clinicians working with hearing impaired adults.

Given the great potential value of lip reading for hearing impaired people, it is perhaps surprising that standard audiological procedures do not routinely include visual and auditory-visual testing. Such testing would appear to offer a more comprehensive view of an individual's overall communication competence. lip reading testing; that is, testing via vision alone, can be criticized on the grounds that it represents a highly artificial situation, as almost all hearing impaired people have at least some acoustic information available to them via hearing aids, cochlear implants, or tactile aids. lip reading testing can, however, determine the limits of visual communication for an individual. Once this 'visual base line' has been determined, the clinician can see whether providing auditory or tactual information leads to an improvement in performance. This is achieved by comparing the subject's unaided (lip reading alone) and the aided (lip reading plus the supplement) performance.

The results of this testing may also assist the clinician in determining appropriate rehabilitative strategies for an individual subject. This can include the choice of sensory modality or modalities to be stressed during training. Such matters are critical in the design of individualized and appropriate training procedures. The effectiveness of various training procedures can also be evaluated by comparing scores obtained pre- and post-training.

Visual and auditory-visual testing may also serve as a valuable demonstration for those hearing impaired individuals who doubt the value of lip reading. The response made by many hearing impaired people to the suggestion that they should attend to visual as well as auditory cues is often; 'It's no use, I can't lip read'. Unfortunately, this judgement is usually based on an experience such as turning off the sound of the television, or attempting to lip read a stranger across a crowded room. A comparison of scores obtained auditory alone and auditory-visually usually results in superior performance in the bisensory condition, especially if the materials are presented in noise. Some hearing impaired people also develop inappropriate listening approaches which may, over time, impede the use of lip reading cues. For example, some people incline their 'good' ear towards the speaker and do not attend to the face of the speaker. Auditory alone and auditory-visual testing can serve to highlight the inherent problems of this strategy.

This chapter is divided into two distinct sections. The first presents a review of tests of visual and auditory-visual speech reception skills. In presenting this review I have tried to cover a wide range of tests suitable for clinical and, to a lesser extent, research purposes. The review is by no means exhaustive, but attempts to present a wide range of test materials. The second section is directly related to clinical issues. It addresses areas such as: test selection, mode(s) of presentation and the use of the test results in determining rehabilitative approaches, targets and effectiveness.

Auditory and auditory-visual tests: a review

The first lip reading tests

The first filmed test of lip reading ability was developed in 1913 by the pioneering lip reading teacher Edward Nitchie. It consisted of the three proverbs — 'Love makes the world go around', 'Spare the rod and spoil the child', and 'Fine feathers make fine birds'. It is not known whether this test was ever used to test the lip reading skills of hearing impaired subjects (O'Neill and Oyer, 1981). It does, however, have some very obvious problems. The materials used are not at all representative of conversational speech. The sentence content is highly predictable and subjects would only have to pick up a few words to guess the rest of the sentence. Finally, the test used too few test items to gain a realistic picture of a person's lip reading skills. Conklin (1917) attempted a more realistic measure of lip reading ability developing a live voice test which assessed a subject's lip reading skills using eight consonants, 52 words, and 20 sentences. The test was presented to a group of adolescents attending the Oregon State School for the Deaf. The test results were highly correlated (0.90) with ratings of the subjects' lip reading abilities made by their teachers (O'Neill and Oyer, 1981).

Studies with children

Although a number of lip reading tests for children were developed over the next 30 years (Day et al., 1928; Heider and Heider, 1940; Mason, 1943) these were not suitable for assessing the lip reading skills of adventitiously hearing impaired adults. The results of two of these studies, however, merit some comment. Day et al. (1928) found that the scores obtained by the children in their study, when the children's teachers read the sentences, were 50–60% better than those obtained when the materials were presented by an outside, and, therefore, presumably unknown, speaker. This result highlights the importance of speaker familiarity for many lip readers. Heider and Heider (1940) found that visual vowel recognition was related to overall lip reading skill. This finding was replicated in a later study by McGrath (1985). Heider and Heider (1940) also found that practice in vowel discrimination led to improvements in lip reading ability.

The development of standardized tests: 1940–1960

It was not until the 1940s that lip reading tests specifically designed for adults started to emerge. The most important of these was the Utley film test — 'How well do you read lips?' (Utley, 1946). In its original version this filmed test consisted of two equivalent forms, each containing a word subtest, a sentence subtest, and a story subtest. The test was standardized using 761 hearing impaired persons ranging in age from 8 to 21 years and was, for many years, generally accepted as the most valid test of lip reading abilities. This was despite detailed criticisms of the test made by DiCarlo and Kataja (1951) who claimed that the test was excessively difficult.

They found that 50% of the test material contributed only 3% to the scores obtained and was therefore non-functional. Jeffers (1967) believed that this excessive difficulty was, to a large part, related to the filmed version of the test. The speaker, 'an attractive, vivacious university co-ed, unaccustomed to speaking to the deaf or hard of hearing' (Utley, 1946) was criticized by DiCarlo and Kataja's (1951) subjects as being excessively difficult to lip read. As a result, many researchers or clinicians preferred to either present the test live voice or record the test using a more suitable speaker. It should be noted that, over time, the test was presented in an abbreviated form, with only the sentence subtests being used. Although the test now appears to be little used, its long-term importance should not be underestimated. The Utley test served as a model for many other, later measures of lip reading skills. Whatever its limitations, it represented a significant step forward in lip reading research.

Morkovin (1974) produced a series of films based on real life situations for lip reading training. One of these, 'The Family Dinner', has been used as a lip reading test. The film showing 'a typical American family at dinner' (Lowell, 1974) was used by DiCarlo and Kataja (1951) in their analysis of the Utley test. They asked subjects 20 questions related to the film's content and found a high correlation (0.77) between this measure and the subjects' Utley test scores. 'The Family Dinner' was also used by Lowell (1975) to evaluate the 'Film Test of Lip Reading' (originally the 'Keaster Film Test of Lip Reading', see Jeffers and Barley, 1971) in studies conducted at the John Tracey Clinic in Los Angeles. This test consisted of two equivalent lists each containing 30 simple, unrelated sentences which were designed to reflect everyday usage. The scores obtained for the two tests resulted in a correlation co-efficient of 0.89 (Lowell,1974).

Recent developments: 1960–the present

The period since 1960 has seen many significant developments in lip reading research and the subsequent development of more appropriate test materials. Two publications, O'Neill and Oyer (1961, 1981) and Jeffers and Barley (1971), provided much of the impetus for this work. Both works provided systematic summaries of current lip reading research, and presented available test materials. Although there have been many studies reported since the publication of these books, they still represent a valuable resource for anyone interested in research into lip reading.

Lip reading tests

A large number of sentence tests of lip reading have been developed over the past 30 years. Although the Utley test was still widely used for both clinical and research purposes as recently as the 1980s, it now seems to have been supplanted by a number of these other measures.

One set of test materials which are now widely used for auditory, visual and auditory-visual testing are the Central institute for the Deaf (CID) everyday sentence lists (Davis and Silverman, 1970). Johnson (1976) for example, reported on the use of the lists to measure the receptive communication abilities of students entering the National Institute of Technology in Rochester, New York. Originally developed for auditory speech perception testing each list consists of 10 unrelated sentences containing 50 key words. The task is to repeat each sentence as it is presented and the subject is scored for the number of key words correctly identified. In a comparative study of lip reading tests, Spitzer et al. (1987) presented all 10 CID lists as a lip reading test. Using the key word scoring system they found that the lists were statistically equivalent. One interesting finding in their study was the relatively low mean score (29.12%) for the CID lists. This is surprising, given the characteristics of the sentence lists, which were designed to mirror everyday sentence content and structures.

Barley (reported in Jeffers and Barley, 1971) selected 40 sentences from the CID corpus and used them in two test lists, each consisting of 20 sentences. In scoring this test — the Barley/CID everyday sentences test — Jeffers did not use the key word method. Rather, the subject received credit for each word correctly identified in each list: Form A presents a total of 125 words, whilst Form B contains 117 words. lip reading testing using these lists revealed that they were statistically equivalent. The mean scores for the two forms were 47.4% correct for Form A and 51.4% correct for Form B. These scores are considerably higher than those reported by Spitzer et al. (1987). The differences in score are probably attributable to a number of factors including live (Barley) vs. recorded (Spitzer et al.) presentations, and the characteristics of the speakers used in the studies. These factors are covered in detail later in this chapter.

Skamris (1974) described a very simple film test in Danish designed to evaluate the lip reading skills of deafened adults. The test consisted of numerals, place names, and a series of short sentences about eating or meals. He found that there was a good correlation between his subjects' scores on this test and a rating of their lip reading skills by therapists, family members and the subjects themselves. One major advantage of this test was the short time taken to administer it — around 3 minutes.

All of the tests described thus far consisted, at least in part, of meaningful materials. In the 1970s, however, a number of tests were developed which assessed the visual recognition of consonants. Binnie et al. (1974) developed a test which consisted of 20 English consonants combined with the vowel [a] to form consonant-vowel (CV) syllables. The test consisted of 100 items with each consonant presented five times in a random order. The test was administered, without sound, to 36 normally hearing adults. Analysis of the subjects' responses indicated that they were able to group the consonants into five visemic (visually distinctive) categories based on consonant place of articulation. Binnie et al. (1974) suggested that the test could be used to identify subjects who were unable to assign the consonants into their appropriate visemic categories. These people, they believed, might benefit from training in consonant recognition at the syllable level. Walden et al. (1977) used a 400-item version of the Binnie et al. (1974) test to evaluate the effects of training on visual consonant recognition. They found that the number of visemic categories their subjects could identify rose from seven pre-training to nine post-training.

The National Acoustic Laboratories' (NAL) lip reading test (Plant and Macrae, 1977, 1981; Plant et al., 1980) consists of two subtests — a consonant subtest and a sentence subtest. In the first subtest the 20 English consonants /p, t, k, b, d, g, f, v, θ, ð, s, ʃ, dʒ, tʃ, w, r, j, l, m, n/ are combined with the vowel /a/ to form CV syllables such as /pa/, /ba/, /ma/, etc. The second subtest consists of 50 simple questions, most of which can be answered by a single word. The questions are divided into five categories:

1. Some questions about you. (What's your name?)
2. Some questions about your family. (How many brothers do you have?)
3. Questions about where you live. (What's the name of your street?)
4. Questions about things you like. (Who's your favourite author?)
5. Questions with easy answers. (What's the opposite of happy?)

The mean score obtained by 30 subjects presented the consonant subtest via lip reading alone (Plant and Macrae, 1977) was 37.3% correct (range 30–46). Analysis of the subjects' responses showed that they were able to differentiate between the various places of articulation, but were unable to differentiate manner of articulation and voicing cues.

The response patterns showed seven distinct confusion clusters which were classified as:

1. Bilabials /p, b, m/.
2. Labiodentals /f, v/.
3. Interdentals /ə, ð/.
4. Rounded labials /w, r/.
5. Alveolar continuants and velar stops /l, n, j, g, k/.
6. Post alveolars /tʃ, dʒ, ʃ/.
7. Alveolar fricatives and stops /s, d, t/.

The sentence subtest was presented to 100 subjects (both normally hearing and hearing impaired) who spoke English as their first language (Plant and Macrae, 1981). The mean score for this subtest (38.9%) was similar to that obtained for the consonant subtest, but there was a much wider performance range (0–88%). Twenty of the hearing impaired subjects in this study were attending lip reading classes. Their teachers were asked to rate the students' lip reading skills, using a five-point scale developed by Skamris (1974). The pupils' scores were then ranked on a five-point scale, and the rank difference correlation coefficient between the two measures was then calculated. This was found to be 0.865, indicating that level of performance on the test is a valid measure of a person's lip reading ability.

The sentence test was also presented to 24 normally hearing adults who spoke English as a second language (Plant et al., 1980). The mean score obtained by this group was only 15% with scores ranging from 2–38%. The difference between the mean score of this group of subjects and that of the subjects who spoke English as their first language, was statistically significant. It was hypothesized that the performance of the English as a second language group resulted from their relatively poor knowledge of the English language. Many parts of speech are ambiguous or absent when transmitted via lip reading, and lip readers have to use their knowledge of the language to supply the missing elements in the lip reading signal.

Spitzer et al. (1987) reported on the NAL/West Haven test, a modification of the NAL lip reading test. The modifications were relatively minor, and involved substituting American idioms for the specifically Australian English items in the original test. Two versions of the NAL/West Haven test were recorded; one by a male speaker and one by a female speaker. The mean scores obtained for the test presented by the male speaker and the female speaker were 63.4% and 65.4% respectively. These scores are considerably higher than the mean score obtained in the Plant and Macrae (1981) study, but no explanation for the differences was given in the Spitzer et al. (1987) paper. Again, factors such as speaker characteristics probably account for the differences in scores for the two studies.

The use of Kalikow, et al. (1977) SPIN test as a lip reading measure was investigated by Plant, et al. (1984). Each list of the SPIN test consists of 50 sentences, with the subject's task being to repeat the last word in each sentence. Half of the sentences presented are designated high predictability items in that cues to the key word are contained within the rest of the sentence. An example of a high predictability item is: 'The boat sailed across the bay'. The remaining sentences offer no such assistance, with the key word being presented in a neutral sentence context. An example of this type of sentence, designated low predictability, is: 'John was talking about the bay'. One of the potential advantages of the SPIN test is that it offers the opportunity to evaluate an individual's speech perception skills, with and without the use of contextual information.

Plant et al. (1984) recorded four lists (Lists A, C, E, G) of the SPIN test on video-tape and presented them to 24 normally hearing subjects as a lip reading task. The mean score for the four lists was only 7.96% (range 0–27%) with only six subjects scoring more than 10% correct. These results indicate that these materials may be excessively difficult for widespread use as a lip reading test. Many hearing impaired people would find the test very discouraging, and it may serve to reinforce already negative attitudes towards the use of visual cues in communication. It may, however, be a useful adjunct to an auditory-visual test battery.

Auditory-visual tests

During the 1970s, tests designed to evaluate the auditory-visual skills of hearing impaired adults started to emerge. The aim of such tests was to provide a measure of the advantage that auditory-visual speech reception gave over lip reading alone or auditory alone performance in quiet or in noise. Special impetus for such tests came with the development of cochlear implants, tactile aids and hearing aids for profoundly deaf adults. Cochlear implants and tactile aids are primarily designed as aids to lip reading and researchers using these devices wanted to determine the difference between aided and unaided lip reading performance.

One of the first tests designed to measure differences between visual, auditory and auditory-visual performance was the HELEN test (Ludvigsen, 1974) developed by an interdisciplinary group of Danish researchers to test 'hearing handicapped persons' perception of speech in a manner which corresponded to the situation in everyday life' (Ludvigsen, 1974). There were eight lists of 25-question sentences, which were presented in a noise background. Within each list there were five broad categories of questions. These were:

1. Sentences with 'before/after' involving numbers, days, or months; 'What day comes after Friday?' 'What number comes after 22?'

2. Sentences with colours; 'What colour is red wine?'
3. Sentences with simple arithmetic computations; 'What is 2 + 4?' 'What is half of 6?'
4. Sentences with opposites; 'What is the opposite of cold?'
5. Miscellaneous questions; 'What language is spoken in Sweden?' 'Which is bigger, an elephant or a mouse?'

The sentences were designed to be relatively simple, to require only a one word response, and to have only one correct response. In a pilot study (Ewertsen, 1974) the test materials were presented auditory only and auditory-visually. Prior to the administration of the test, the signal-to-noise ratio (SNR) which resulted in an auditory alone score of 50% or worse was determined. The test lists were then presented auditory alone and auditory-visually with the SNR held constant at the predetermined 50% point. The aim of the study was to determine the improvement that resulted when the materials were presented auditory-visually. Eighteen hard-of-hearing subjects were tested and showed improvements ranging from 6–38 percentage points (mean = 23.4%) when the materials were presented auditory-visually.

Plant, et al. (1982) used an English translation of the first four lists of the HELEN test to measure the visual, auditory and auditory-visual performance of 48 elderly hearing aid users. The mean scores obtained in the three presentation conditions were; visual alone—17.1%, auditory alone—82.3% and auditory-visual—90.8%. Clearly, the differences between the visual alone condition and the other two presentation conditions were highly significant. The difference between the auditory alone and auditory-visual was also significant (at better than the 1% level). The amount of improvement, however (8.5 percentage points), appeared to be an overly pessimistic indication of the value of visual cues to speech perception by hearing aid users. This small improvement was due to the high auditory alone score obtained by almost all of the subjects.

The HELEN lists were then presented in a noise background (four speaker babble at –3 dB SNR) to a group of 12 elderly hearing aid users. The scores obtained for this testing were: visual alone—39.2%, auditory alone—31.25% and auditory-visual—81.7%. Two-way analysis of variance revealed no significant differences between the auditory alone and the visual alone conditions. The score for the auditory-visual condition, however, was significantly better than those obtained for the other two conditions.

Walden et al. (1981) described a sentence test designed to be presented auditory-visually in noise. The test consisted of 38 sentences (100 key words) related to a common theme — the US Army's drill sergeant program. This was considered appropriate, as the subjects in the study were either serving, or had served, in the US Army. The subjects were instructed to repeat each sentence as it was presented, and were scored on the percentage of key words correctly identified. The SNR required to reduce each subject's auditory-visual score to 40–50% correct was determined prior to testing, and the test was then presented at that level. Testing was conducted pre- and post-training at the same SNR to determine whether subjects had derived benefit from the training procedures adopted.

MacLeod and Summerfield (1987, 1990) reported on the use of Bench and Bamford's (1979) BKB sentences as a means of determining the advantage visual cues afford to speech reception in noise. In both studies, normally hearing subjects' speech reception thresholds (SRT — defined in these studies as the level at which all three key words in a sentence were correctly identified) in noise were obtained in two conditions — auditory alone, and auditory-visually. In the first study the mean auditory-visual benefit was +11 dB. That is, the subjects' mean auditory-visual SRT was –22.8 dB SNR compared to –11.8 dB SNR for the auditory only condition. The major drawback in this first study was that the method used took an excessive amount of time and was too cumbersome for clinical use.

In the 1990 study the authors used an adaptive technique involving increasing or decreasing the level of the speech signal in 2 dB steps to determine an individual subject's SRT. The results of this testing revealed a mean auditory only SRT of –16.8 dB S/N and a mean auditory-visual SRT of –23.2 dB SNR. That is, a visual benefit of +6.4 dB SNR. In both studies, MacLeod and Summerfield reported that the subjects who were the best lip readers gained the most benefit in the auditory-visual condition. MacLeod and Summerfield (1990) concluded that the adaptive technique was most suitable for clinical use. They suggest that two lists (each consisting of 15 sentences) were sufficient in each condition to obtain a valid SRT measure.

Boothroyd, et al. (1985) described a set of 48 sentence lists —The City University of New York (CUNY) sentences — to be used testing lip reading alone and lip reading supplemented by fundamental frequency (F_0) information.

Each list consisted of 12 sentences typical of everyday conversation, and ranged in length from three to 14 words. There were a total of 102 words in each of the lists, and subjects were scored for the number of words correctly identified. Four of the sentences were statements, four were commands and four were questions. Each of the sentences within a list were related to a specific topic such as food ('Have you eaten yet?'), sport ('Don't try to run unless you have good shoes'), weather ('Take an umbrella'), and health ('Cover your mouth when you cough'). The same 12 topics were used in each list, and the subjects were cued as to the topic prior to the presentation of each sentence. Testing of three normally hearing subjects via lip reading supplemented by F_0 showed only small difference between the individual lists. There was, however, strong evidence for short-term learning of the task. That is, the subjects' scores showed marked improvements for the first eight or nine lists. The authors suggested that naive subjects should be administered 10 sentence lists before the lists were used to contrast various presentation conditions.

The CUNY sentence lists have been used in a number of studies investigating auditory and tactile supplements to lip reading (Boothroyd, et al., 1988; Hanin, et al., 1988; Boothroyd, et al., 1992). The set of sentences has subsequently been increased to 72 lists (Boothroyd, 1991) using the design criteria outlined above. These lists have been recorded on video-disc with the full acoustical signal on one audio channel and the output from an electroglottograph on the other. The large number of available lists makes this test an extremely valuable resource for visual and auditory-visual testing. The problems of test familiarity are reduced to a large extent, and sufficient numbers of lists are available to ensure that any short-term learning effects can be eliminated by provision of practice lists. A number of lists can also be presented in each of the sensory conditions being tested, providing a more valid measure of performance differences.

Another test material available on video-disc is Tyler, Preece and Tye-Murray's (1987) Iowa audiovisual speech perception tests. This test consists of sentence materials, vowels presented for identification in an [hVd] format and consonants in an [iCi] environment. The sentence test consists of 100 sentences presented by 20 different speakers (20 speakers × five sentences each). The sentences are relatively short, have simple grammatical structures, and draw their vocabulary from Bench and Bamford's (1979) BKB sentences. The use of laser disc technology enables randomized presentations of the test materials.

The use of Kalikow, Stevens and Elliott's (1977) SPIN test as a lip reading test has already been covered. Although the test appears to be too difficult for widespread use as a lip reading test, there may be a place for its use in auditory-visual testing. Plant et al. (1984) also presented the test with minimal auditory cues (speech low-pass filtered (LPF) at 200 Hz, or a fixed frequency signal at 115 Hz presenting voice intensity cues) supplementing lip reading. A control group was presented with the materials via lip reading alone. The mean scores for the three subject groups were: lip reading alone, 12.6% (range 0.5–27%); lip reading plus voice intensity cues, 23.5% (range 4–41%) and lip reading plus LPF speech, 41.5% (range 14–65%). These results indicate that the SPIN lists may be suitable for auditory-visual testing especially if the subject being evaluated is a very good lip reader. The highest score obtained via lip reading in the study by Plant, et al. (1984) study was 27%. This subject's score for the NAL lip reading test (Plant and Macrae, 1981) was 76%. If the NAL lip reading test was re-presented to this subject with supplementary cues the scope for improvement would be severely limited as performance via lip reading alone is at near ceiling level. The use of a more complex lip reading alone material in this case would offer a better opportunity to see how performance is affected when supplementary information is provided.

Consonants in nonsense syllable formats such as [aCa] and [Ca] have also been used for comparing aided and unaided lip reading performance. This is especially true of studies evaluating performance with cochlear implants and tactile aids. The aim of such studies is to determine whether the auditory or tactile cues provided by the aid(s) lead to improvements in consonant perception. Although there are around 24 consonants in English, most studies have used a reduced set of 12 items: /p, t, k, b, d, g, f, v, s, z, m, n/. This set has been chosen because it provides voicing, manner of articulation (stops, sibilant and non-sibilant fricatives and nasals), and place of articulation (bilabials, labio-dentals, alveolars and velars) contrasts.

Such testing can provide very useful insights into the subject's performance in the aided and unaided conditions. The percentage correct score is only one measure which can be obtained. The subject's responses can be analysed for feature perception to determine whether, for example, the aid is providing information enabling the subject to detect voicing or nasality cues. For example, in a recent study Plant and Gnosspelius (1994) looked at the consonant perception of a deaf man who supplements lip reading by 'tactiling'; that is, by placing his thumb lightly on the side of a speaker's throat to pick up the vibrations which accompany speech (Öhngren, 1992; Söderlund, 1992). The twelve consonants listed above were used as the stimulus materials in an [aCa] environment. Lists of 60 items (12 consonants × five random presentations) were presented via lip reading alone and lip reading + tactiling. The subject's responses were then analysed to determine how well he was able to correctly identify consonantal features in the aided and unaided conditions. The results of this analysis are presented in Table 11.1. These show an improvement of almost 40 percentage points when lip reading is supplemented by tactiling. This is an improvement of 80.6% due to enhanced perception of voicing and manner of articulation contrasts.

Table 11.1 Overall percentage correct and percent correct feature recognition for the consonants /p, t, k, b, d, g, f, v, s, z, m, n/ in a [aCa] frame presented via lip reading alone and lip reading plus tactiling

	Lip Reading Only (%)	Lip Reading Plus Tactiling (%)
Overall	47.5	85.8
Voicing	66.7	97.5
Manner of Articulation		
Stops	73.3	96.7
Nasals	65.0	80.0
Fricatives	100	100
Sibilants	40.0	75.0
Overall Manner	70.8	90.8

Although the information provided by such testing is very useful, the use of such a limited set can lead to an overly optimistic view of an aid's capabilities. Table 11.2 presents the results of testing (Plant et al., 1995) carried out using an expanded set of consonants: /p, t, k, b, d, g, f, v, s, z, h, m, n, ʃ, w, r, l, y, tʃ, dʒ/, with the subject in the Plant and Gnosspelius (1994) study. Both studies used the same speaker and the same vowel environment.

Table 11.2 Overall percentage correct and percent correct feature recognition for the consonants/p, t, k, b, d, g, f, v, s, z, h, m, n, ʒ, w, r, l, y, tʃ, dʒ/ in a [aCa] frame presented via lip reading alone and lip reading plus tactiling

	Lip Reading Only (%)	Lip Reading Plus Tactiling (%)
Overall	42.9	64.3
Voicing	76.2	98.8
Manner of Articulation		
Stops	54.2	83.3
Nasals	41.7	50.0
Fricatives	100	100
Sibilants	75.0	50.0
Semi-vowels	68.7	81.2
Affricates	0	37.5
Overall Manner	59.5	71.4

The improvement in the lip reading plus tactiling condition was only around 20 percentage points in this case. This represents an improvement of 49.9%, which is considerably less than that found when the testing involved only 12 consonants. Voicing continued to be identified at a very high rate in the combined condition but the scores for stops, nasals, and sibilants were considerably lower. Adding nine consonants to the stimulus set created many more potential error responses for the subject. The addition of the semi-vowels and affricates created many more errors in perception of the stops and nasals than had been found in the previous study. For example, in eight presentations of the velar nasal it was correctly identified only twice, being mis-identified as /l/ three times and /g/ twice. These results indicate that a larger set may be a more valid measure of consonant perception in the aided and unaided conditions. This should be taken into account in selecting sets for testing and when evaluating claims made for various supplementary approaches to lip reading such as tactile aids and cochlear implants.

A criticism that can be made of all of the tests covered so far is that they are not truly representative of everyday conversations. This is especially true of syllable and word level tests, but it can also be applied to many sentence materials. Typical conversations consist of connected discourse involving groups of interrelated sentences. This provides opportunities for understanding — through the use of context and collocation for example — which are not found in conventional speech test materials.

Speech tracking (connected discourse tracking) developed by De Filippo and Scott (1978) represents an attempt to measure speech reception skills using connected discourse materials. In this procedure the sender (the talker) reads from a prepared text segment-by-segment, with the receiver asked to repeat exactly what was said. If the subject responds correctly the next segment is presented for identification. If the receiver does not repeat the segment correctly, however, the sender uses either repeats, paraphrases, or uses some other strategy until all the words are correctly identified. Any deviation from the prepared text is unacceptable. At the end of a pre-determined time period (usually 5 or 10 minutes), the number of words correctly identified is tallied and divided by the time elapsed to derive a words-per-minute (wpm) score. For example, a receiver may correctly repeat back 295 words in a 10 minute tracking session, yielding a tracking rate of 29.5 words per minute (wpm).

Since its introduction in 1978, speech tracking has become a key element in many aural rehabilitation programmes for adventitiously hearing-impaired adults. It has been used for evaluating the performance of subjects fitted with cochlear implants (Martin, Tong and Clark, 1981; Dowell, Brown, Seligman and Clark,1985; Levitt, Waltzman, Shapiro and Cohen, 1986), tactile aids (De Fillippo, 1984; Brooks, Frost, Mason and Gibson, 1986; Cholewiak and Sherrick, 1986; Plant, 1988; Cowan, Blamey, Sarant, Galvin, Alcantara, Whifford and Clark, 1991), and 'natural' tactile approaches such as Tadoma (Reed et al., 1992) and Tactiling (Plant and Spens, 1986; Öhngren, 1992). Typically, a number of tracking sessions are conducted in the aided and the unaided conditions and the tracking rates are compared. For example, Plant and Spens (1986) found that their subject's tracking score rose from around 40 wpm lip reading alone to over 60 wpm when lip reading was supplemented by tactiling.

Despite its wide spread acceptance by research groups, there have been criticisms of the use of speech tracking as a test procedure. The most detailed of these criticisms is that of Tye-Murray and Tyler (1988) who argue that 'speech tracking is an effective aural rehabilitation strategy but inappropriate as a test procedure' (Tye-Murray and Tyler, 1988; p.226). They cite a number of extraneous variables which they believe are extremely difficult, if not impossible, to control. These include: speaker variables such as speaking style, articulator movements and proficiency in providing repair strategies; receiver characteristics such as assertiveness and language skills and the type and complexity of the text used.

Many of these criticisms can be resolved, to some extent, by the use of recorded materials. Computer-based systems using recorded materials have been developed by a number of research groups. These include Boothroyd's (1987) computer-assisted speechreading perception evaluation and training program (CASPER) and Dempsey, Levitt, Josephson and Porazzo's (1992) computer-assisted tracking simulation (CATS). These enable control of speaker variables, and allow the use of a strict hierarchy of response and repair strategies. Unfortunately, the systems do have some disadvantages. The most obvious problem is the cost of the equipment — which includes video or laser disc players, monitors and a computer — to present the materials and record the subject's response. Such equipment may not be available to many clinicians who use tracking as an integral part of their rehabilitative approach, and wish to use their subjects' scores to evaluate performance change with training and/or the fitting of alternative supplementary aids.

The KTH tracking procedure (Gnosspelius and Spens, 1992) represents a compromise between the use of recorded materials and live-voice presentation. The text is presented live voice, but the segment length is pre-determined and the use of only one repair strategy is permitted. The text to be used is entered into a computer line-by-line. The segments should be grammatically and logically correct, and should neither be too long nor too short, as both can contribute to blockages. The only repair strategy allowed with this approach is for the sender to repeat any word(s) not correctly identified. The number of repeats is pre-determined and once that number is reached the receiver is shown the word via an LED display or a computer monitor.

Prior to the tracking session the sender sets the session duration and the number of repeats allowed before a word will be displayed on the screen or the monitor. The sender starts the session by pressing a mouse button and reading the first segment on the monitor. If the segment is repeated correctly the sender clicks onto the next segment. If the response is incorrect the sender clicks on the first blocked word and repeats it in isolation or in combination with some or all of the remaining words in the segment. Once the receiver has correctly identified all the words in the segment, with or without written prompts, the sender moves on to the next segment. This procedure continues until the predetermined testing time has elapsed.

At the end of the session data on the tracking session are stored in a file. These include the subject's tracking rate and ceiling rate. The ceiling rate is the time taken on segments that are correctly identified on the first presentation. This measure can vary considerably, as the sender may vary the presentation speed to a rate that seems to be appropriate to an individual subject's receptive skills. The subject's response time may also vary depending upon how confident the subject is that the response is correct. The programme also stores the number of words repeated, the number of times each is repeated, and the number of words presented via the LED screen or the monitor. These data are used to calculate the proportion of blocked words in a particular session.

The KTH tracking procedure provides the opportunity to measure a subject's aided and unaided lip reading performance over time to determine whether a supplementary aid is providing useful supplementary information. As an example, data from a project involving the use of the Tactaid VII— a seven channel vibrotactile aid — by an adventitiously deaf adult will be presented. The subject was provided with systematic training including 'speech tracking' using the KTH procedure. The duration of each tracking session was 5 minutes, and the text used was a children's novel 'The Brothers Lionheart' by Astrid Lindgren. For the first 50 sessions, lip reading was always supplemented by the tactile aid. The aim of this initial training was to build up the subject's confidence in the tracking task. The subject's mean scores for these 50 sessions were: tracking rate, 31.4 wpm; ceiling rate, 75.8 wpm; proportion of blocked words, 0.29; number of words displayed on the monitor, 7.8.

Twenty-five 5-minute sessions were then provided in two sensory conditions lip reading alone and lip reading plus the Tactaid VII. The mean results for these sessions are presented in Table 11.3. These show an advantage of 6.1 wpm (around 20%) in the subject's tracking rate. This score could, of course, be obtained using conventional tracking The remaining scores, however, are unique to the KTH procedure. The ceiling rates are almost identical indicating that the sender and the receiver were operating at similar rates in the two conditions. This is an important finding, as variations in the ceiling rate can lead to differences in tracking rates (Plant, et al., 1994). There are differences between aided and unaided performance in the proportion of blocked words and the number of words presented via the monitor. These indicate that the subject is receiving useful supplementary information in the aided condition.

Table 11.3 Mean tracking rates, ceiling rates, proportions of blocked words and number of words transmitted in a written form for 25 5-minute sessions presented via lip reading alone (L only) and lip reading plus the Tactaid VII (L + TVII)

	Tracking Rate (wpm)	Ceiling Rate (wpm)	Proportion Blocked Words	Words Displayed on Monitor
L only	31.5	80.1	0.31	8.1
L + TVII	37.6	82.1	0.24	5.3

Summary

The tests and procedures reviewed cover a wide range of approaches to evaluating visual and auditory-visual speech perception skills. Test stimuli ranging in complexity from nonsense syllables to connected discourse have been used and highlight the need to provide a range of materials to gain an overall view of an individual's strengths and weaknesses. A subject's aided and unaided consonant perception scores may provide much useful information on the phonetic information available in the two modalities, but the scores are probably a very poor indicator of performance with sentence and connected discourse materials.

The wide range of scores found in most studies also indicates that no one test is suitable for use with all subjects. Test materials which are excessively easy or excessively difficult may not provide adequate measures of a subject's abilities, as they may introduce unwanted ceiling or floor effects.

The clinical use of visual and auditory-visual tests

The aim of this section is to provide suggestions for the clinical use of visual and auditory-visual test materials. Before considering which of the tests reviewed are most suitable for clinical use, four important factors need to be considered. These are the use of recorded vs. live tests, dialectical appropriateness of the test materials, the speaker's dialect and the presentation conditions for testing.

Live vs. recorded tests

An important consideration in visual and auditory-visual testing is whether the materials should be presented 'live', or whether a recorded version should be used. The use of live voice testing does appear to have a number of advantages, the most obvious being that it does not require the use of any special equipment. The importance of this factor has diminished considerably, however, as video recorders have become more and more common in clinical settings. A second advantage of live voice presentation is 'its greater fidelity to a three dimensional real-life situation' (Elphick, 1984). This factor, however, does not appear to be of critical importance. A study by McCormick (1979b) comparing live and video-taped presentations of the same test materials concluded 'that there was strong evidence to support the hypothesis that the loss of the third dimension does not degrade lip reading scores if all other variables are carefully controlled'. A final advantage of live voice testing is that it allows access to a wide range of materials. The tester merely has to have the scripts of various tests and can choose the material(s) most appropriate to assess the performance of a particular individual.

The most important advantage of a recorded test is that it provides consistency of presentation. No speaker can be reasonably expected to replicate his or her articulatory patterns across numerous presentations of the same test. A recorded test presents the same material time after time without the subtle differences that occur when live voice presentation is used. Recorded tests also eliminate the problem of speaker differences. Martony (1974) found rather large variations between speakers presenting non-labial Swedish consonants and vowels as a lip reading test. The scores for individual speakers ranged from 19.8% to 33.3% with a mean score of 27.4%. A second study involving both vowel and consonant tests revealed significant differences between the speakers who had been hardest and easiest to lip read in the first study.

Recorded tests allow an unfamiliar speaker to be used for evaluation. When a therapist acts as both the test speaker and the trainer there is always a danger that post-training scores may reflect familiarity with the speaker rather than any real improvement in performance. A recorded test allows ease of presentation of materials without voice. When a speaker attempts to present lip reading materials without voice, this may unintentionally provide exaggerated non-normal articulatory patterns. There is also the possibility that the speaker may provide some auditory cues. A recorded test allows the speaker to use normal voice and articulatory patterns, and the audio signal to be removed during test presentation.

Recorded tests allow for better control of the level of the audio signal in a noise background. Although a trained speaker may be able to maintain a relatively stable SNR with the aid of a sound level meter, this is a very difficult task. Speakers in noisy situations normally raise their voice level in a consistent fashion (the Lombard effect) and it is difficult to override this effect. A final factor which needs to be considered is that recorded tests 'don't look back'. As Summerfield (1983) has noted, the use of recorded materials may be beneficial for some hearing impaired people who find it difficult to interact with a live speaker. This, of course, may lead to unrealistically high scores with some people who normally avoid watching the speaker's face. Under these circumstances, however, the score reflects the person's 'visual potential' and could be used to encourage attention to the speaker's face and lips during conversations.

In summary, the arguments in favour of recorded tests appear to outweigh those for live voice testing. Recorded tests allow much greater control of test materials and consistency of presentation. This, of course, presupposes the existence of recorded test materials. If appropriate recorded test materials are not available the clinician should use live voice presentation. Testing of visual and auditory-visual performance is a very important part of determining a person's communication competence and should be a standard part of an audiological evaluation.

Dialectical appropriateness of the test materials

Test materials should reflect the dialectical variations of the subject's linguistic community. For example, tests using American English expressions should not be used in Australian or British conditions. Before test materials are used in a specific dialectical community the texts should be checked for their appropriateness. Consider the following sentence taken from Boothroyd, Hanin and Hnath's (1985) CUNY sentence; 'We're going trick or treating on Halloween'. This sentence would be quite inappropriate for use in Australian conditions. Firstly, Halloween is not widely observed in Australia, and the references to 'trick or treating' or even the holiday itself may be lost on many people. Secondly, the use of the preposition 'on' is inappropriate in this context for Australian conditions where 'at' would be used. This need to carefully consider vocabulary, colloquial expression and usage patterns should not be seen as pedantic 'nit-picking'. If test materials do not reflect local usages the subject may be penalized not for reduced perceptual skills but rather for the unfamiliar nature of the test materials.

The speaker's dialect

There is a certain irony in this item, given that the author is an Australian currently living and working in the United States. This can create some problems in communication with both hearing and hearing impaired people. General Australian English differs greatly in its pronunciation and in its usage patterns from American English. Even small differences such as [nyu] rather than [nu] for 'new' can cause communication breakdowns with some deaf people. I know of no studies looking at the effects of dialect on visual and auditory-visual communication, but the anecdotal evidence is overwhelming. Hearing impaired people very often comment on the difficulties they have in understanding different dialects. This is especially true for those who speak English as a second language. As a result it is very important that when recorded tests are used they should be presented by a native speaker of the predominant local dialect. This is probably easier done in a country such as Australia where general Australian English is the predominant variety spoken throughout the country. Countries with much wider dialectical ranges such as the UK or the US may create greater problems. Again, however, the test materials should reflect the subject's communication skills, not familiarity with dialectical variations.

Presentation conditions

Differences in test conditions can result in wide variations in performance. Consequently, clinicians should attempt to use the same test protocols with all subjects. Care should be taken that the same instructions are given to each subject, even if this means using a written cue card. The use of practice items will also help ensure that the subject understands the task prior to the presentation of the test materials. The distance from the television monitor or the live speaker should also remain constant. The image on the monitor should approximate life size and the subject should be seated directly in front of the screen (or speaker) at a distance of around 2 metres. The materials should be presented in a quiet but not necessarily sound treated test room. This applies not only to auditory-visual presentations but also to the visual only condition. Background noise, especially speech, can interfere with lip reading performance and lead to reduced performance.

   In clinical situations it is probably best to present the acoustic speech signal via a loudspeaker mounted directly in front of the subject. The signal should be presented at a level which approximates real life situations. At a distance of 2 metres from the loudspeaker the signal peaks should occur at around 70 dB SPL. This level should be measured using a sound level meter at the subject's ear level. The use of a short audio recording of connected discourse recorded at the same level as the test materials can be used to calibrate the test system. This can also allow the subject to set the hearing aid(s) to the preferred listening level.

   Where auditory and/or auditory-visual testing is being carried out in noise, two factors need to be considered: the type of noise to be used and, the level of the noise. Although white noise can be used for testing (see MacLeod and Summerfield, 1990 for example) continuous speech babble has been widely used in both experimental and clinical environments, and would appear to be the noise signal with the best face validity. Hearing impaired people typically report that they experience most difficulties understanding speech at parties, clubs, noisy meetings etc. Further, the spectrum of speech babble corresponds to that of the speech signal and provides appropriate masking effects.

There would appear to be two options for testing in noise. One is to present the speech material at a pre-determined SNR and evaluate what effect this has on the subject's performance. Auditory-visual and/or auditory testing can be carried out in quiet and in noise to determine what, if any, effects this has on performance. Plant, et al. (1982) for example, presented the HELEN test at a +3 dB SNR. The second alternative is to change the SNR level until the subject attains some pre-determined criterion. For example, MacLeod and Summerfield (1987, 1990) altered the noise level until they found the SNR at which their subjects were able to identify all three key words in a sentence. Other researchers have altered the noise level to locate the SNR at which the subject is able to identify 50% of the syllables in a sentence (Middelweerd and Plomp, 1987) or 50% of key words (Walden et al., 1981). The availability of equipment will determine in part whether a varied or pre-set SNR level is used for testing. If the choice is for varying the SNR until some pre-set performance criterion is attained, it is strongly suggested that the speech level (the signal) be held constant, and the noise level raised and lowered.

Clinical tests

Clinicians working with hearing impaired people on a regular basis require access to a variety of test procedures that will enable them to evaluate the auditory, visual and auditory-visual skills of their clients. If a measure of a client's lip reading skills is required, it is suggested that the use of the NAL lip reading test (Plant and Macrae, 1981) should be considered. Testing in both Australia (Plant and Macrae, 1981) and the US (Spitzer, et al., 1987) has indicated that the test provides a reliable measure of lip reading performance. Some changes to the test sentences will be needed to meet local dialectical forms, but these will probably be relatively minor. The modified test can then be recorded and presented to a range of control subjects for standardization. Once this has been completed a subject's score can be compared to the control group scores for an estimate of performance level. If this test proves to be excessively difficult for subjects the use of an easier test material such as the HELEN test (Plant, et al., 1982) may be more appropriate.

For screening of visual alone, auditory alone and auditory-visual performance, Boothroyd, Hanin and Hnath's (1985) CUNY sentences are recommended. A major advantage of this test is the large number of lists, enabling multiple presentations without repeating test items. A recorded version of the test is available for use in the US, and this should be used where appropriate. In other English speaking countries, consideration should be given to adapting the CUNY sentences and then recording them using an appropriate speaker. The sentences can be used for testing in quiet or with a noise background. For clients with mild, moderate, or severe hearing losses it may be necessary to test auditory and auditory-visual performance in a noise background. If it is feasible, the noise level should be adjusted until the subject scores around 50% for auditory only presentations of the sentence lists. Once this level has been determined the test should be presented auditory-visually to determine what, if any, benefit the subject receives from lip reading cues.

The CUNY sentences can also be used with profoundly hearing-impaired subjects. In these cases the test conditions will need to be adapted to meet the auditory skills of the client. Some profoundly deaf subjects will be able to cope with materials presented via audition alone in quiet or in noise. Others will be unable to identify any words in this condition. In these latter cases, testing should be confined to lists presented via lip reading alone and lip reading plus the acoustic signal presented at 70 dB SPL. The client should set the aid(s) to the preferred signal level.

The clinician should also have access to supplementary materials for use with clients who find the CUNY sentences either excessively easy or excessively difficult. The HELEN sentences can be used with clients who find the CUNY sentences overly difficult whilst the SPIN lists are relatively complex materials that should challenge almost all lip readers. Again, it is preferable that these materials be recorded but if the facilities and resources are not available to do this, live voice testing can be used.

Using test results for rehabilitative planning

The results of this testing can be used to help develop individualized training plans for clients needing rehabilitative intervention. In these cases, the use of other, supplementary, test materials should also be considered. At the analytic level, testing of a client's ability to identify consonants in the aided and unaided conditions can provide extremely valuable information. If VCV syllables are used for testing, all of the consonants can be presented for identification. The client can be given a sheet setting out the test alternatives and asked to point to the consonant she or he thinks has been presented. The only difficulty with this approach is that at least four of the consonants, /θ, ʒ, ʃ, ð/, are difficult to present orthographically and clients may have difficulty understanding the task. For this reason it is suggested that the following 20 consonants be used for testing: /p, t, k, b, d, g, f, v, s, z, ʃ, tʃ, dʒ, j, m, n, l, r, w, y/. It is further suggested that three different vowel environments, [aCa], [iCi] and [uCu], be used, as vowel lip shape can influence performance. Lists of 60 items should be prepared presenting each of the consonants in each of the three vowel contexts.

The subject's error responses in the various sensory conditions should be analysed to determine how well he or she is able to perceive consonantal features. These should include: voicing; manner of articulation features — stops /p, t, k, b, d, g/, nasals /m, n/, fricatives /f, v, h/, sibilants /s, z, ʃ/, semi-vowels /w, r, l, y/, affricates /tʃ, dʒ/; and place of articulation features — bilabials /p, b, m/, rounded labials /w, r/ labio-dentals /f, v/, alveolars /t, d, n, s, z, l/, post-alveolars /ʃ, tʃ, j/, palatal /y/, velars /k, g/ and glottal /h/. The subject's results can help determine whether analytic training is needed and, if it is, the sensory modality(ies) in which it should be provided.

The CUNY sentences can also be used for more in-depth testing at the sentence level. Blocks of at least five lists can be presented in each of the test conditions to gain an accurate picture of the subject's performance. The testing modalities (auditory, visual and auditory-visual) and presentation conditions (quiet or noise) will be determined by the capabilities of the individual subject. Prior to the testing a simpler test material, such as the HELEN test can be used to help in the choice of modalities and test conditions. The SPIN sentence lists can also provide valuable insights into an individual's use of synthetic/global (syntactic, semantic, contextual etc.) and analytic (phonetic, acoustic) cues, and this information can assist in the planning of rehabilitative programmes. If the clinician wishes to assess a subject's performance with connected discourse materials, speech tracking, despite the limitations cited above, would appear to be the best available method.

The KTH tracking procedure appears to overcome many of the problems of speech tracking but some variables, such as speaker and receiver characteristics, are extremely difficult, if not impossible, to control. If the clinician does not have access to the KTH procedure, she or he should develop protocols that ensure consistency from presentation to condition. For example, the clinician may decide that the only strategy used in the event of blockage will be to repeat the word a maximum of three times. If the subject still fails to respond correctly, the blocked word should be written down and shown to the subject. At the completion of the tracking session the tracking rate should be calculated and the number of words presented in a written form appended; for example 33.4 wpm (seven blockages).

The subject's scores for sentence and connected discourse materials will also provide very useful insights for planning an individualized therapy programme. Valuable information on: (a) the relative complexity of training materials, (b) the modalities to be used in training and (c) the appropriateness of using noise masking can all be obtained from a comprehensive visual and auditory-visual test battery.

In testing, an important consideration should be to locate an appropriate level of complexity for training. For example, if the client experiences difficulty with the CUNY sentences auditory-visually, the therapist should consider the use of an easier test material such as the HELEN sentences. If these also prove to be excessively difficult an informal test procedure using closed set materials can be considered. For example, the subject may be given a set of pictures and the therapist asks a series of questions about each picture. This can help assess whether context leads to improved performance. The insights gained from such testing can ensure that the client experiences success in therapy sessions. Based on the results of testing the therapist can select materials that challenge, but do not defeat the client. As the subject's performance improves the materials used for training can become progressively more and more complex. The aim of training should be to show what the client CAN DO not what she or he CAN'T DO.

Other clients may be able to perform very well auditory-visually in quiet but have great difficulty when materials are presented visually alone or auditory-visually in the presence of background noise. The therapist may decide to provide a training programme that focuses on enhancing the use of visual cues. The test results can determine the SNR at which performance starts to be affected, and this can be the starting point for training. As performance improves, the level of noise can be increased. The level of complexity of the training materials can also be determined to a large extent by the test results. Similarly, clients with good auditory alone performance but only a small gain in the auditory-visual mode may benefit from bisensory training with a distorted auditory signal, to force them to attend more closely to the visual signal. This can be achieved through the use of auditory masking, low-pass filtering (Plant, Macrae, Dillon and Pentecost, 1984), intensity gating (Montgomery, Walden, Schwartz and Prosek, 1984), or by the extraction and prevention of one speech feature such as F_0.

Conclusion

The tests and procedures covered in this chapter highlight the need for visual and auditory-visual testing to be an integral part of the overall aural rehabilitation process. Testing should provide an accurate measure of a person's communication competence. Testing with pure tones and monosyllabic words provides valuable information on the subject's audiological status, but may not accurately reflect communicative performance in everyday life. An added benefit of visual and auditory-visual testing is that it enables the therapist to provide training at an appropriate level and in the appropriate modality or modalities. Much work remains to be done in this area, but tests and procedures do exist which can be used to obtain a comprehensive picture of an individual's communication competence. Audiologists and other therapists working with hearing impaired people need to utilize the materials currently available and use the information gained to enhance the overall quality of aural rehabilitation.

Chapter 12
Speech audiometry in the USA

BARBARA KRUGER and FREDERICK M KRUGER

This review of speech audiometry in the United States of America updates the material presented in the previous edition. Current clinical practices will be discussed and compared with previously reported clinical practices. Some additional speech audiometry tests and procedures are introduced, particularly as applications for paediatric audiometry, rehabilitative audiometry and assessment of the intelligibility of communication systems.

Speech audiometry provides a means of assessing communication ability: speech recognition ability or the ability to understand speech. In the USA, the primary use of speech audiometry is as an integral component of the differential diagnostic hearing evaluation. Speech audiometry, as it is practised today, refers to determining a 'speech recognition threshold' and a 'speech recognition score' i.e. a 'word or sentence recognition score'.

As a principal component of the basic audiologic evaluation, speech audiometry plays an important role in differential diagnosis, to identify and isolate conductive hearing losses as opposed to sensorineural or mixed losses. These and other speech audiometry tests are still used in differential diagnosis, less for assessment of retrocochlear involvement, or assessment of functional hearing loss and more for assessment of central auditory nervous system involvement or rehabilitative audiology.

The application of speech audiometry to the selection and fitting of hearing aids continues to be secondary, but it is expanding. The growing use of speech-in-noise tests will be discussed. The newer applications of speech audiometry continue to be for the prediction or assessment of hearing aid performance, in prognostic and rehabilitative evaluation of communication ability and handicap, and in communication training of individuals and communication systems.

Terminology

The terminology used in speech audiometry continues to be imprecise. For example, the terms 'speech reception threshold', 'spondee threshold' and 'speech recognition threshold' are frequently used interchangeably. Commonly used speech audiometry terms are defined below.

A *psychometric function* describes the relation between some measure of performance and a stimulus dimension. In the case of speech audiometry, a typical psychometric function displays the percentage correct identification of the speech stimulus as a function of stimulus intensity. Today, this is often called a *performance-intensity* (P-I) *function*. Figure 12.1 illustrates the psychometric functions for recognition of 36 spondees (curve a); 50 monosyllables (curves b, c, d, f); and synthetic sentences (curve e). The average slope of the function for Central Institute for the Deaf (CID) W-1 spondees is 10% per curve dB over the range of 20–80%. The average slope for CID W-22 monosyllables is 4% per dB, not as steep as the slope for spondees. In general, a steeper psychometric function results when the task is simpler, the stimuli are more familiar, or more homogeneous and the subject is more experienced. Although the average psychometric function should best predict the slope of an individual subject's psychometric function and, therefore, predict a subject's performance at a given level, it is important to remember that each individual's psychometric function is unique and can be quite different from the average function.

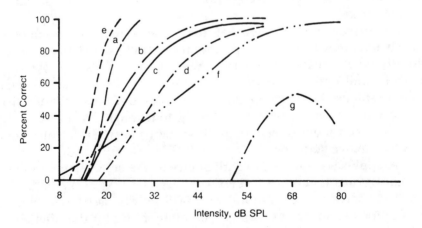

Figure 12.1 Performance-intensity functions for a variety of speech stimuli. Modified from Wilson and Margolis (1983) and Olsen and Matkin (1979). (a) CID W-1, 36 spondees; (b) CID W-22; (c) NU-6; (d) PAL PB-50; (e) SSI (closed set); (f) CCT (closed set); (g) CID W-22, sensorineural listeners.

The P-I function is currently used to describe what was previously called an *articulation-gain function*. It is simply a psychometric function that describes the percentage correct word recognition or identification as a function of intensity. *Articulation*, as it is used today, refers to speech production. The only exception is the use of 'articulation' in the *articulation index* (AI), where 'articulation' refers to the relative prediction of intelligibility under a wide range of listening situations (French and Steinberg, 1947; Kryter 1962a,b). Current adaptations of the AI will be discussed later under speech audiometry applications for rehabilitation.

Threshold is the statistical point on a psychometric function that specifies the intensity level (in dB) at which a patient correctly identified the stimulus a predetermined percentage of the time. This percentage (probability of responses) is between chance performance and perfect performance. For example, one might select 50%, or 70% correct stimulus identification to define the threshold.

Threshold performance clearly differs with the type of response required by a particular test. A threshold based on *detection* requires a judgement of stimulus presence or absence. This is called a *detection threshold*. The subject's familiarity with the stimulus often lowers (i.e. improves) the threshold. A threshold based on recognition requires a judgement made not only on stimulus presence or absence, but also on the correct stimulus identification from a set (open or closed) of possible stimuli. This is called a *recognition threshold*. Recognition is a more difficult task than detection. Therefore, recognition thresholds are higher (poorer), that is, they require more energy than detection thresholds. Recognition is not only a threshold measure. A recognition judgement may be made at supra-threshold levels, e.g. 'speech discrimination or word recognition testing', as well as at threshold levels, e.g. 'speech reception threshold' now called a 'speech recognition threshold' (SRT).

The American Speech-Language-Hearing Association (ASHA) 'Guidelines for Determining Threshold Level for Speech' (1988) define 'speech threshold audiometry' as the procedure used in the assessment of an individual's threshold for speech. The speech recognition threshold is the minimum hearing level for speech at which an individual can recognize 50% of the speech material. These current ASHA practice guidelines indicate that 'speech recognition threshold' is the preferred terminology, and that it is synonymous with the traditional term 'speech reception threshold'. The previously recommended practice (ASHA, 1979) was to use terminology that specified the speech material, e.g. 'spondee threshold' (ST) if the standard test materials — spondaic words (two-syllable equal-emphasis words) — were used. The ASHA 1988 guidelines indicate that the term spondee threshold is not preferred. Today, the term most often used to describe both the speech reception threshold or the spondee threshold is 'speech recognition threshold'. The speech material assumed is spondaic words; if other materials are used they should be stated. 'Speech recognition threshold', however, remains the most commonly used term, as it is shorter to say, and could mean either the more traditional term of speech reception threshold or the more current correct term of speech recognition threshold.

The term speech reception threshold originally referred to the intelligibility of sentences (Hughson and Thompson, 1942), and has evolved to refer to the threshold for a non-specified speech stimulus. More important, the problem with using the term speech reception threshold is that it does not accurately describe the performance required of the patient. The speech recognition threshold task requires that the speech stimulus (spondee) must be heard, recognized and repeated, although not necessarily understood. The more appropriate general term recommended for a speech threshold is speech recognition threshold (Feldmann, 1960; Bilger and Wang, 1976; Olsen and Matkin, 1979; Wilson and Margolis, 1983). Throughout this chapter SRT is used as the abbreviation for speech *recognition* threshold, and not for speech *reception* threshold.

A *speech detection threshold* (SDT) describes the minimum level at which an individual can just discern the presence of a speech material 50% of the time (ASHA, 1988). The speech signal need not be identified. Although the term speech awareness threshold (SAT) is used interchangeably with SDT, SDT is still recommended, since awareness suggests the psychological preparedness of the listener while SDT is task specific.

Intelligibility is a term used to describe how well speech is understood. It originally referred to how well speech was transmitted over a communication system and thus was understood by an observer. It has come to mean how well everyday-speech or other speech-like material are understood by a listener whose hearing may or may not be impaired. Intelligibility is most often described by an individual's performance on a word recognition task, i.e. the percentage of words correctly recognized at a particular intensity level. Therefore, today the terms intelligibility and recognition are used interchangeably. Recognition does not necessarily imply understanding. To make matters worse, *discrimination* has incorrectly been used as a synonym for both intelligibility and recognition, to describe supra-threshold word recognition ability. Although many audiologists in the United States continue to refer to this recognition task as 'word discrimination' or 'speech discrimination' testing, there is increased usage of 'speech recognition' testing. For the purpose of clarity in this chapter, a supra-threshold intelligibility test is considered a recognition task and is described by the type of speech material used, e.g. word recognition, nonsense recognition, or sentence recognition test. The performance score on the word recognition test is abbreviated WRS for *word recognition scores*.

Discrimination is a judgement based on the comparison of two or more stimuli. The judgement can be made at threshold or at supra-threshold levels. Classical psychophysics distinguished between absolute or detection thresholds and discrimination or difference thresholds. Modern psychophysics does not make this distinction, since for both there is a background noise against which the stimulus must be differentiated.

Current clinical practices

Most audiologists in the USA currently obtain both an SRT and a WRS for every patient undergoing a basic audiologic evaluation. Each is discussed separately under the headings of Speech Recognition Threshold and Supra-threshold Speech Recognition Tests. The information on current practice in speech audiometry presented herein reflects the findings of a recent survey of audiometric practices (Martin, Armstrong and Champlin, 1994), of four older surveys (Martin and Pennington, 1971; Martin and Forbis, 1978; Martin and Sides, 1985; Martin and Morris, 1989) and of recent relevant literature.

Speech recognition threshold (SRT)

Purpose of speech recognition thresholds

The primary reason that an SRT or spondee threshold (ST) is considered a valuable part of a diagnostic audiologic evaluation is that it lends validity to pure-tone thresholds (ASHA, 1988). There is generally good correspondence between speech and pure-tone thresholds both for normals (Fletcher, 1929) and those with hearing loss (Fletcher, 1929; Hughson and Thompson, 1942; Fletcher, 1950; Carhart and Porter, 1971; Wilson et al., 1973). The other very common reason for determining a speech threshold is its use as a reference level for supra-threshold recognition tests. Additional reasons include its reliability with the difficult-to-test patient, and the apparent face validity of using speech stimuli to assess sensitivity since communication depends upon listening to speech rather than pure tones.

Test materials

The commercially available speech threshold materials are listed in Table 12.1. The most commonly used test material is the CID auditory test W-1 (Hirsh et al., 1952). The CID auditory test W-2 is no longer commonly used. Other materials such as speech babble, running speech, or familiar words can be adopted when clinical situations require modification of the standardized spondaic lists (ASHA, 1988).

Table 12.1 Speech test materials used to obtain a Speech Recognition Threshold (SRT)

	Surveys on Audiometric Practice								
	Martin and Pennington (1971)		Martin and Forbis (1978)		Martin and Sides (1985)		Martin and Morris (1989)		Martin, Armstrong and Champlin (1994)	
Speech Material	Number	%	Number	%	Number	%	Number	%	Number	%
CID Auditory Test W-1	161	57.9	179	61.3	118	55.9	260	59.6	244	97
CID Auditory Test W-2	40	14.4	63	21.6	47	22.2	111	25.5		
PAL Auditory Test No. 9	11	4.0	15	5.1	5	2.4	—	—	—	—
PAL Auditory Test No. 14	1	0.4	0	0	2	0.9	—	—	—	—
Children's spondees	22	7.9	—	—	—	—	—	—	—	—
Connected discourse	2	0.7	1	0.3	0	0.0	—	—	—	—
Other	15	5.4	26	9.0	40	18.9	65	14.9	—	—
More than one response	26	9.5	8	2.7	—	—	—	—	—	—
(Number of respondents)	(278)		(302)		(212)		(436)		(252)	

CID Auditory Test W-1 Revised (ASHA, 1988)[1].
CID Auditory Test W-2 Revised Half Lists (ASHA 1988)[1].
Streamlined Spondaic Word List for Adults[2].
Children's Picture Spondaic Word List[3].

1 Revised to emphasize the criteria of dissimilarity and homogeneity of audibility (ASHA, 1979)
2 Printed in ASHA 1988 and suggested by Young et al., 1982.
3 Frank, 1980.

Auditory Tests No. 9 and No. 14 (the original spondaic word lists developed at the Harvard Psycho-Acoustic Laboratory (PAL) by Hudgins et al., 1947) are hardly used clinically any more. Each of these two lists consists of six randomizations of 42 words; there are 84 different spondees. In the former recording (PAL No.9), each six word set is attenuated 4 dB below the previous set for a total attenuation range of 24 dB. The latter recording (PAL No. 14), has a constant presentation level relative to the carrier phrase.

The more widely used CID W-1 list and rarely used W-2 lists (Hirsh, et al., 1952) consist of the 36 more familiar spondaic words: the W-1 recording attenuates the spondee 10 dB relative to the carrier phrase 'say the word....'; and the W-2 recording is progressively attenuated 3 dB for each block of three words. In the most recent survey of audiometric practices, Martin, Armstrong and Champlin (1994) stated that 98% of the respondents reported that they administer SRT tests, and that 97% of these respondents use the CID spondaic words, as recommended by ASHA (1988). The typical clinical presentation mode is monitored live voice (MLV), rather than the described recorded modes. The surveys reflect an increasing consensus on use of spondaic words as test stimuli (Martin and Pennington, 1971; Martin and Forbis, 1977; Martin and Sides, 1985; Kruger and Mazor, 1987; Martin and Morris, 1989; Martin et al., 1994).

The primary impetus to revise the PAL recordings was to achieve better homogeneity of audibility. The CID recordings were adjusted to be homogeneous within ±2 dB, for mean recognition thresholds of 20 dB SPL for experienced listeners and 21 dB SPL for inexperienced listeners. The variability in the physical characteristics of speech and the variability introduced by use of a VU meter to monitor the presentation of recorded spondee tests, make it impossible to achieve perfect homogeneity. Clinicians need to be aware of the expected sources of increased variability (Wilson and Margolis, 1983).

Recorded vs. monitored live voice presentation

The clinician typically presents spondee test materials using MLV in preference to using recorded materials (Martin and Pennington, 1971; ASHA, 1979; Martin and Sides, 1985; Martin and Morris, 1989; Martin et al., 1994). The most recent survey of audiometric practices (Martin et al., 1994) reported that percentage of audiologists using MLV had not changed since 1985 (Martin and Sides, 1985): 90% of the respondents use MLV, 6% use commercial tape and 4% used compact disc (CD). There is an increased use of CD since 1989, when no use was made of this medium. The ASHA (1988) guidelines state that either recorded or MLV presentation is acceptable, but prefers using recorded speech for standardized and consistent presentation of test material.

The MLV mode is selected primarily because it offers greater flexibility. MLV permits modifications to suit the patient's capability and the available test time: it permits either faster or slower presentation, omission of the carrier phrase, and/or use of selected words. The use of MLV presentation of the test materials is often indicated by the clinical situation, e.g. testing very young children, difficult-to-test children or adults, or some elderly patients. It should be remembered, however, that a speech test is not a list, but an utterance that varies with the speaker or recording (Kruel et al., 1969). Therefore, when MLV presentation is used and standardized stimulus materials must be sacrificed, the clinician should keep in mind that other sources of variability are introduced. The use of the VU meter to monitor the presentation level is then very important in order to achieve maximal homogeneity of audibility for each talker.

For either recorded or MLV presentation, the level, in dB SPL, at which the speech stimuli are equivalent to 0 dB HL is dependent upon the output transducer used. Typically spondees and other speech stimuli are presented through the standard audiometric earphone, TDH 39 or 49, mounted on an MX41/AR cushion American National Standards Institute (ANSI S3.6, 1989), or through an ER-3A insert earphone (Wilber, Kruger and Killian, 1988; ANSI S3.6, 1989). In this stimulus presentation mode (earphone), 20 dB SPL is the reference for speech stimuli. Current standards for audiometer calibration (ANSI S3.6, 1989) recommended calibration of speech by adjusting the rms SPL of a 1 kHz signal so that the VU meter deflection is equal to the average peak VU meter deflection produced by the speech.

Sound field conditions are indicated when difficult-to-test children, or adults, will not accept earphones, or when aided and unaided SRTs are compared, in quiet or in noise, as a part of the hearing aid selection and fitting process. Loudspeaker calibration must consider the orientation of the listener to the loudspeaker in the sound field. In this stimulus presentation mode (sound field), the sound field should be calibrated to 16.5 dB SPL for 0 degrees azimuth and 12.5 dB SPL for 45 degrees azimuth (Dirks et al., 1972). The complexity of specifying the sound pressure level of speech is emphasized by the fact that speech calibration techniques are still being researched. Although standards exist for earphone testing, sound field calibration standards are still in the development phase.

Increment and response criterion

According to Martin et al., (1994), most (87%) of recent survey respondents use a 5 dB increment size to obtain the ST, although the second most common step size was 2 dB (7.5%) (see Table 12.2). There has been an increase in the use of 5 dB step size from 40% in 1971 (Martin and Pennington), to 57% in 1978 (Martin and Forbis), to 78% in 1985

(Martin and Sides), to 84% in 1989, to 87% in 1994. The practice of using a 5 dB increment appears to have stabilized at about 85%. The literature supports this practice in that there is little difference in SRTs obtained with either step size (Chaiklin et al., 1964, 1967). The ASHA 1988 guidelines do not specify a recommended increment size.

Table 12.2 Increment size used to obtain a speech recognition threshold (SRT)

	Surveys on Audiometric Practice								
	Martin and Pennington (1971)		Martin and Forbis (1978)		Martin and Sides (1985)		Martin and Morris (1989)		Martin, Armstrong and Champlin (1994)
Step size (dB)	Number	%	Number	%	Number	%	Number	%	Number	%
2	144	49.8	100	33.1	38	17.5	60	13.5	19	7.5
4	15	5.2	13	4.3	5	2.3	3	0.7	0	0
5	117	40.5	172	57.0	170	78.3	374	84.0	219	86.9
Other	8	2.8	8	2.6	5	1.7	8	1.8	14	5.6
More than one response	5	1.7	9	3.0	—	—	—	—	—	—
(Number of respondents)	(289)		(302)		(217)		(445)		(252)	

As can be seen in Table 12.3, the largest number of audiologists responding (40%) use a response criterion of two out of three correct responses to determine the SRT. The second most common criterion, used by 32% of the respondents, is two out of four correct responses. This has remained stable for the 1989 and 1994 practice surveys. There is a trend towards using only two correct responses out of either three or four responses. These criteria account for 72% of the respondents in 1994 (Martin et al.), compared with the 66% in 1985 (Martin and Sides), and with the earliest two surveys where the response criteria were fairly equally distributed; 49.5% in 1978 (Martin and Forbis) and 52.1% in 1971 (Martin and Pennington). Still, many other criteria are in use, which highlights the fact that many different methods are still used to obtain an SRT. The response criteria most commonly used in clinical practice are not consistent with the ASHA (1988) guidelines, which specify a response criterion of five of the last six spondees presented, in a descending series, using a 50% criterion for SRT.

Table 12.3 Response criteria used to obtain a speech recognition threshold (SRT)

	Surveys on Audiometric Practice								
	Martin and Pennington (1971)		Martin and Forbis (1978)		Martin and Sides (1985)		Martin and Morris (1989)		Martin, Armstrong and Champlin (1994)	
Response Criteria	Number	%	Number	%	Number	%	Number	%	Number	%
2 out of 3	72	25.2	82	27.1	93	43.4	181	40.8	100	39.8
2 out of 4	77	26.9	68	22.4	50	23.4	142	32.0	81	30.3
3 out of 4	15	5.2	16	5.2	16	7.4	31	7.0	16	0.6
3 out of 5	26	9.1	21	7.0	12	5.6	37	8.3	18	0.7
3 out of 6	52	18.2	64	21.0	21	9.8	—	—	—	—
Lowest level with 3 correct responses	27	9.4	30	10.0	13	6.1	34	7.7	21	0.8
5 out of 6 (ASHA 1988)	—	—	—	—	—	—	—	—	5	0.2
Other	17	5.9	17	6.0	9	4.2	19	4.3	10	0.4
More than one response	—	—	4	1.3	—	—	—	—	—	—
(Number of respondents)	(289)		(302)		(217)		(444)		(251)	

Familiarization

Recognition of the importance of familiarity with the speech stimulus material dates back to Hudgins et al. (1947) and has been reinforced by Hirsh et al. (1952), by ASHA (1979, 1988) and by many other studies (for example, see Olsen and Matkin, 1979; Wilson and Margolis, 1983). In addition, most methods stress the importance of familiarizing the patient with the spondees face-to-face, or through the speech audiometer, but without visual cues. Despite the fact that familiarization can improve threshold, reduce variability, and control for the effects of prior knowledge, few clinicians take the time to familiarize the patient with the stimuli prior to obtaining an SRT. In the recent clinical practice survey (Martin et al., 1994), 53% of the respondents reportedly familiarized their patients compared to 51% according to Martin and Morris in 1989 and 55% according to Martin and Sides (1985). This most recent number is probably an over-estimate (ASHA, 1979). The percentage of audiologists who employ familiarization prior to SRT determination has remained essentially the same from 1971 to the present. The importance of familiarization is stressed in the ASHA 1988 guidelines.

Carrier phrase

When obtaining an SRT in clinical practice, the carrier phrase is often omitted. As previously reported, according to Martin and Sides (1985) more than half of the audiologists disregard the carrier phrase. This practice had remained the same since 1971 (Martin and Forbis, 1977; Martin and Pennington, 1971). According to the more recent surveys, the practice of omitting the carrier phrase has remained the same, at less than 40 – 50% (40%, Martin and Morris, 1989; 45%, Martin et al., 1994). Of those who use a carrier phrase, 44.4% use 'say the word'. Eighty-one per cent present the carrier phrase and the stimulus word at the same hearing presentation level, thereby helping the patient to define the listening level. The contribution of a carrier phrase is as redundant as spondees.

Test methods

A number of clinical methods have evolved to obtain SRTs. Currently, there is no commonly used clinical method, despite the standardized method recommended by the ASHA guidelines (1988). Concise summaries of the differences in the various procedures can be found in Olsen and Matkin (1979) and in Kruger and Mazor (1987). In spite of the lack of uniformity of procedure in practice, variants of Chaiklin and Ventry's (1964) protocol are commonly used.

As with pure-tone threshold assessment, a modified method of limits is used to determine the SRT. In contrast, however, the SRT is most commonly obtained using a descending method rather than an ascending method. Assessment begins at a level above the expected threshold, to familiarize the listener with the words and the task. The level is then decreased in 5 dB steps, presenting one to three words at each level until a word is missed. At this point the stimulus level is raised 10 dB and then lowered in 5 dB steps, presenting three to six spondees with each change in stimulus level. The level at which 50% of the spondees are correctly repeated is recorded as the SRT.

Evolution of the ASHA 1988 'recommended descending method'

In the earlier (1987) version of this chapter, three methods were discussed. There were two different descending procedures for obtaining an SRT (one using a 2 dB step size, and the other using a 5 dB step size), and an ascending method (ASHA, 1979) that had been proposed. Neither of the descending methods had come into common usage, but the 5 dB increment version of the descending method (Huff and Nerbonne, 1982; Wilson and Margolis, 1983; Wall, Davis and Myers, 1984) held promise.

The ASHA guidelines (1988) now specify the descending procedure recommended by Wilson et al. (1973) and Tillman and Olsen (1973). ASHA has adopted the two different descending procedures for obtaining an SRT. The procedure represents a methodological revival of the SRT technique of Hudgins et al. (1947). The procedure requires familiarization of the patient with the spondees presented at a most comfortable listening level and elimination of any familiar or incorrectly identified words. The preliminary phase is used to obtain the starting level for the test phase. The initial presentation level is 30 – 40 dB above the expected SRT (if the individual does not respond, the level is increased in 20 dB steps until a correct response is obtained (Martin and Staufer, 1975)). As the level is decreased in 10 dB steps, one or two words are presented at each level. When two words are missed, the presentation level is raised 10 dB. This begins the test phase. The test descent is begun again in 2 dB steps. For every 2 dB decrement two words are presented. Threshold criterion is reached when five of six words are missed. The SRT is the number of correct words minus the starting level plus a correction factor of half the attenuation rate (1 dB). The simplified ASHA 1988 descending method calls for 5 dB decrements, five words per decrement, termination when all five words at an intensity level are missed, and use of a 2 dB correction factor. This method was based on ease of administration using then current clinical audiometers and had been recommended by Wilson and Margolis (1983) and Wall et al. (1984).

In a comparison (Wall et al., 1984) of two descending methods (Chaiklin and Ventry, 1967) and two ascending methods (Chaiklin and Ventry, 1967; ASHA, 1979) it was found that: there were no significant differences among the SRTs using the four methods; the descending methods were the most sensitive (lowest thresholds) and were equivalent in time consumption and test–retest reliability; but the ascending methods agreed best with a three frequency pure-tone average (PTA). The ASHA (1979) method was the most time consuming. The ascending method, which had been recommended previously by ASHA (1979), (see review in Kruger and Mazor, 1987), has been abandoned in favour of the descending methods, because the ASHA 1979 ascending method was more awkward and time consuming than either descending method, especially the simplified descending method (Wall et al., 1984). Time will determine whether the ASHA 1988 recommended descending methods will be accepted for clinical use.

Relationships between pure-tone thresholds and speech thresholds

A clinical value often ascribed to the SRT is its correspondence to pure-tone thresholds. The SRT can be predicted with some precision from an average of selected pure-tone thresholds. For flat and gradually sloping losses, a three-frequency PTA of the thresholds obtained at 500 Hz, 1kHz and 2kHz optimally predicts the SRT (Fletcher, 1929; Carhart, 1946a,b). Although the three-frequency PTA is the most popular prediction method, it can overestimate the SRT, especially for patients with sloping high frequency losses. For steeply sloping losses, the average of the two best pure-tone thresholds is a better predictor of the SRT (Fletcher, 1950). Also, Carhart and Porter (1971) have recommended averaging the thresholds at 500 Hz and 1 kHz minus 2 dB, since that average adequately predicts the SRT from most audiometric configurations (see also Carhart, 1946a).

In clinical practice, the audiologist considers an agreement between the SRT and PTA of ±6 dB (to as much as ±10 dB) to be within acceptable limits (Olsen and Matkin, 1979). If the SRT is significantly lower (better) than the PTA, results are most often considered pathognomonic of pseudohypoacusis. It suggests that the pure-tone results are suspect and that additional testing is indicated. However, a discrepancy of 10 dB or greater can also be obtained from very young children or difficult-to-test adults (e.g. psychiatric or mentally retarded patients). This discrepancy is thought to result from the patient responding to the loudness of speech and does not reflect a threshold for speech (Ventry, 1976). Although less common, a disparity of 10 dB or greater where the PTA is lower (better) than the SRT, can be obtained from patients with severe communication or word finding difficulties (e.g. retrocochlear lesions).

The relationship between the speech threshold and the PTA is dependent not only on the speech materials, the presentation method and the configurations of the loss, but also on the type of speech threshold obtained. An SDT requires less energy than an SRT, thus the SDT is typically at levels 8 – 9 dB lower (better) than the SRT or the PTA (Chaiklin, 1959; Beattie, Edgerton and Svihovec, 1975; Beattie, Svihovec and Edgerton 1975). Often, better agreement is found between the SDT and the 250 Hz pure-tone threshold. Either the SRT or the SDT may be used to indicate agreement with pure-tone thresholds.

Masking

Often during speech audiometry, acoustic signals presented to the test ear are sufficiently intense that they can be perceived in the non-test ear.

In practice, most audiologists mask when cross-hearing is suspected, but they do not apply a uniformly accepted masking criterion for determination of the SRT. Rather, there are two masking criteria which are used quite widely during SRT testing (Martin and Sides, 1985; Martin et al., 1994). Table 12.4 illustrates the various changes in masking in clinical practice. Most audiologists (54.7%, Martin et al., 1994) use a specific difference criterion between the SRTs of each ear to indicate the need for masking for SRT testing. The preferred criterion difference is 40 dB, but it ranges from 15 to 60 dB. The use of this method has increased from 41% (Martin and Sides, 1985).

The masking criterion of a 40 dB or greater difference between the SRT of the test ear and the best bone-conduction threshold of the non-test ear is used by more than a third of the respondents (35.5%, Martin, Armstrong and Champlin, 1994). The preferred criterion difference is 40 dB, but it ranges from 0 to 60 dB. Acceptance of the former technique (SRT of the test ear re: the non-test ear's best bone-conduction threshold) seems to have decreased somewhat (48%) since the last reported surveys by Martin and Sides (1985) and Martin and Morris (1989), although it had increased in use since the earliest surveys (Martin and Pennington, 1971; Martin and Forbis, 1978).

This division in approaches to masking criteria for SRT testing is consistent with the recommendations of the ASHA guidelines (1979, 1988) which specify two criteria: masking of the contralateral non-test ear is indicated when either the SRT of the test ear exceeds the SRT of the non-test ear by 40 dB or more, or the SRT of the test ear exceeds the pure-tone bone-conduction thresholds of the non-test ear at 500 Hz, 1 kHz, or 2 kHz by 40 dB or more. Fewer than 9% never mask, or always mask when obtaining an SRT.

The masking practices are somewhat conservative but in agreement with the critical interaural differences for air-conducted stimuli presented to the poorer ear, with a standard supra-aural earphone and the better ear's bone conduction thresholds (Zwislocki, 1953; Liden, 1954). The masking practices are quite conservative for air conducted stimuli presented to the poorer ear with an insert earphone, and the better ear's bone-conduction thresholds (Zwislocki, 1953; Liden, 1954; Killion, Wilbur, and Gudmundsen, 1985; Wilber et al., 1988). The amount of masking introduced into the non-test ear (Table 12.5) is determined by several methods including many variants of the plateau method that are used by most of the respondents (56.9%, Martin et al., 1994). Some used an arbitrary starting level (8.8%), with a safety factor of 10 – 60 dB before beginning to plateau. The most recent survey reports that some 37.1% indicated using an 'other' amount of masking, an increase from 21% (Martin and Sides, 1985).

Table 12.4 Masking criteria used to obtain a speech recognition threshold (SRT)

Masking Criteria	Surveys on Audiometric Practice									
	Martin and Pennington (1971)		Martin and Forbis (1978)		Martin and Sides (1985)		Martin and Morris (1989)		Martin, Armstrong and Champlin (1994)	
	Number	%	Number	%	Number	%	Number	%	Number	%
Mask all SRTs	—	1	1	0.3	4	1.8	—	3	—	1.2
Patient hears speech in non-test ear or in middle of the head	11	43.7	5	1.6	50	22.0	4	0.9	1	0.4
40 dB or greater difference between SRTs of each ear	115	43.7	97	31.1	92	40.5	207	45.4	134	54.7
40 dB or greater difference between SRT of the test ear and the best bone conduction threshold of the non-test ear	93	35.4	169	54.2	109	48.0	221	48.5	87	35.5
Never	·	–	17	5.4	6	2.6	20	4.4	20	8.2
Other	18	6.8	7	2.2	12	5.3	—	—	—	—
More than one response	26	9.9	16	5.2	—	—	—	—	—	—
(Number of respondents)	(263)		(312)		(227)		(456)		(245)	

Table 12.5 Amount of masking used to obtain a speech recognition threshold (SRT)

Amount of Masking	Surveys on Audiometric Practice									
	Martin and Pennington (1971)		Martin and Forbis (1978)		Martin and Sides (1985)		Martin and Morris (1989)		Martin, Armstrong and Champlin (1994)	
	Number	%	Number	%	Number	%	Number	%	Number	%
SRT of opposite ear then plateau.	—	—	125	41.9	109	50.0	47	12.6	29	12.1
AC threshold ± dB then plateau.	—	—	—	—	—	—	40	10.7	44	18.3
AC threshold ± dB	—	—	—	—	—	—	91	24.3	36	15.0
Arbitrary level	—	—	—	—	—	—	22	5.9	21	8.8
Arbitrary beginning then plateau	—	—	96	32.3	63	28.9	—	—	—	—
Equal to or - dB below presentation level	—	—	—	—	—	—	28	7.5	—	—
AC threshold ± dB + OE then plateau	—	—	—	—	—	—	—	—	21	8.8
Other	—	—	77	25.8	46	21.1	146	39.0	89	37.1
(Number of respondents)	—		(298)		(218)		(374)		(240)	

Bone conduction

In the typical practice of audiology, an SRT or SDT is most often determined with air-conducted signals. However, at times it may be clinically advisable to determine bone-conducted speech thresholds. Bone-conducted speech is used to assist in confirming the presence of an air–bone gap, as well as the estimation of the air–bone gap. This provides useful information for the medical management of the difficult-to-test patient. Bone-conducted speech threshold correlates with either 500 – 1000 Hz, for an SRT, or 250 Hz for an SDT.

Re-evaluation of the use of the SRT

Most audiologists customarily obtain an SRT for every patient. In fact, it is often clinical protocol to obtain an SRT prior to assessing pure-tone air-conduction thresholds because the task of repeating spondees is easy for most patients. The SRT is an admittedly helpful clinical check on the correctness of pure-tone thresholds. The SRT appears to assess communication ability of the patient. According to the procedures commonly used to obtain an SRT (discussed above), many short-cuts and compromises are introduced in a busy clinic practice with only minimal changes in the obtained level of the SRT. Thus, some re-evaluation of the rationale for the wide use of the SRT may be indicated. Wilson and Margolis (1983) have suggested that the routine use of the SRT for patients who have been tested before and who have reliable pure-tone thresholds is redundant and not cost effective. They have suggested that perhaps the SRT only be determined when there is a question of unreliable pure-tone thresholds (pseudohypoacusis) and for difficult-to-test patients.

Clinical resistance to the selective use of the SRT rests with one of the primary reasons an audiologist gives for obtaining an SRT. That is, to determine a reference level for supra-threshold speech recognition tests. The supra-threshold speech test is typically presented at some specified number of decibels in sensation level, relative to the SRT. This sensation level is based on the mean psychometric function or P-I function for the test material thought to indicate the level at which the maximum recognition is attained. The inference that the mean level for maximum recognition is appropriate for the individual patient under test is questionable (see Supra-threshold Recognition Testing below). More important, sensation level implies that the same stimulus is used for both the threshold and the supra-threshold test. This is not so in practice. Less variability is introduced when the presentation level for the supra-threshold test is referenced to a pure-tone detection threshold since the reference psychometric function is steeper. Wilson and Margolis (1983) suggest that an appropriate PTA provides an adequate and efficient means of determining the reference level for supra-threshold speech recognition tests.

Further, comparison of two SRTs obtained under two different test situations (pre-post-treatment) confounds the clinical conclusion. Each SRT represents a point on a psychometric function for the individual. The two points (levels) may differ if two different recordings were used and especially if MLV presentation of two different lists was administered by two different talkers. These differences may be exaggerated by any intervening treatment (medication or amplification) thus changing the slope of the psychometric function.

Most clinicians recognize that the validity of the SRT is questionable. Clinically, the use of speech stimuli to obtain an estimate of auditory sensitivity was considered an appealing and valid approach to the understanding of communication disability. However, the SRT has only an apparent face validity since neither the spondee nor the recognition task are directly related to the communication process. In addition, the specification of speech stimuli is difficult, and its resultant threshold is not frequency specific. Pure-tone thresholds, however, provide a valid estimate of auditory sensitivity.

Difficult-to-test

The SRT continues to be used clinically for testing children, psychiatric patients, and some limited-function geriatric patients. However, it is sometimes difficult to obtain an SRT from patients with limited or unintelligible speech (e.g. young children), those with mental retardation, profoundly hearing-impaired individuals, or deaf patients. Simple modification of test procedure may be sufficient. Typically, the audiologist changes the response mode by having the patient point to pictures or toys that illustrate the spoken spondee words rather than repeating the spondee heard. Flexibility of administration may include use of a modified carrier phrase (e.g. 'show me'), MLV presentation, selected spondees, children's spondees (Newby, 1958; Frank, 1980; ASHA, 1988), or monosyllables (TIP) (Siegenthaler and Haspiel, 1966). When it is impossible to determine an SRT by any means, most difficult-to-test patients will perform an SDT test with spondees, or simple, more familiar words, such as 'go' or 'mama'. Modification of behavioural techniques used to obtain the SDT include visual reinforcement audiometry (VRA), conditioned orienting response audiometry (COR), and tangible reinforcement operant conditioning audiometry (TROCA) under earphones or in the sound field.

Supra-threshold speech recognition testing

Test materials and their purposes

Some of the available speech recognition tests are listed in Table 12.6. The word recognition tests used most often in the USA (Martin and

Table 12.6 Speech test materials used to obtain word recognition scores (WRS)

Speech Material	Surveys on Audiometric Practice									
	Martin and Pennington 1971		Martin and Forbis 1978		Martin and Sides 1985		Martin and Morris 1989		Martin, Armstrong & Champlin 1994	
	Number	%	Number	%	Number	%	Number	%	Number	%
CID Auditory Test W-22	202	71.6	217	70.7	113	61.0	246	54.2	132	53.2
CNC Word Lists	9	3.2	37	12.0	10	46.0	—	—	—	—
PAL PB-50 Word Lists	25	8.9	22	7.2	4	1.5	—	—	—	—
Modification of Fairbanks Rhyme Test	2	0.7	—	—	—	—	—	—	—	—
Synthetic Sentences	—	—	—	—	—	—	10.2	—	20.8	—
Northwestern Univ. No. 6	—	—	—	—	51	23.4	170	37.5	103	41.5
CHABA or CID sentences	—	—	—	—	—	—	10.2	·	20.8	—
Other	28	9.9	17	5.5	20	9.2	36	7.9	11	4.4
More than one response	16	5.7	14	4.6	—	—	—	—	—	—
(Number of respondents)	(282)		(307)		(218)		(454)		(248)	

Pennington, 1971; Martin and Forbis, 1978; Martin and Sides, 1985; Martin and Morris, 1989; Martin et al., 1994)) are the CID Auditory Test W-22 (Hirsh et al., 1952) and the Northwestern University No. 6 (Tillman and Carhart, 1966). Today, in clinical practice, there is very little use of the CNC word lists (Peterson and Lehiste, 1962) and the PAL PB-50 word lists (Egan, 1948).

Each of these word lists consists of 50 open-set monosyllables. For each word correctly understood the patient receives a score of 2%. Normal hearing patients and patients with conductive hearing loss generally score 90 – 100%, whereas patients with sensorineural or mixed hearing loss generally score less than 90%. Patients with central auditory problems usually have no difficulty with the word recognition test and score normally in the routine battery.

Thus, the word recognition test can be used for differential diagnosis by helping to determine the site of lesion of peripheral and central auditory pathologies. In addition, this measure is useful to the physician in determining surgical candidacy. The WRS is also used by audiologists in hearing aid assessment and in planning aural rehabilitation programmes. Aural rehabilitation applications will be discussed later in this chapter.

Since the overwhelming majority of audiologists use open set monosyllabic word lists (see Table 12.6), our summary of available clinical speech recognition tests begins with those types of stimulus materials. Some other types of speech materials used primarily in aural rehabilitation applications and in research are also presented below: nonsense syllables, open set as well as closed set monosyllables and sentences.

Open set monosyllables

PAL PB-50 monosyllables

The PB-50 monosyllables were the first speech materials used in the evaluation of the hearing impaired. These speech tests were originally designed to assess the efficiency of communication systems. It was for this purpose that, during the Second World War, Egan developed the PB-50 monosyllables (1948). They were designed in order to meet the following criteria: all of the sounds of English speech should be represented with a relative frequency of occurrence which reflects their common usage, test items should have an equal average difficulty and equal range of difficulty. Twenty 50-word lists of familiar monosyllables were constructed. Unfortunately, these lists did not satisfy the criteria as well as expected. The phonetic balance was not exact, and words used were not all equally familiar. Eight of the original 20 lists were recorded at the CID by Rush Hughes and are currently referred to as the Rush Hughes PB-SOs. Contrary to the original design criteria, these recordings are noted for their low reliability and for their difficulty; an important variable was the speech production of the speaker. The resultant recordings are so poor that even a normal listener cannot achieve a perfect score. Although these lists are not commonly used for basic audiologic evaluation, audiologists do use these recordings when difficult material is needed, e.g. central auditory testing.

CID W-22 monosyllables

In an effort to overcome the poor reliability and difficulty of the PB-50 word lists and to improve phonetic balance Hirsh et al. (1952) developed the CID W-22 lists. Word difficulty was reduced and phonetic balance was improved. Reliability was improved through the use of magnetic tape recording, and more recently, has been further improved by CD recording. The CID W-22 word lists are still the most popular lists used by clinicians in the USA today (53%), but use of the NU-6 word lists (see below) have increased to 42% (Martin et al., 1994). The CID W-22 word recognition tests consist of four 50-word lists with six randomizations of each list. These are available commercially on both records and tape from Auditec of St Louis (330 Selma Avenue, St Louis, MO 63119, USA, tel (314) 781-8890, fax (314) 781-4946.

Consonant-nucleus-consonant (CNC) monosyllables

The CNC lists employ phonemic, rather than phonetic balance (Lehiste and Peterson, 1959). In order to achieve this phonemic balance Lehiste and Peterson used CNC monosyllables in which each initial consonant, each vowel and each final consonant appears with the same frequency of occurrence within each list. Lehiste and Peterson argue that phonetics is concerned with the physiological and acoustical properties of speech, i.e. speech production, whereas phonemics is 'perceptual phonetics'. As the speech signal is not acoustically invariant, it would be impossible to achieve phonetic balance, therefore, intelligibility measures should use materials which are instead phonemically balanced. The original 10 lists were revised (Peterson and Lehiste, 1962) in order to reduce the frequency of usage problem which occurred in the earlier lists. There are ten 50-word lists with five randomizations of each list in the commercially available CNC test.

Northwestern University auditory tests No.4 and No.6 (NU-4, NU-6)

The NU-4 test (Tillman, Carhart and Wilber 1963) was developed from the CNC lists (Peterson and Lehiste, 1962). The two NU-4 lists have high test–retest reliability and conform better to Lehiste and Peterson's plan for phonemic balance. The NU-6 lists (Tillman and Carhart, 1966) are an expansion of the NU-4 CNC lists; there are four lists available, instead of two, with four scramblings of each list. The NU-6 word lists had achieved some popularity among clinicians by 1985 (23%, Martin and Sides 1985) and have continued to increase in popularity (42%, Martin et al., 1994), as can be seen in Table 12.6.

Isophonemic CNC word lists

Boothroyd (1968) published additional CNC lists which he described as isophonemic word lists. There are only 10 words per list, and each of 15 lists is phonemically balanced. Each of the three phonemes in a word is scored as correct or incorrect allowing for a phoneme-error score rather than a word-error score. In addition to allowing for phoneme error analysis, these short word lists have the advantage of being faster to administer. Nonetheless, they have not achieved clinical popularity in word recognition testing in the USA.

Nonsense syllables

The primary advantage of using nonsense syllables for the speech recognition test is that they permit detailed analysis of the types of phonemic errors made by the listener. In addition, nonsense syllables ensure that both word familiarity and memory effects are reduced. On the other hand, because of their inherent non-meaningfulness and resultant lack of intelligibility (Lehiste and Peterson, 1959) which increase the difficulty of the task for the listener, these stimuli are not usually used as part of the routine evaluation. A more appropriate use for these words is in hearing aid assessment and aural rehabilitation, at which time phoneme error analysis may be important.

Nonsense syllable test (NST)

The NST was developed for hearing aid assessment and aural rehabilitation (Resnick et al., 1975; Levitt et al., 1978). This test is a closed set response test made up of consonant-vowel (CV) and vowel consonant (VC) syllables. There are seven test modules with nine syllables in each module. There are three vowel contexts representing the extremes of the vowel triangle: /i/, /a/ and /u/. Consonants in each module are either voiced or unvoiced so that errors in voicing cannot be made. Levitt and his co-workers made no attempt at phonetic balance but were more concerned with the most frequent perceptual confusions made by both normal hearing listeners (Miller and Nicely, 1955; Wang and Bilger, 1973), and hearing impaired listeners (Owens, Benedict and Schubert, 1972). The estimated reliability of the NST is 0.93 for 91 items (Dubno and Dirks, 1982). They suggest that the high reliability of these word lists make the NST a good choice when comparison scores are needed such as in hearing aid assessment and aural rehabilitation treatment programmes (Dubno, Dirks and Langhofer, 1982).

Closed set monosyllables

Traditional open set testing paradigms have at least two disadvantages; they do not control for the subject's previous linguistic experience and the extent to which that experience may affect the responses and subject response error scoring is difficult. Most closed set tests are not commonly used in clinical practice.

Rhyme tests

The rhyme test was developed by Fairbanks (1958) in order to reduce linguistic confounds and to provide a test of 'phonemic differentiation'. This test is of the fill-in type in which the subject responds by filling in only the initial consonant from a set of five rhyming monosyllabic words. The rhyme test was later modified to include words in the forms CVC, VC, and CV, and called the modified rhyme test (MRT) (House et al., 1963). A multiple choice type test, the subject chooses from six possible alternatives. The MRT has the advantage of assessing both initial and final consonants. Kreul et al. (1968) adapted the MRT to make it more clinically useful. Changes were made in recording technique, speaker control, carrier phrase, noise levels for masking the speech, instructions, test forms and signal-to-noise ratio (SNR) levels for each of three individual speakers. However, this test is not often used clinically.

The diagnostic rhyme test (DRT) is a two-choice, 'minimal contrasts' test based on a phonemic taxonomy derived from the distinctive features systems of Miller and Nicely (1955) and of Jakobson, Fant and Halle (1952) which was developed for the overall evaluation of speech intelligibility over communication systems and devices (Voiers, 1977), but is now beginning to find application for the hearing impaired and deaf (Milner and Flevaris-Phillips, 1985). In this test, each item involves two rhyming words, the initial consonants of which differ by a single distinctive feature of six possible features. It is the listener's task to judge which of the two words has been spoken, implicitly indicating whether or not they have apprehended the speaker's implicit intent with respect to the critical feature. It is designed for phonemic analysis of the initial consonant. A further discussion of the use of speech tests in the overall evaluation of communication systems and devices is found below.

Multiple choice discrimination test (MCDT)

The MCDT uses the CID W-22 words in a closed message response set (Schultz and Schubert, 1969). Unlike the MRT confusions in the MCDT can be made between either initial or final consonants within the same response set.

California consonant test (CCT)

Owens and Schubert (1968) published the CCT using a format similar to the MCDT. There are 100 test words with three foils in each response set, and like the MCDT, both initial and final positions are assessed. Although this test is time consuming, by 1987 it had gained some popularity for use in hearing aid evaluation and aural rehabilitation. However, as with most closed set tests that are time consuming, it has not found its way into clinical practice.

Sentence materials

Sentence tests are not typically used clinically to assess word recognition. It can be argued, however, that clinicians should use larger linguistic units such as sentences, rather than single words, to assess intelligibility. The sentence is a much better representation of a sample of spoken communication and allows for linguistic features such as intonation patterns and co-articulatory effects not possible to achieve with a single word utterance. Although sentences are still not frequently used by American audiologists for word recognition testing, they do deserve mention. They will probably gain in popularity in the future, because they are useful in certain clinical situations, especially aural rehabilitation. There are a few more recent tests, mentioned below, that may gain clinical acceptance.

CID everyday sentences

The sentences most frequently used to assess speech intelligibility are commonly referred to in the USA as the 'CID everyday sentences' or the 'CHABA sentences' (Silverman and Hirsh, 1955). There are 10 sentences with a total of 50 key words. The subject must respond by repeating the entire sentence, but is scored only for each correct key word. They are particularly useful for evaluation of the patient with severe recognition problems, such as the limited geriatric patient.

Synthetic sentence identification test (SSI)

This is a closed set sentence test which consists of third-order approximations of syntactically correct English sentences (Speaks and Jerger, 1965). The listener's task is to identify the test sentence from a group of 10 sentences on a response sheet. A message-to-competition ratio (MCR) of 0 (the competing message is a discourse on the life of Davey Crockett) results in P-I functions which are equivalent to P-I functions for PB words (Jerger, Speaks and Trammell, 1968). The SSI is currently used as part of the central auditory test battery and is sometimes used in hearing aid system assessment. For these applications the MCR is varied, e.g. from –30 dB to +10 dB for ipsilateral presentation, from –40 dB to 0 dB for contralateral presentation.

The speech perception in noise (SPIN) test

The SPIN test utilizes the predictability of words in context as a factor in word recognition testing (Kalikow et al., 1977). There are eight sets of 50 sentences presented in a background of speech babble. Half the sentences contain high predictability test items and half contain low predictability test items. The subject's task is to identify the last word in each sentence. An overall score is derived from the difference between the scores on high and low predictability items This test is beginning to gain clinical acceptance, especially for aural rehabilitation.

Connected speech test (CST)

The CST is an 'everyday conversational-speech' recognition test; available in two versions (Cox et al., 1988, 1987). The first version of the CST, (CSTvl), consists of 57 passages of connected speech (nine for practice and 48 for test), containing 10 simple seven to 10 word sentences, with a six-talker babble as a competing signal (Cox et al., 1987). Each passage is about a familiar topic, presented one sentence at a time, and the repetition is scored on 25 key words (five words/level of difficulty). The percentage correct scores are transformed into rationalized arcsine units (rau) (Studebaker, 1982); the SBR function (passage score as a function of level) is 12 rau/dB for normal hearing listeners. CSTv1 was developed to be equally intelligible for the average normal hearing listener. The second version of the CST (CSTv2) consists of 28 passages of connected speech (four pairs for practice and 24 pairs for test), recorded on two optical laser disks: 12 pairs/disk (Cox et al., 1988). It was developed to be equally intelligible to both the hearing impaired and the average normal hearing listener. The mean proportion of key word consonants in various phonetic categories (nasals, voiceless plosives, voiced plosives, voiceless fricatives, voiced fricatives and other — l, r, j, w, h) was controlled to be similar to proportions in conversation, but to provide equivalence across passages.

Using specific passage-pairs reduces variability. Performance on the CST is based on two passage pairs: the 95% critical difference for SDT scores is 15.5 rau; the SBR function is less (8.5 rau/dB) for hearing impaired listeners than for normal hearing listeners. The test passages were presented at normal conversational speech levels (55 dB Leq, or integrated A-weighting, beside the listener's head which is equivalent to 61 dB Leq at the eardrum) plus SRT/2, to represent the hearing aid gain. The CSTv2, using CST scores based on two passage pairs, permits detection of changes in intelligibility equal to a 2 dB change in SBR. The CSTv2 was developed to have equivalent intelligibility for all hearing losses, except rising and severe sharply sloping configurations. The everyday language is probably too difficult for those individuals with congenitally profound hearing loss or deafness. Since the CSTv2 has high content validity, a large number of equivalent forms and a small error of measurement, it is appropriate to measure hearing aid benefit.

Speech in noise (SIN) test

The SIN test is a new sentence test (Fikret-Pasa, 1993; Killion and Villchur, 1993). The test material is a DAT recording of the IEEE sentences (72 lists of 10 sentences each) spoken by a woman. The noise is DAT recordings of a four-talker babble (three women and one man). The SIN test consists of 40 sentences arranged as two sub-blocks (A and B) of 20 sentences; each sub-block is a series of five sentences recorded at each of four decreasing, positive SNRs: 15 dB, 10 dB, 5 dB and 0 dB. Sub-block B is presented 30 dB below the level in sub-block A; i.e. with the first sub-block presented at 70 dB HL, while the second sub-block is presented at 40 dB HL (the original work used 65 dB HL and 35 dB HL). The levels are intended to represent 'fairly loud speech', commonly found at parties (Teder, 1990), and 'fairly soft speech'. The patients are told that they are at a party 'which starts in the next room and gets closer ...' (Killion and Villchur, 1993). Each sentence has five key words that are scored; answers that are close to correct are given half-credit. The test was designed to efficiently evaluate and compare the benefit an individual receives from of a pair of hearing aids; two 40-sentence test blocks should take about 24 minutes. The test is available in DAT and CD form (from Auditec of St Louis) and comes with a spreadsheet program (SINSHEET) to facilitate the graphic display of test results.

Hearing in noise (HINT) test

The HINT test is a new sentence test designed to measure sentence speech reception thresholds (SSRTs) in quiet and noise (Nilsson et al., 1990, 1991; Nilsson et al., 1994; Soli and Nilsson, 1994). It is based on the original work of Plomp and Mimpen (1979) which measured SRT for sentences in noise; i.e. SRT expressed in SNR for 50% correct sentences for noise with a spectrum equal to the long-term spectrum of the sentences and the speech level, in Leq, based on long-term sentence intensity. The HINT test consists of 240 sentences (six to eight words in length, recorded by a male talker), grouped into 10, or 20, phonemically-balanced sentence lists. There can be 24 lists of 10 sentences, or 12 lists of 20 sentences. The spectrum of the masking noise matches the long-term average spectrum of the sentences. The noise level is fixed, while the levels of the sentences are adaptively adjusted until the listener can recognize and repeat the sentences 50% of the time; resulting in 78% intelligibility at threshold. A 1 dB SNR change corresponds to a 8.5% change in intelligibility.

The test was designed to efficiently and reliably evaluate speech intelligibility in noise. The administration time is reportedly short: a 10-sentence list can take 2 minutes, a 20-sentence list can take 3 – 4 minutes. It can assess binaural advantage or directional hearing with the signal at 0 degrees and the noise at 0, +90 and –90 degrees. The relation between the performance of the individual under test (with or without hearing loss) and the normal hearing individual can be expressed as dB threshold elevation, as estimated percent intelligibility based on the relation between change in SNR and the change in percent intelligibility, or as percentile rank corresponding to the elevated threshold, and can be used to estimate possible communication handicap.

Methods

The most frequently used clinical method for assessing word recognition ability in the USA today includes the use of CID W-22 monosyllables, in an open set paradigm (Table 12.6). The NU-6 lists are a close second in popularity. Most clinicians use only half-lists (25 words) instead of full lists (50 words) (see Table 12.7).

Table 12.7 Number of words used to obtain a word recognition score (WRS)

	Surveys on Audiometric Practice								
	Martin and Pennington (1971)		Martin and Forbis (1978)		Martin and Sides (1985)		Martin and Morris (1989)		Martin, Armstrong and Champlin (1994)	
Number of Words	Number	%	Number	%	Number	%	Number	%	Number	%
50 for all patients	—	—	50	16.9	12	17.5	27	5.9	8	3.2
25 if patient answers first 25 correctly	—	—	125	40.8	70	31.7	113	24.8	24	9.5
25 for all patients	—	—	99	32.5	118	53.4	259	56.9	151	59.9
Other	—	—	30	9.8	21	9.5	56	12.3	19	7.5
More than one response	—	—	20.7	—	—	—	—	—	—	—
(Number of respondents)			(306)		(221)		(455)		(252)	

The majority of audiologists continue to use the SRT as the reference level for determining the level at which to administer the word recognition test (Table 12.8). This has increased to 75% from 65% (Martin et al., 1994).

Table 12.8 Level at which to obtain a word recognition score (WRS)

| | Surveys on Audiometric Practice | | | | | | | | | |
| Presentation Level | Martin and Pennington (1971) | | Martin and Forbis (1978) | | Martin and Sides (1985) | | Martin and Morris (1989) | | Martin, Armstrong and Champlin (1994) | |
	Number	%	Number	%	Number	%	Number	%	Number	%
dB SL re: SRT	147	52.9	207	68.0	142	64.8	337	74.2	191	75.5
dB HL	25	9.0	5	1.6	5	2.3	15	3.4	11	4.3
MCL	45	16.2	49	16.1	47	21.5	—	—	—	—
dB SPL	—	—	—	—	—	—	2	0.4	—	—
Obtain a P-I Function	9	3.2	15	4.9	8	3.7	—	—	—	—
Other	7	2.5	4	1.2	17	7.8	100	22.0	51	20.2
More than one response	45	16.2	25	8.2	—	—	—	—	—	—
(Number of respondents)	(278)		(305)		(219)		(454)		(253)	

The words are usually administered MLV, and each word is generally preceded by the carrier phrase 'say the word...'. Contralateral masking (of the non-test ear) is typically employed with speech weighted noise as the masker (Table 12.9).

These clinical methods, and their limitations, are discussed below. In addition, methods used for the evaluation of the paediatric population are also discussed, although there are no reported data on frequency of usage for paediatric procedures.

Half-lists vs. whole lists and the binomial distribution

The majority of audiologists (60%) use 25-word lists (see Table 12.7) with all patients regardless of the number of errors made in that half-list (Martin et al., 1994). In 1978 Martin and Forbis reported that 40.8% of audiologists responding were qualifying their use of 25-word lists by presenting a full 50-word list if the patient missed a certain number of words in the first half of the list. That figure dropped to 31.7% in the Martin and Sides (1985) report, and has continued to drop markedly to 9.5% in the most recent Martin et al., (1994) report.

Table 12.9 Masking criteria used to obtain a word recognition score (WRS)

Masking Criteria	Surveys on Audiometric Practice									
	Martin and Pennington (1971)		Martin and Forbis (1978)		Martin and Sides (1985)		Martin and Morris (1989)		Martin, Armstrong and Champlin (1994)	
	Number	%	Number	%	Number	%	Number	%	Number	%
Mask all WR tests	—	—	14	4.5	16	7.1	33	7.3	26	10.7
Patient hears speech in non-test ear or in middle of the head	10	3.9	6	1.9	4	1.8	5	1.2	2	0.8
40 dB or greater difference between SRTs of each ear	66	25.7	188	61.0	53	23.7	103	22.8	71	29.2
40 dB or greater difference between presentation level of test ear and the bone conduction threshold of the non-test ear	132	51.4	51	16.6	117	52.2	255	56.4	114	46.9
Never	—	—	31	10.2	6	2.7	19	4.2	10	4.1
Other	23	8.9	6	1.9	28	12.5	37	8.1	20	8.2
More than one response	26	10.1	12	3.9	—	—	—	—	—	—
(Number of respondents)	(257)		(308)		(224)		(452)		(243)	

We regret that there has been a significant move towards the use of half-lists without qualification. By applying the binomial distribution to the WRS, Thornton and Raffin (1978) have demonstrated the need for frequent use of full lists. Studebaker (1982) suggests that lists even longer than 50 words may be necessary for reliable test scores. The formula for the standard deviation of a binomial distribution shows that when we increase the sample size (i.e. length of the word list), we decrease the standard deviation, or increase reliability.

Specifically, a doubling of the number of words used, e.g. 50 instead of 25 words, results in a decrease in the standard deviation by the square root of two. In other words, variability is reduced by using full lists. What is also determined by the binomial distribution is that the largest standard deviations occur for WRSs in the mid-range, around 50%. It is true, therefore, that WRSs at either the upper limits (90 – 100%) or lower limits (0 – 10%) are the most reliable scores, so audiologists may have greater confidence in those scores after only 25 words are presented.

What we should have learned from considering speech recognition as a binomial distribution is that the audiologist should use careful judgement in order to determine what is an acceptable score with regard to a 'critical difference' as described by Thornton and Raffin (1978). For example, a large sample size, or longer word lists, may be necessary in order to determine if hearing aids differ in their ability to provide optimum speech intelligibility. Indeed, Studebaker (1982) showed that if a performance difference of 10% is obtained when comparing results of two word recognition tests, e.g. scores obtained with two different hearing aids, then 135 words must be presented in order to have an error rate no greater than 5%. In other words, in order to have 95% confidence that the two scores are different by 10%, 135 words must be presented. Furthermore, to achieve the accepted criterion difference of 6% with 95% confidence, 376 words must be presented (when comparing two WRSs for normal listeners). To make matters worse, if comparisons are made with more than two aids, the error rate increases further necessitating the use of still longer word lists.

The fact that audiologists in the USA have continued to move toward the more frequent use of half-lists reflects a lack of understanding of the implications of Thornton and Raffin's application of the binomial distribution. Thus, the impact of their contribution appears to have been ignored. Hopefully, clinical practice will soon benefit from the application of well-demonstrated theory.

Presentation level

The majority of audiologists continue to use the SRT as a reference level for determining the level at which to present the word recognition test (see

Table 12.8); this has increased to 75% from 65% (Martin et al., 1994). The most comfortable loudness (MCL) was the next most frequently used level in the 1985 report (Martin and Sides), but today appears to have fallen into disuse. Sometimes, although less frequently, clinicians report the determination of the WRS at a specific hearing level, e.g. 50 dB HL), or the determination of a P-I function for each patient. There are problems introduced by using any one of these particular methods to determine the presentation level. These problems can be reduced, however, if the factors which affect the WRS are understood by the clinician.

When examining the P-I functions in Figure 12.1, the practice of using the SRT as a reference level seems reasonable for normal hearing/conductive impaired listeners. For those patients, the average maximum score using CID W-22 monosyllables appears to be reached at 25 – 30 dB re SRT; above that level the function plateaus. However, the average optimum level changes for different stimuli, lists, recordings, etc. For example, the plateau (PB_{max}) for PB-50 monosyllables is reached at a higher level of approximately 33 dB. Knowledge of the psychometric function for the different materials available is thus essential in choosing a presentation level. It should be remembered, however, that average psychometric functions do not predict individual psychometric functions; individual P-I functions would be best.

Still, audiologists typically use SRT plus 25 – 40 dB as the presentation level since that level assumedly reaches plateau or maximum WRS (at least for persons with normal hearing or conductive hearing loss). Secondarily, the choice of SRT plus 25 – 40 dB is made to reduce cross-hearing and thus reduce the need to mask the contralateral ear.

If we examine the P-I function for patients with sensorineural hearing loss, we can see that the use of any fixed reference level is not appropriate. The psychometric function for the sensorineural impaired listeners illustrates the decrement in performance that can occur at sound pressure levels greater than their level of maximum performance. The thoughtful audiologist will perform the word recognition test at more than one level if it is believed that the optimum score was not obtained. Still better, an individual P-I function should be obtained. This is rarely done in general clinical practice due to the limited time available. Perhaps a better use of clinic and patient time might be to omit the SRT, and obtain pure-tone thresholds and a complete P-I function.

Of course the audiologist must also keep in mind the relevance of the binomial distribution when comparing scores between tests presented at different levels. First, the WRS for the sensorineural patient is likely to be less than normal, or less than 90%. Therefore, the variability of that score will be greater (Thornton and Raffin, 1978) than for scores of 90% or higher. For example, a patient who scores 50% on the first word recognition test must achieve a score on the second test which differs by more than 20% in order for that score to be considered statistically different within 95% confidence limits. Second, variability will increase as the number of comparison tests increases by the square root of the number of comparisons.

Another consideration when testing a patient with a sensorineural hearing loss is the configuration of the hearing loss. For persons with high frequency sensorineural hearing loss, we recommend accounting for the pure-tone threshold at either 2 or 3 kHz, since those frequencies are critical to consonant understanding. If possible, that is if not too uncomfortable for the patient and if hearing sensitivity permits, the word recognition test should be administered approximately 5 dB above the threshold of either of those frequencies. Optimally, obtaining a P-I function will assure that the maximum discrimination score under earphones has been obtained. Time constraints in a busy clinic, however, may prevent the audiologist from obtaining the complete P-I function.

The use of MCL for speech as a strict determinant in choosing presentation level is not recommended since the level of maximum word recognition need not be equivalent to MCL in hearing impaired patients (Posner and Ventry, 1977). For patients with recruitment ears, the severely limited dynamic range of which results in tolerance problems, the audiologist may have no choice but to deliver the speech stimuli at a comfortable level. It should be noted on the audiogram that the MCL was chosen for that reason.

Recorded vs. live voice presentation

Most audiologists use MLV presentation for word recognition testing (Martin and Pennington, 1971; Martin and Forbis, 1978; Martin and Sides, 1985; Martin and Morris, 1989; Martin et al., 1994), since, as discussed earlier, MLV presentation does allow the audiologist greater flexibility during the evaluation. Because of the important use of the WRS as it relates to differential diagnosis, surgery related decisions and amplification/aural rehabilitation, the audiologist is cautioned regarding the greater need for the standardization offered by recorded test materials, in order to reduce variability.

Inherent in the WRS is poor test–retest reliability. Variability can be as much as 48% in a patient with a sensorineural hearing loss whose WRS is reduced to a mid-range score (Thornton and Raffin, 1978). When variability is a critical issue, it can be reduced by careful attention to test parameters, such as the selection of recorded over MLV presentation for the word recognition test.

Carrier phrase

A majority of clinicians (51%) in the USA do use a carrier phrase for word recognition testing with MLV presentation. 'Say the word...' is preferred by the majority (45%) of those who use a carrier phrase (Martin et al., 1994). There are arguments in the literature both for and against the use of a carrier phrase (Martin, Hawkins and Bailey, 1962; Gladstone and Sieganthaler, 1971; Gelfand, 1975; Lynn and Brotman, 1981). In practice, the clinician chooses to use or not use a carrier phrase in accordance with the needs of the clinical situation and the patient. For example, some children or geriatrics may be confused by the carrier phrase. On the other hand, some of these patients may require the carrier phrase as an alerting device. Indeed, some patients are annoyed by the carrier phrase.

Masking

The majority of audiologists use contralateral masking when there is a specific difference in ears (threshold). The criterion still most often used (Table 12.9) is a 40 dB difference between the test presentation level and the best bone-conduction threshold of the non-test ear (Martin and Pennington, 1971; Martin and Sides, 1985; Martin and Morris, 1989; Martin et al., 1994). Today a greater number of audiologists continue to use speech noise as the contralateral masker. According to Martin et al., (1994), 95% of audiologists are using speech noise as a masker compared to 1985 when Martin and Sides reported that 75% of audiologists were using speech noise as a masker. There are no specific guidelines set forth by ASHA for determining the amount of noise necessary for supra-threshold masking.

Clinicians in the USA typically assume 40 to 50 dB as the amount of interaural attenuation for speech. They subtract the interaural attenuation value from the hearing level of the non-test ear and then add the largest air-bone gap of the non-test ear (Martin and Forbis, 1978; Martin and Sides, 1985; Martin, et al., 1994). Simply stated, enough noise should be used to effectively mask out the amount of speech that may possibly cross over to the non-test ear, using the best bone-conduction threshold of the non-test ear as a reference.

Word recognition tests for children

Choosing an appropriate word recognition test for a child is difficult because of the many factors that can affect the child's performance. Of primary importance are the child's receptive vocabulary, the response modality and reinforcement techniques. Response set definition and vocabulary restriction are important principles in the development of speech audiometric tests for children (Jerger, 1983). We must be particularly careful in test selection for a child who has a significant hearing loss, since we cannot be certain to what extent the hearing loss has contributed to language delay. Thus test scores may not reflect the child's auditory perceptual capabilities alone. There are, however, a few popular paediatric tests available which attempt to reduce the pragmatic and developmental problems inherent in this population. The primary focus of speech recognition tests for children is the same as for adults. Some of these tests have also been applied to retrocochlear differential diagnosis and central auditory processing evaluation (Jerger, 1987; Jerger et al., 1988; Jerger and Zeller, 1989; Connolly et al., 1992). Although there are more paediatric tests available than are mentioned here, we have tried to present those which we believe are either commonly used or may be gaining in clinical popularity.

PBK-50 word lists

To overcome word familiarity problems imposed by adult PB monosyllables, PBK word lists were devised by Haskins (1949). They are composed of phonetically-balanced monosyllables selected from vocabulary word lists representative of kindergarten children's language. Use of this test is limited to children over 3.5 years old, since younger normal hearing children do not achieve a maximum score (Sanderson-Leepa and Rintelmann, 1976).

Word intelligibility by picture identification (WIPI) test

The WIPI test was developed in a closed set format to permit an alternate response mode for children (or any other difficult to-test population) who have difficulty responding verbally (Lerman, Ross and McLauchlin, 1965). The test has gained popularity in the USA because it provides the audiologist with four monosyllabic word lists that are easy to administer and score. The child must simply point to one of six pictures on a page. Pictures are colourful and, for the most part, easy to identify. Although vocabulary items were chosen for the paediatric population, this test (similar to the PBK word lists) is most appropriate for children whose receptive vocabulary is age 4 years or older. Clinically, we have observed that some of the test items are culturally biased (e.g. church, farm, barn). In spite of its limitations, the WIPI appears to have greater clinical popularity than other picture tests such as the DIP (Siegenthaler and Haspiel, 1966), NU-CHIPS (Katz and Elliott, 1978; Elliot and Katz, 1980) and PSI (Jerger et al., 1980; Jerger, Jerger and Lewis, 1981).

Discrimination by identification of pictures (DIP) test

The DIP test is a closed set picture test. Limitations of this test are word familiarity problems and the small size of the closed set — a two picture matrix.

Northwestern University children's perception of speech (NU-CHIPS) test

The NU-CHIPS test (Katz and Elliot, 1978; Elliot and Katz, 1980) test was developed to assess the receptive vocabulary of 3-year-old inner-city children. It is also a closed set picture test of monosyllabic words. It has the advantage of being appropriate for children as young as 3 years of age.

Newer paediatric speech intelligibility (PSI) test

The PSI test is a picture test which uses 20 monosyllabic words and 10 competing-message sentence materials (Jerger, et al., 1980). It is a closed-set test picture identification task in which the child must point to one of five pictures. Sentences are broken into two groups: Format I sentences are for children with low receptive language ability and Format II sentences are for children with high receptive language ability. There is an apparent advantage in controlling for the linguistic capabilities of the child.

Sound effects recognition test (SERT)

The SERT is a non-linguistic test (Finitzo-Hieber, Gerlin, Matkin and Chernow-Skalka, 1980). This test, although not truly a word recognition test, was designed to assess the ability of the kindergarten child to recognize 30 environmental sounds within their own spontaneous language. It is a closed set test in which the child must point to one of four pictures.

Auditory numbers test (ANT)

The ANT (Erber, 1980) is a simple verbal test. The speech materials are numbers one to five. It is a closed set test in which the child must point to one of five pictures.

Nonsense syllable discrimination test (NSDT)

The NSDT (Kelly and Pillow, 1979) is a simplified verbal test. The speech materials are 50 syllable pairs. It is a closed set test in which the child must indicate whether the syllables are the same or different.

Summary

Paediatric word and sentence recognition tests control the effect of language by using appropriately age-based receptive and expressive language. The SERT, the ANT and the NSDT control the effect of receptive language by using either non-verbal or simple verbal materials.

Paediatric speech recognition procedures are presented as either unspecified, unrestricted or restricted response domains. Unrestricted responses (which do not specify the target item) and restricted responses (which do specify the target items but not the foil items) are closed set message set procedures. Unspecified target responses are open set message set procedures.

Methods

Presentation of test materials to children is usually performed using MLV, if test materials permit. This format allows for the greater flexibility needed when working with a child. The audiologist can reinforce when indicated, use encouragement, change instructions, and otherwise do what is necessary to elicit responses. Obviously, certain tests, such as the SERT and PSI require recorded materials.

Informal assessment of word recognition by young children is also achieved by asking the youngster to point to various body parts. This can be done with a simple command or question or by playing the game 'Simple Simon says'.

Applications of speech audiometry to aural rehabilitation

Hearing aid evaluation and selection

Traditionally the SRT and WRS have been used in hearing aid evaluation and selection (Carhart, 1946a,b). This approach was practised widely throughout the 1970s (Smaldino and Hoene, 1981) and even into the mid-1980s (Martin and Morris, 1989). Today, the SRT is rarely used to choose the amount of gain of a hearing aid, since using the SRT can lead to over amplification, especially in low frequencies. Pre- and post-evaluation comparisons of WRS are still used, but they are used to verify benefit from a selected hearing aid, rather than to select the hearing aid system providing the maximum speech intelligibility as had been specified by Carhart (1946a). Despite the fact that the WRS did not adequately discriminate one hearing aid from another (Shore, Bilger and Hirsch, 1960), the Carhart method (1946a) dominated clinical practice for over 40 years (Studebaker, 1980).

This domination probably continued because improved speech recognition remains as a primary goal of hearing aid selection. Fortunately, there has been a considerable move away from using WRSs as a major determinant in hearing aid system selection. This move can be attributed to several factors (Kruger and Kruger, 1993): greater understanding of the binomial distribution as it relates to reliability and paired comparison variability issues (Thornton and Raffin, 1978; Studebaker, 1982), research clarifying the external ear and its resonance characteristics (Shaw, 1974, 1975, 1980,) and eardrum impedance (Zwislocki, 1971; Djupesland and Zwislocki, 1972; Rabinowitz, 1981), the development of prescriptive hearing aid fitting targets, and the development of clinical real-ear probe microphone measurement equipment.

Currently, clinicians are using real-ear frequency specific methods of hearing aid system selection and verification. Hearing aid system selection procedures now emphasize comparison of unaided and aided real-ear probe microphone responses (insertion gain), and less often, unaided and aided narrow-band or warbled pure-tone thresholds (functional gain). The application of prescriptive methods has grown (Gengel, 1971; Pascoe, 1975; Byrne and Tonnison, 1976; Shapiro, 1976; Berger, Hagberg and Rane, 1977; Byrne 1978; Pascoe, 1978; Cox, 1983, 1985, 1988; McCandless and Lyregaard, 1983; Skinner and Miller, 1983; Libby, 1985, 1988; Seewald, Ross and Spiro, 1985; Byrne and Dillon, 1986; Skinner, 1988), and mushroomed in popularity in the late 1980s and early 1990s (Seewald et al., 1990, 1992), as prescription rules were implemented in real-ear probe-tube microphone measurement instrumentation and the precursors of contemporary and future 'universal fitting systems' have appeared.

Prescriptive methods and speech-based comparison methods using WRSs have alternated in favour as hearing aid fitting strategies (Pascoe, 1985; Humes and Houghton, 1992; Northern, 1992; Humes and Halling, 1993). Today, along with acceptance of prescriptive methods, there is now a re-emergence of the use of speech materials for: (1) the selection/verification of optimal hearing aid response (e.g. Cox, and McDaniel, 1984; Hodgson, 1986; Cox, Alexander, and Gilmore, 1987; Cox and Moore, 1988; Nilsson et al., 1990; Fikret-Pasa, 1993; Killion and Villchur, 1993; Soli and Nilsson, 1994; Nilsson et al., 1994;); (2) the prediction of optimal speech intelligibility based on AI (Pavlovic, 1988, 1991; Humes and Houghton, 1992); and (3) the evaluation of hearing aid benefit/quality (Punch and Beck, 1980; Hagerman and Gabrielsson, 1984; Walden, Demorest, and Helper, 1984; Liejon, Lindkvist, Ringdahl and Isreaelsson, 1990, 1991; Cox and Alexander, 1991a, 1992; Gatehouse and Killion, 1993; Gatehouse, 1994). It is anticipated that prescriptive methods, real-ear probe measurements, speech-based comparative methods, and benefit determination methods will all be integrated into future hearing aid selection, fitting and verification procedures and systems (Kruger and Kruger, 1993).

Some of the newer speech materials, like the SIN (Killion and Villchur, 1993), the HIN (Nilsson et al., 1990; Soli and Nilsson, 1994; Nilsson et al., 1994), and the CSTv2 (Cox et al., 1987), have sufficient reliability and validity to be used for evaluation of hearing aid performance and hearing aid benefit. Although both the traditional WRS tests and the newer key words-in-sentences-in-noise (KISIN) tests will continue to be used to study hearing aid benefit, it is hoped that the KISIN tests will gain in popularity.

They are relevant to both the diagnostic evaluation, and the prognostic process for hearing aid selection and rehabilitation of persons with hearing impairment. Clinically, we need to know how a person with hearing loss functions in noise both with and without amplification. The utility or clinical efficiency of the newer speech recognition (KISIN) tests, i.e. administration time, ease of presentation, scoring and interpretation, will determine which of these tests (or other evolving test/procedures) gains acceptance in practice. These tests will be applied to present and future clinical and research issues relating to the strategies for selecting and verifying hearing aid fittings (Valente, 1994), with both traditional linear, and particularly non-linear conventional and digitally programmable circuitry; and to measurement and prediction of the performance with, and the benefit from, these hearing aid fittings.

Rehabilitation

The rehabilitation process is beginning to receive serious attention from both the clinical and research audiologist. Traditional approaches to rehabilitation focused on speech reading, emphasizing both phonetic and synthetic analysis of speech. Rehabilitation now covers a broader scope. It includes counselling, speech reading and training to optimize the individual's ability to synthesize both auditory and visual cues. The development of new training techniques and new devices which enhance training continue to help improve the impaired listener's ability to make more and more complex phonemic distinctions.

Phoneme recognition

The use of monosyllabic word tests in aural rehabilitation is limited because they do not accurately reflect the individual's everyday communication ability. Other factors such as motivation, speech reading ability, intelligence and language skill contribute to the individual's communication success in real life situations. Most clinicians still use the CID W-22, or the NU-6 monosyllabic word lists, with MLV presentation, in order to assess word recognition ability. However, these lists, used in their traditional open set format, do not allow for easy phoneme error analysis. As mentioned earlier, other word recognition tests such as the MRT, the CCT, the isophonemic CNC word lists and the NST can be used when it is necessary to eliminate the problem of word familiarity and reduce memory effects.

On the other hand, when highly contextual material is needed, sentence materials such as the CHABA sentences are available. The newer speech in noise test, i.e. 'KISIN' tests like the SIN, HIN and CSTv2 are available to evaluate the individual's ability to understand in noise without and with their hearing aids. The errors can provide targets for modification of hearing aid performance or for rehabilitation (e.g. speech reading). The SPIN test provides the clinician with a sentence test which varies the amount of contextual cues offering both high- and low-predictability items.

Research on phonemic recognition (e.g. Miller and Nicely, 1955; Walden and Montgomery, 1975; Bilger and Wang, 1976) has revealed that certain distinctive features facilitate intelligibility: nasality, sonorance, voicing. Some consonants are more easily confused than others. Training programmes are being developed which focus on making same–different discriminations of consonant sounds in different word and sentence contexts, adjusting the level of complexity of the confusions to maximize learning (Kopra et al., 1985).

More recently the major aim of an aural rehabilitation programme is towards synthetic analysis of connected discourse. Attention is still given to auditory and visual training using a more analytic approach but with the understanding that these two modalities are complimentary. Visual cues which are not distinguishable from each other, i.e. within group visemes (Woodward and Barber, 1960; Binnie et al., 1974) can be processed with the aid of auditory cues. On the other hand, auditory cues which are homophonous result in within-group confusions (Miller and Nicely, 1955) which can be resolved with visual input. For example, the homophones /p, t, k/ are visually recognizable due to differences in place of articulation, whereas the visemes /p, b, m/ are more easily differentiated auditorily.

Thus, an aural rehabilitation programme must include phoneme recognition work to train across homophone and viseme boundaries. In addition, training must extend beyond phonemic recognition to include recognition of contextual, situational and pragmatic features of the communication process using both the auditory and visual modalities. The rehabilitation programme moves from easy or highly contextual materials, such as sentence materials, to more difficult of less contextual materials, such as monosyllables.

Fundamental speech skills test (FSST)

The FSST (Levitt et al., 1990) is a new speech test which assesses production skills, pitch control, suprasegmentals and spontaneous speech production. The production skills assessed include breath stream capacity, basic articulation, pitch control, syllabification, stress and intonation contours. The pitch control skills assessed include variability in voice pitch, repeated and alternated syllables and average voice pitch monosyllabic words. Suprasegmental aspects of speech include syllable number, syllable accent, word stress and intonation contours. The spontaneous speech sample is assessed for pitch variation, average pitch, intensity control and intelligibility. Administration time is about 25 minutes. Rating and scoring is simple. The results of the test can be used to develop therapy protocols for persons with severe to profound hearing loss.

Speech tracking

A more recent approach, which emphasizes the need for simultaneous analysis of visual and auditory cues, is speech 'tracking' (De Filippo and Scott, 1978; Owens and Telleen, 1981). In this method the speaker and listener sit face-to face so that the hearing-impaired patient is able to receive auditory, visual and kinaesthetic cues. The task of the patient is to repeat short segments of connected discourse spoken by the talker. Improvement is measured as an increase in speed of recognition in words per minute, or increased percentage of words correctly identified. Passages are repeated at subsequent therapy sessions. The technique is gaining in popularity for the profoundly hearing impaired/deaf. The limitations to the procedure include no standardized materials or procedure, live voice presentation, and tester/ therapist dependent modes of cueing the patient to repeat the connected discourse correctly.

Minimal auditory capabilities (MAC) battery

Another new series of tests has been developed for use with the severe-to-profound population. The MAC battery (Owens et al., 1980, 1981; revision: Owens et al., 1985) is currently being used to evaluate potential candidates for a cochlear implant. The MAC battery consists of 14 subtests (13 auditory and one lip reading) which include recognition of environmental sounds, phonemes, words and sentences. These tests were designed to assess the auditory capabilities of those patients for whom routine speech recognition material is too difficult and to provide a profile of those patients' speech recognition abilities that could be useful in the determination of an appropriate rehabilitation programme.

Self-assessment inventories

Interest in evaluating a patient's communication impairment in everyday life has led to the development of numerous hearing handicap inventories (Rupp, Higgins and Maurer, 1977; Alpiner, 1978; Giolas et al., 1979; Ventry and Weinstein, 1982; Weinstein and Ventry, 1982). A short description is presented of two useful scales, the hearing performance inventory (HPI) and the hearing handicap inventory for the elderly (HHIE).

The HPI is a questionnaire which permits the self-assessment of speech reception abilities (Giolas et al., 1979). The individual is able to assess his or her own ability to understand speech in a variety of listening situations including speech in quiet, speech in noise and speech with only auditory (no visual) cues available. Test items are divided into six categories: understanding of speech, intensity, response, social, personal and occupational. The subject rates his or her behaviour in a particular everyday situation. Results from the HPI provide insight into the individual's own perception of a communicative handicap, but do not necessarily correlate well with speech recognition performance measures (Rowland et al., 1985).

The HHIE examines the patient's communication difficulties as well the psychosocial effects of hearing loss on the patient's daily activities. A sample question on the HHIE is: 'Does a hearing problem cause you to visit friends, relatives, or neighbours less often than you would like?' (Ventry and Weinstein, 1982; Weinstein and Ventry, 1982; Weinstein, Spitzer and Ventry, 1986; Weinstein, 1993). The HHIE provides a subjective evaluation of the patient's degree of handicap and can thus be helpful in predicting successful hearing aid use. More recently the Hearing Handicap Inventory for Adults (HHIA) was introduced; this is a version of the HHIE appropriate for use with adults (Newman et al., 1990, 1991).

Profile of hearing aid benefit (PHAB) and the abbreviated profile of hearing aid benefit (APHAB)

The PHAB is a 66-item self-assessment questionnaire (Cox and Rivera, 1992). It is a disability-based inventory. The PHAB is used to determine the predictability or reliability of hearing aid benefit. It may be used to document the outcome of a hearing aid fitting, or to compare several fittings or the same fitting over time. The PHAB, however, is more applicable to research due to its length and administration time. The APHAB, is a new short version (Cox and Alexander, 1994). It consists of 24 items, scored in four six-item subscales: ease of communication (EC), reverberation (RV), background noise (BN), and aversiveness (AV). Administration is 10 minutes. The items are statements about communication ability of perception of sound in everyday life. Each subscale results in a score for unaided performance, for aided performance and for hearing aid benefit.

Speech audiometry instruments as engineering tools

Most of the discussion to this point has been specifically directed toward clinical speech audiometry. At this point we want to deviate somewhat in order to provide a brief discussion of the use of speech audiometry instruments for the evaluation of communications devices and systems. 'But isn't the hearing aid a communications device?' you may ask. Yes it is. It is actually a particular type of communications system with an input transducer, a communications channel (here an amplifier) and an output transducer. In all of the earlier discussions, we considered the human subject's performance evaluation in terms of whether or not the hearing aid helped to improve the performance on a given test instrument (i.e. did use of the (hearing aid) communications system raise the test subject's score?).

To adapt a different point of view; try now to imagine that the test subject is a detector. The role of the test subject is to receive and respond to the above threshold audiological test items. The critical question is now whether the use of the communication system improves, leaves unaltered, or reduces the intelligibility of the presented communications. In other words, has the introduction of the communications system enhanced or hurt the intelligibility of the desired communication?

Several of the tests discussed earlier are used frequently for the evaluation of communications systems other than hearing aids — even though the same block diagram of input transducer, communications channel and output transducer is used. For example both the MRT (House et al., 1963; Kruel et al., 1968) and the DRT (Voiers, 1977) are frequently used to evaluate the performance of new communications devices (intercom systems, radios, telephones, etc.) and the value of the speech transmission index (STI) (Steeneken and Houtgast, 1980) in estimating the speech intelligibility of a communications channel has been demonstrated. Sometimes, it is only the microphone, the electronic processing circuitry, the earphones, or the loudspeaker which is being evaluated, with all other components kept constant.

As we enter the age of true digital processing of signals within hearing aids, we need to know whether intelligibility suffers as the desired speech signals are acted upon by these elegant circuits and noise is stripped, or an echo in a reverberant room is cancelled. The three tests mentioned above and some of the other tests, such as the SIN test, and the HIN test, will help to provide these answers. It is not engineering elegance alone that will serve the hearing impaired person. It is the proper clinical use of these tests during instrument development and, again, during the fitting process that will assure client benefits.

These tests are only tools, however. The skilled clinicians who use these tools (and the sophisticated software/hardware fitting systems) to evaluate and properly fit these new engineering marvels will contribute greatly to the improvement of client life style.

Research directions

Research in speech intelligibility will remain multifaceted. Some research will focus on the issues of validation and reliability of newly developed speech recognition tests for the diagnostic assessment of auditory sensitivity and of the ability to understand speech. Greater research efforts will pursue the development of speech recognition tests with special focus on hearing aid assessment and aural rehabilitation. Research will continue to refine the application of the AI to predict the benefit of amplified speech understanding. The AI has been, and will continue to be studied for its predictive ability to estimate the speech recognition ability of hearing impaired individuals without and with hearing aids (Pavlovic and Studebaker, 1984; Pavlovic, 1985, 1987, 1988, 1989, 1991; Pavlovic, Studebaker and Sherbecoe, 1985; Marincovich and Studebaker, 1985; Marincovich, 1987; Mueller and Killion, 1990; Pavlovic, 1991; Rankovic, 1991; ANSI S3.5 1994 proposed revision of 1989 edition).

The AI is also being compared with other prediction schemes such as the speech transmission index (STI) as predictors of speech recognition performance of normal listeners (Steeneken and Houtgast, 1980; Humes, Boney and Ahlstrom, 1985) and of hearing impaired listeners (Humes, 1991; Humes, 1993) in quiet and in various listening environments (Kruger and Kruger, 1994).

Along with the prediction of speech recognition performance comes the estimation of the speech intelligibility of a communications channel. The STI, as originally developed and described by Steeneken and Houtgast (1980), provided an objective physical measure of the quality of a speech communications channel. The index value is calculated from the modulation transfer function using an artificial speechlike test signal. The values generated (the STI) had a predictable relationship to speech intelligibility. Since the original STI development work was validated for the Dutch language, there was some question of the validity of its use in evaluating communications systems proposed for use with the English language. The STI method was validated in the USA by using the STIDAS II-D device (described by Steeneken and Agterhuis, 1982) under various test conditions and then comparing the test results with intelligibility scores obtained using Harvard PB work lists (Anderson, Wayne and Kalb, 1987). The correlation is not perfect, however, and caution must be exercised in extrapolating from STI to human subject intelligibility test data. The STIDAS device yields an STI reading in a few minutes and has been used in various types of measurements on radio communication links, as well as in measurements of room acoustics.

Further investigations using the STI will provide additional data regarding the robustness of STI-based intelligibility predictions. As a result of the development of the STI, several new test tools based on the modulation transfer function have evolved to aid in the evaluation of the intelligibility of new communications systems (e.g. the Bruel & Kjaer RASTI system). Some of these tools promise to be quite usable; even when various digital speech compression schemes are integrated into the communications system.

Research interest will continue to develop high technology applications of speech recognition/intelligibility assessment. There is ongoing research in the application of computers to clinical and educational programmes, particularly in the area of aural rehabilitation and real-ear hearing aid fitting (Aitken and Bianco, 1985; Traynor et al., 1985). We will see continued increases in the application of the laser video disc and CD ROM technology as an interactive system for computer-assisted instruction in aural rehabilitation including speech reading and voice training (e.g. Show, Bolsora, Smedley and Whitcomb, 1993; Tait, 1993). Computer use for the scoring of traditional word recognition tests will continue. We will probably see the computer applied to both the presentation and scoring of adaptively adjusted SPIN materials. We are already beginning to see the computer used as an integral part of clinical evaluation/hearing aid fitting and programming systems.

The expanded use of speech materials, and assessment profiles will continue to modify the hearing aid assessment procedures (Cox and Riviera, 1992; Cox and Alexander, 1994; Cox et al., 1994a; Cox et al., 1994b). Considerable attention will be devoted to development and validation of KISIN tests, and of databases of everyday listening environments, at varied levels, for the evaluation of speech recognition with amplification and of hearing aid benefit. The increased importance of the performance of individuals, and of hearing aids at different speech and noise levels will continue (Kruger and Kruger, 1994; IHAFF, 1994; Kuk, Harper and Doubek, 1994).

Selection and fitting strategies will be used to specify and set (programme) hearing aid gain as a function of input level for various input signal levels to match the individual's auditory area or dynamic range. The AI will be used in the prediction of benefit derived from amplified speech and the KISIN materials will be used in the verification of benefit derived from amplified speech in various listening systems. This will be accomplished with the advent of universal fitting systems with virtual reality databases of speech samples in different listening environments (Kruger and Kruger, 1994).

Research continues on the development and application of self-assessment scales. The psychometric adequacy of self-assessment scales has been addressed by Demorest and DeHaven (1993). The use and validation of self-assessment scales has been assessed as an outcome measure in hearing aid fitting (Weinstein, 1993), as a measure of communication strategies (Tye-Murray et al., 1993), as a measure of cochlear implant and profoundly hearing impaired patients (Spitzer, 1993), as a measure of balance function (Newman and Jacobson, 1993) and as a measure of tinnitus disability (Tyler, 1993).

A plethora of assistive listening devices continue to emerge on the market for hearing impaired listeners. Some are directly coupled to the individual's hearing aid and others are independent. Research is beginning in areas of the calibration, selection and fitting of these devices, as well as in their use during therapy. We will see the continued development and evaluation of the recognition ability and efficiency of assistive listening devices for both the classroom (Lewis, 1994a,b) and for everyday life.

In addition, the development of new sensory aids for the severe and profoundly hearing impaired/deaf will continue. The clinical research with cochlear implants will remain an impetus for a significant amount of speech recognition research (e.g. McKay and McDermott, 1993). Aural rehabilitation will focus on determination of, and training of, the linguistic aspects of auditory processing of speech (e.g. Jerger et al., 1994), and the oral communication skills of normal hearing and hearing impaired children (e.g. Elfenbein, Hardin-Jones and Davis, 1994).

It is still hoped that more research will be directed towards the development of clinical branching strategies which will improve the efficiency of speech audiometry procedures. Such strategies might include: more selective use of the SRT, appropriate use of pure-tone estimates of levels at which to present supra-threshold speech recognition materials and increased use of P-I functions to assess speech intelligibility.

Chapter 13
The Swedish approach to speech audiometry

STIG ARLINGER and BJÖRN HAGERMAN

The purpose of this review is to present the main aspects of speech audiometric testing being used in audiologic clinics in Sweden today. This includes speech test material as well as equipment and principles for calibration. In addition, some scientific projects concerning speech audiometry and the development of new methods are discussed.

Routine diagnostic testing

Speech recognition threshold

For the determination of speech recognition threshold (SRT), the test material used is bisyllabic words, or spondees. Three lists are available, each containing 24 words. The test words are presented alone without any carrier phrase. The interval between successive words is about 5 seconds. The test lists used today were originally developed by Lidén in his 1954 dissertation, with the original version recorded on gramophone records. In 1965 a revision was made by the Department of Technical Audiology, Karolinska Institute, Stockholm. In this revision a number of test words were discarded as being semantically too difficult for many hearing impaired listeners. New recordings were made, this time on magnetic tape. The master tapes were stored at the Department of Technical Audiology, where all official copies were produced.

However, when magnetic cassette recordings became popular, many clinics started to do their own copying. This meant that the quality of the recordings could not be controlled any longer, an obvious step backwards. So when compact disc (CD) technology became available at a reasonable cost it was an obvious choice of medium for the recordings. Today, essentially all clinics use only the CD recordings.

The standardized test procedure used in Sweden starts with the introduction of the test words at a level approximately 20 dB above the listener's pure-tone average hearing threshold level (average of 500 Hz,

1 kHz and 2 kHz). After presenting a few test words, the level is reduced in steps of 5 dB until the patient starts failing to repeat the words correctly. Ten test words are then presented on that level. If five or more of these words are repeated correctly, the level is reduced by 5 dB and another set of 10 test words is presented, until a score of less than five out of 10 is obtained. The SRT, defined as the level corresponding to a score of 50%, is determined by means of linear interpolation.

When contralateral masking is required in order to avoid the risk of cross-hearing, the standardized weighted noise from the clinical audiometer is used. The masking level required, expressed in terms of effective masking level, is calculated as the speech level in the test ear minus 40 dB for the skull attenuation plus the average air–bone gap (500 Hz, 1 kHz and 2 kHz) for the masked ear. Thus, when the speech level is changed during the testing, the masking level also has to be changed.

Maximum speech recognition

For the determination of maximum speech recognition score, monosyllabic test words are used. Twelve lists are available, also originating from Lidén's basic work (1954). Each list contains 50 test words preceded by a carrier phrase: 'Now you'll hear ....'. Each list is phonetically balanced (hence the common abbreviation PB list) and equalized. Experience has shown that there are slight differences in the degree of difficulty between the lists.

The normal test procedure recommends a first test level that the patient finds comfortable, typically about 30 dB above the patient's SRT for the test ear. A complete list of 50 test words is presented at the level chosen and the number of correctly repeated test words is counted, each word corresponding to 2% of the score. If the score is less than 70%, it is essential to use other test levels also to determine the maximum score and the shape of the psychometric function. On each other level, another complete test list is presented.

Since each complete list of 50 words is phonetically balanced, it is not recommended that only part of a list is used. However, if after the first 25 words of a list the patient has missed at most one word, it is permissible to stop the test there in order to save time. The possible error is considered negligible.

When contralateral masking is required, the same rules apply as for SRT testing. When very high masking levels have to be used, giving rise to risk for overmasking, insert masking is recommended to reduce the risk. If the insert earphone is calibrated in terms of effective masking level for the speech weighted noise used as a masker, the masking level required is calculated using the same formula as for SRT testing. If an uncalibrated insert earphone is used, the correct setting of the masking level attenuator can be calculated by replacing the air-conduction threshold levels with the attenuator settings corresponding to hearing thresholds, determined with the particular insert earphone, minus bone-conduction thresholds for the air–bone gap.

Distorted speech tests

In 1973, Margareta Korsan-Bengtsen published her dissertation on distorted speech audiometry. She applied several types of distortion on her test material, consisting of sentences of four to eight words each with four key words on which the scoring was based:

- Interrupted speech with interruption rates of 4, 7 and 10 per second and 50% duty cycle.
- Frequency-distorted speech with a pass-band from 445 to 900 Hz.
- Time-compressed speech with speech rates at 220 and 290 words per minute.

In addition she studied the effect of competing speech, in which each test sentence was presented to the test ear simultaneously with the presentation to the contralateral ear of a monosyllabic word and its carrier phrase from the standard PB-lists.

In subjects with normal hearing she found age to be a significant factor, which thus has to be taken into account in the clinical interpretation of distorted speech tests. The main diagnostic aim of these is to detect central disorders that influence the information processing in the auditory pathways. Korsan-Bengtsen showed significantly reduced speech recognition scores in patients with temporal lobe lesions involving the auditory cortex and with brainstem tumours involving the cochlear nuclei. She found interrupted speech and time-compressed speech to be the most sensitive test materials.

In a Swedish study on subjects with long-term occupational exposure to industrial organic solvents, Ödkvist et al. (1987) found recognition of distorted speech to be one of the few audio-vestibular tests that yielded pathological results. A significant reduction of speech recognition for interrupted speech was seen, interpreted as indicating central neurological damage caused by solvent exposure.

Speech audiometry in rehabilitation

Since speech perception is such an essential part of human life and interaction with other human beings, there is a very obvious interest in using measures of speech recognition to evaluate the degree of disability caused by hearing loss and the effect of intervention such as the fitting of hearing aids, the use of a cochlear implant or reconstructive middle ear surgery. However, conventional speech tests with the test material presented in quiet have usually shown a very low sensitivity and therefore have not been widely used. By presenting the speech test material in a background of noise, test sensitivity has increased at least to a degree which makes it possible to show significant differences between group means. One example of such a study is the comparison of in-the-ear and behind-the ear hearing aids reported by Jerivall et al. (1983).

An increasing interest in developing new speech test material and alternative, improved test methods will probably gradually increase the use of speech audiometry in audiological rehabilitation.

Auditory tests

The difficulty in hearing weak sounds due to impaired auditory sensitivity is described well by the pure-tone audiogram, and the reduction of this component of the disability by the hearing aid can be assessed by measuring the real-ear gain as insertion gain or functional gain.

However, almost every patient, regardless of degree of hearing impairment, has problems in recognizing speech in noisy environments. Therefore, most efforts over the last decade to use speech audiometry for functional diagnosis have been directed to measuring speech recognition in noise. In most applications, the speech stimulus and the competing noise are presented through loudspeakers in a sound field rather than through headphones. Although an international standard is now available giving details of loudspeaker placement (ISO 8253-3 1996), a consensus between clinics has yet to be established. Arrangements span from one loudspeaker for both the speech and the noise, up to five loudspeakers.

Regarding speech material and methods used, the set of sentence lists by Hagerman (1982) is probably the most commonly used material in Sweden. It is recorded on the same CD as the PB-lists. Twelve lists are available on the CD, each list made up of 10 five-word sentences. Each sentence contains one name, one verb, one digit, one adjective and one substantive, e.g. 'Gustav took 18 black boxes'. Each list contains exactly the same words as those originally recorded, but in different combinations. Each list has a fairly good phonemic balance. Since the material is based on 50 words which all occur in all lists with the same original recording, the lists are as equivalent as is possible. For children there is also a four word version with the adjective omitted and a three word version with the first two words omitted.

A very high sensitivity is obtained by presenting the word lists in a background of slightly amplitude modulated noise, with a spectrum identical to that of the long term average of the speech signal. The background level is varied, scoring is done word by word, and the signal-to-noise ratio (SNR) that gives a 50% correct score is determined (Hagerman, 1982, 1984; Hageman and Kinnefors 1995). For normal hearing subjects he found a maximum slope of the psychometric function of about 25% per dB change in SNR and a standard deviation of 0.44 dB for repeated measurements of the SNR-threshold. These results were obtained for SRT in noise with monaural earphone presentation using two test lists requiring less than 4 minutes of test time.

The ordinary PB lists are also used at some clinics for the purpose of determining speech recognition in noise, using a random noise masker low-pass filtered with a slope of 12 dB per octave from 1 kHz. This noise is recorded on the same CD as the word lists. With this speech material a fixed SNR is usually chosen and the result is presented as a percentage score.

For both these methods a speech level in the range 60–70 dB SPL is used, corresponding to a normal conversation level at a distance of 1 metre.

Hearing impaired listeners with severe impairment may have difficulties in analysing speech sounds even in quiet and even if the sounds are sufficiently amplified to be audible. The PB lists presented in quiet can be useful to estimate this ability. For patients with a hearing loss too severe to allow the speech-in-noise test to be performed this might be a suitable alternative.

Audio-visual tests

There are no standardized audio-visual tests in Sweden. Various recordings exist at several clinics, some of them have been in use for about 20 years, although none have been scientifically evaluated regarding, for example, list equivalence. Originally they were used mostly for training in lip reading and for assessment of the results of such training. However, there is increasing interest in their use for evaluating the benefit of hearing aids and cochlear implants.

Quality assurance in hearing aid fitting

Recently, considerable interest has been devoted to the development of systematic quality assurance in hearing aid fitting. In Sweden, a national working group has just finished a document defining an acceptable strategy for this purpose, this is gradually being introduced into Swedish hearing centres (Arlinger, 1993). In the assessment of the results of hearing aid fitting, aided speech recognition in noise in comparison with unaided speech recognition is defined as one of the three variables to be measured (the other two are real-ear gain and subjective benefit). In an acceptable hearing aid fitting, aided speech recognition is expected to be equal to or better than unaided.

Testing is based on the presentation of speech (speech level 65 dB measured as equivalent C-weighted sound pressure level) against a background of broad-band speech spectrum noise. Three alternative test procedures with different types of test material are offered. One is based on the determination of the SRT in noise, expressed as the SNR using Hagerman's test sentences (1982). In an adaptive procedure the noise level is varied in 1 dB steps and one or preferably two test lists are used for the calculation of the SNR, Hagerman and Kinnefors (1995).

A second alternative makes use of the PB-test lists with monosyllabic test words and is based on determining a speech recognition score at a fixed SNR, typically in the range 0–10 dB. The best value to use depends on the test room acoustics, placement of loudspeaker(s), exact spectrum of background noise etc. and should be determined according to the local conditions.

The third alternative is called 'just follow conversation' (JFC) (Hawkins et al., 1988; Hygge et al., 1992; Larsby and Arlinger, 1994). This is a method of adjustment, using a recording of continuous normal connected speech. The task of the listener is to adjust the noise level to an SNR at which they can just follow what is being said — an occasional word will be missed but the general message understood. On several occasions during a 3 minute speech passage, the tester changes the noise level abruptly by 10–20 dB and the listener has to readjust the noise level to the stated criterion. The average of these repeated SNR-settings is taken as the test result. The JFC method is very attractive to use for the assessment of the effect of hearing aid fitting on speech recognition because of its subjective character, being a method of adjustment, and its use of normal continuous speech as the test signal — these characteristics giving it high validity. The test–retest reliability seems to be equivalent to that of more conventional speech recognition test methods. However, the clinical experience is still limited.

Speech audiometry for children

Speech audiometry for children is naturally more difficult, since they are still developing their language skills, and thus the possibilities for the construction of test material become rather more limited than with adult patients. Phonetic and linguistic requirements usually have to be adjusted and more emphasis placed on the test words being simple and easy.

No phonetically standardized test material for children exists in Sweden. The test material for paediatric use included on the CD for speech audiometry in Swedish are lists of three digit combinations and very simple mono- and bisyllabic test words. Phonetic balance and equalization are not controlled.

Research and development

The recordings of spondee lists and PB lists used today are almost 30 years old, but there are no plans to re-record them. The technical quality is still acceptable for its general audiological purpose, although not up to date. The main reason for making new lists would be the need to replace some words which have now fallen from common usage. A more urgent requirement, however, is to obtain modern speech test material for children.

Since speech tests are time consuming to perform, an attempt has been made to evaluate their efficiency (Hagerman, 1993). The efficiency is defined by the following formula:

$$E = (v_b / v_w - 1) / T$$

where v_b is the variance between subjects of a relevant population of patients, v_w is the variance within subjects for the same population and T is the time required for a single test. This formula allows the comparison of the efficiency of various speech tests (and other audiological tests), and also takes the time required to perform the test into consideration.

To further enhance the efficiency of Hagerman's sentences, an adaptive method was recently designed to be used with this test material (Hagerman and Kinnefors, 1995). This gave at least 20% improved test–retest reliability for hearing impaired subjects, compared to the figure given earlier.

At the Department of Technical Audiology of the Karolinska Institute, a computer-controlled rhyme word test has been developed. The speech material consists of six consonant lists, testing voiceless initial consonants, and four vowel lists, testing vowels, each list with 40–46 logatoms, i.e. consonant-vowel-consonant combinations without verbal meaning. The speech sounds are stored on the hard disk of a PC. It is a very flexible test and provides several options for testing, e.g. with or without auditive and/or written feedback, or by choosing partial lists with a selected group of phonemes. It can be used for functional diagnosis, hearing aid fitting and auditory training. Hearing impaired users of this material have been very positive about the possibility of auditory training on their own, without any test leader to cause them stress.

The JFC method of adjustment has been the subject of several studies (Risberg and Öhngren, 1989; Hygge et al., 1992; Larsby and Arlinger, 1994). Of special interest is the correlation between results obtained with the JFC method with other methods. Risberg and Öhngren in a study on 13 hearing impaired subjects found no correlation between SRT in noise, using Hagerman's lists, and the SNR for JFC with random noise as masking. In Larsby and Arlinger's study, also comparing SRT using Hagerman's test lists and SNR for JFC but with different types of masking, no significant correlation was found for random noise as masking. However, with speech as masking, presented either in forward or reverse mode, a significant correlation was found. This study was performed on 12 normal hearing and 12 hearing impaired subjects. We may thus conclude that under certain circumstances the speech recognition threshold in noise and the adjustment method (JFC) show some correlation but there are also clearly different mechanisms involved.

At the Department of Speech Transmission and Music Acoustics of the Royal Institute of Technology in Stockholm some work has been done to record new audio-visual tests. The BKB-sentences (Bench and Bamford, 1979) have been translated into Swedish. However, the final editing as a result of the evaluation has not yet been performed. A material designed for interactive training and testing has also been developed. It is stored on an optical disc for the purpose of demonstration. It contains consonants, vowels, rhyme words, various kinds of prosodic distinctions, spondees, everyday sentences, topic-related words and sentences, questions, dialogue, running speech, and, finally, various examples of the mouth-hand system and sign language. However, it does not contain complete, evaluated tests, with alternative lists of equal difficulty.

Technical equipment

Since 1988 the test material used in most clinical applications of speech audiometry in Sweden has been available as a CD. This recording technology, being based on optical detection of digital information, provides a very wide dynamic range, low noise and negligible loss of quality with repeated use.

The Swedish CD for speech audiometry contains the spondee lists used for SRT determinations, the PB- monosyllabic test lists for determining maximum speech recognition scores, test lists for children and 10 sentence lists as produced by Hagerman (1982). Three test lists with interrupted speech (seven interruptions per second; Korsan-Bengtsen, 1973) are also included. In addition, five test lists with bisyllabic test words in Finnish (Jauhiainen, 1974) are recorded, since a considerable number of people with Finnish as their native language live in Sweden. Finally, a frequency sweep is included to provide a means for checking the frequency response of the complete equipment for speech audiometry.

Today, equipment is available which makes it possible to record a small number of CDs in a local laboratory. This gives access to the same technical advantages as the general CD technology for special applications and for the recording of speech test material with more limited applications.

Calibration

A well known problem in speech audiometry is calibration, i.e. the exact measurement of the levels used, both of the speech signal and of the competing noise sound. On the Swedish CD for speech audiometry, the calibration signal recorded at the beginning of the CD is used to measure the sound level. The relation between this signal and the various speech test lists then provides the correction needed to calculate the true speech level.

Within the International Organization for Standardization, (ISO), Technical Committee 43, a working group has addressed the task of formulating an ISO-standard on speech audiometry. A standard has just been approved and published (ISO 8253-3, 1996). Unfortunately, the definitions of speech level and competing sound level are not as specific as desirable. Speech level is defined as 'The sound pressure level or the vibratory force level of the speech signal as measured in an appropriate coupler, artificial ear or sound field with specified frequency weighting and specified time weighting'. However, no recommendation has been agreed with regard to which frequency and time weighting to use.

In Sweden an informal trend can be seen towards the use of C-weighting for the frequency weighting and the use of the equivalent sound pressure level over the relevant time with silent pauses of significant duration omitted from the measurement time. This is based on the absence of evidence for any weighting to have superior correlation with speech recognition. The C-weighting is then a rather arbitrary choice — with the alternative being A-weighting. The equivalent level or long term integration has the advantage of not requiring any visual averaging and therefore provides good reproducibility of the speech level measured (Ludvigsen, 1992). Hopefully, this choice of weightings will gradually spread, and so facilitate inter-laboratory comparisons.

Chapter 14
Speech audiometry in Australia

JOHN BENCH

In writing for a book on speech audiometry which has a marked international flavour, it is worth taking a little space to comment on some general characteristics of Australia and its population. Such characteristics will set a context for a discussion of Australian work in speech audiometry, which has developed very considerably in recent years, and thereby assist the reader to appreciate the discussion which follows.

It is well known internationally that Australia occupies a very large land mass, which approaches the size of the United States of America. It is also well known that much of the country is desert or semi-desert (colloquial reference is made to the 'red centre'), which is sparsely populated. Most of the population lives close to the coast, especially the east and south-east coasts, which have hilly or mountainous regions close by (the Great Dividing Range), attract reasonable rainfall, and hence can support a population, which now totals some 18 million souls. The most recent specific figure, for 1992, is 17.5 million (Castles, 1994).

What is much less well known is that about 64% of the Australian population is concentrated in the major eight city areas, which have grown up alongside the few great rivers, and a further significant proportion is based in the smaller towns, many recently developed on the east coast. Hence the Australian population is heavily urbanized. About 85% of the people lead an urban or suburban existence. They visit the deep country or desert areas relatively rarely, and then mainly for leisure purposes. The provision of audiological services is thus not greatly affected by issues of distance for the great majority of Australians. However, Australia does have other special problems.

Immigration and ethnicity

Population has always been an issue in Australia (Birrell and Birrell, 1981: Palmer and Short, 1989), usually on the grounds that there were not enough people, or that the rate of expansion of the population was too slow, or that the birthrate was falling. Australia has had a generous attitude to immigration and to refugees, and this attitude is reflected in its ethnic diversity and its population growth. The population has more than doubled from the 7.6 million of 1947 (Birrell and Birrell, 1981), in large part due to the encouragement of immigration, which has in recent years accounted for about half of the population growth (Castles, 1994). Since the Second World War, this emphasis on immigration has increasingly emphasized immigration from Europe other than the UK and Eire. More recently a large proportion of immigrants has been taken from north-east and south-east Asia. Thus about 20% of the Australian population was born overseas and around 14% does not have English as a first language.

There is then a large minority of non-Anglo-Australians comprised of ethnic groups. These ethnic people (and often their children) do not have English as their first language. This situation may not be appreciated by the non-Australian reader, who may have been led to expect that any lack of familiarity with English would be limited to the Aboriginal population (Aboriginals and Torres Strait Islanders). The latter population is, however, small (Castles, 1994) albeit with a high prevalence of middle ear disease, especially amongst its young children (Lewis, 1979; Boswell et al.,1994). It amounts to around 1.5% of the total population, and most of its members speak good or fair English. Aboriginal Health Workers are aware of the value of assessing and remediating hearing problems in children (Anderson, 1988).

It might be thought that special efforts would have been made to develop materials and techniques in speech audiometry for the relatively large ethnic population, and to train ethnic staff to administer and assess the results of such special speech audiometric tests. Such developments have frequently been discussed by audiologists and some teachers of the deaf. But these developments are only beginning to be explored in a systematic way. The main reason is that the Anglo-Australians are by far the dominant social and cultural group, and ethnic or cultural pluralism ('multiculturalism') as government policy is a relatively recent phenomenon (Martin, 1978; Palmer and Short, 1989).

In this context, one of the first published Australian studies to illustrate the nature of the problem (Smith et al., 1987) compared the performance on the widely used open set Boothroyd (1968) word lists (Australian voice recording) of normally hearing monolingual Greek, monolingual Australian English and bilingual Greek/Australian English adults.

The test materials were presented to one ear at 75 dB HTL, with masking of the contralateral ear at 45 dB HTL. Results showed that, although a few bilingual subjects performed as well as the native English speakers, overall both groups of non-native speakers performed significantly poorer than the native speakers. Elliot and Doyle (1994) recently obtained similar results with Boothroyd words and BKB/A sentence lists (Bench and Doyle, 1979) for monolingual Italian, monolingual Australian-English, and bilingual Italian/Australian-English speakers. The poorer scores of the ethnic groups occurred mainly because of reduced familiarity with both the English consonants and vowels used — of which, for example, up to 30% do not exist or do not exactly match those in Greek. The findings suggested that it is not realistic to re-standardize open set English speech audiometry tests on non-native English speakers, but that such groups should be assessed in their native language, or that purpose-designed tests should be developed for them (Danhauer et al., 1984). Such a purpose-designed test could be constructed as a nonsense syllable test, probably best presented in closed set format (Preston, 1991), containing phonemes with equal frequency of occurrence in the two languages.

The provision of audiological and aural rehabilitation services

A useful recent publication of the Australian Bureau of Statistics (1993) indicated the prevalence of hearing disability in Australia at around 2–3% of the population, the second highest disabling condition after arthritis/musculoskeletal diseases. However, the figure of 2–3% has been criticized as far too low (e.g. Deafness Forum, 1994) with indications that up to 20% may be a more valid figure. Earlier Australian Bureau of Statistics surveys (1979, 1980) themselves gave prevalence data of up to 10%, suggesting variation in survey technique. The two earlier surveys covered hearing problems by age, sex, cause, age at first occurrence, surgical operations, possession of a hearing aid, prices of aids, types of aids, use and non-use of aids, recency of tests and types of tests (with or without an audiometer, but it is not possible to discover from the reports how many of the audiometric tests involved speech audiometry).

The main national agency for the provision of audiological services is the Australian Hearing Services (AHS), formerly the National Acoustic Laboratories (NAL). AHS has its main base in Sydney, where its techniques are researched in what are still called the National Acoustic Laboratories, and clinical centres in the major cities throughout the several states of the country. The very large cities, such as Melbourne and Sydney, may have several AHS centres. AHS has been active for many years in audiological diagnostics, including speech audiometry and in the design and development of hearing aids. There has been recently increased emphasis on rehabilitation and counselling. AHS services are free for those under 21 years, over retiring age, or otherwise in receipt of a pension or in a special category, but adults of working age must pay for their hearing aids. Other main agencies providing audiological services include hospitals (especially the larger hospitals), but there are a large number of other agencies which provide some audiological services, the sum total of which is far from negligible (cf. Bench and Duerdoth, 1983).

These agencies make a considerable contribution to aural rehabilitation, covering counselling, education, training and advice, as well as those aspects of aural rehabilitation immediately related to hearing impairment (e.g. how to get the best performance from a hearing aid). The provision of services through these agencies is a complex operation involving a large number of professional, semi-professional, ancillary and volunteer personnel (Bench and Duerdoth, 1983). Also, the types of agencies are quite different, involving public, private and charitable organizations. This results in the potential for communication problems between agencies and possible confusion for patients. To avoid such problems, most agencies are members of (or, in some cases, have observer status in) the Deafness Forum, a government-assisted body which offers a coordinating umbrella function for all concerned with hearing impairment and services to hearing impaired people in Australia.

Speech audiometry and Australian English usage

The assessment of hearing for speech is clearly dependent on the familiarity of the speech material to the listener. This means that the English content of material for speech audiometry in Australia should reflect Australian English usage. Australian English has a basic similarity to English as spoken in the UK, but increasingly reflects North American English usage, besides containing some expressions, phrases, and word usages which are essentially Australian (e.g. 'milk bar', very roughly equivalent to the American 'drug store' or the English 'corner shop'). Standard Australian English is very similar to standard English as regards grammar, but a minority of words (especially nouns or noun phrases and some verbs) as used in English may have a somewhat different meaning in Australia (Bench and Doyle, 1979). Thus whereas in Australia one 'barracks for' (i.e. expresses support), in the UK one 'barracks against' (i.e. decries), a team or group. Interestingly, the verb 'to barrack' in the sense of 'decry' or 'jeer' as used in the UK is Aboriginal Australian in origin, whereas, used in the sense of support, it is Irish in origin ('MacQuarie Dictionary'). There has been something of a cross-over in usage between the two hemispheres. For the reader who may wish to consider these matters further, the style and usages of Australian English have been reported by Blair (1977) and Mitchell and Delbridge (1965a,b).

Word and phoneme tests and their usage

The major audiological centres (AHS and audiology departments in the larger hospitals and in tertiary education institutions) make use of a variety of word and phoneme tests for clinical speech audiometry, most of which will be familiar to audiologists in English-speaking countries. Many of the more esoteric tests are used as screening tests for the more difficult-to-test patients, and as adjuncts to the clinical assessment of patients with central auditory processing problems, or hearing difficulties associated with ageing (Erber, 1992; Lee and Dermody, 1994).

In earlier work, Upfold and Smither (1981) outlined the use of the CUNY nonsense syllable test (Levitt and Resnik, 1978), the modified rhyme test, the Norton HRRC rhyme test (see later), the monosyllable-trochee-spondee test (Erber and Alencewicz, 1976), and the SPIN test (Kalikow et al., 1977, adapted for Australian speech characteristics) in a systematic hearing aid fitting protocol. This set of tests was designed for demonstration, counselling, training and potential verification of phonetic correlates of aided pure-tone information.

Probably the most commonly used test (especially as an initial speech audiometry test) is the Boothroyd word lists (Boothroyd, 1968), usually scored by whole words reported correctly. The lists are available in Australia from recordings spoken with a general Australian accent. Boothroyd's word lists are popular clinically because of their long history of usage, familiarity to all audiologists, convenient length and convenience of scoring. Other tests currently used include the Kendall toy test (Kendall, 1956), the word intelligibility by picture identification (WIPI) test (Ross and Lerman, 1970), the paediatric speech intelligibility test (Jerger and Jerger, 1984), the modified rhyme test (House et al., 1965), the HRRC rhyme test (Eisenberg et al., 1977), various nonsense syllable tests and the PLOTT test (Australian: Plant, 1984b). The CAL-PBM word lists (Australian: Macrae et al., 1963) and the Clark PB word lists (Australian: Clark, 1981) are no longer frequently used (see later).

Of these the PLOTT test, as developed by Plant and his colleagues in Sydney, represents an attempt to devise a comprehensive speech perception test. It consists of nine subtests for phoneme detection; number patterns; monosyllable, trochee, spondee and polysyllable distinctions; a picture vocabulary test; vowel length discrimination; vowel discrimination; initial voiced and voiceless stop consonant discrimination; consonant manner of articulation discrimination; and discrimination of place of articulation for consonants. The PLOTT test helps in deciding whether a severely to profoundly hearing impaired person can perceive spectral information, or only time and intensity cues. Many children with hearing losses greater than 100 dB (ISO) were found by Plant (1984b) to use spectral information in speech perception, and even those children who seemed to be limited to the use of time/intensity cues were able to distinguish between a number of vowel and consonant contrasts. A clinically significant drawback of the PLOTT test is that it is lengthy to administer, typically taking 1 to 2 hours. Partly as a result, Martin and Gillies (1994) have suggested that the subtests of the PLOTT test be used in a selective way, depending on the information sought and the abilities of the child.

It is of interest that the CAL-PBMs and the Clark lists were especially designed for Australian usage, yet they are now infrequently used. Why should this be so? The CAL-PBM lists consist of 12 lists each of 25 monosyllables, designed to be phonemically balanced across lists and to reflect common occurrence in Australian speech. However, Grant (1980) showed that, although 34% of the phonemes correlated well, 44% did not correlate well, with a sample of Australian speech. Further, across the lists, 29% of phonemes showed a wide range of occurrence, but 66% of phonemes did not occur in one or more lists. She concluded that the CAL-PBM lists could not be considered to be phonemically balanced.

Clark's word lists were derived from the Northwestern University auditory test No.6 (NU-6), but were specially designed for Australian English. Clark's criteria for the design were: (1) monosyllabic consonent-vowel-consonent word structure; (2) exact interlist phonological balance; (3) minimal intralist phonotactic redundancy; (4) high lexical familiarity; and (5) phonological distribution generally compatible with that for monosyllabic words in Australian English. Clark's lists do not appear to have been taken up by Australian audiologists to any great extent, despite their apparent virtues. The main reasons are clear: there are too few lists and each list is rather long (there are only four lists, each of 50 monosyllables). It seems then that the CAL-PBM lists are phonemically suspect, and each list is relatively long (25 monosyllables compared with Boothroyd's 12 monosyllables), while the Clark lists are much too few, and each list is too long, for regular clinical use.

Byrne (1983) in Sydney has reviewed the area of word intelligibility in speech audiometry as it affects the assessment of speech hearing in children. Byrne noted that a basic principle in designing word intelligibility tests is that the words should be familiar to the youngest age group for which the test is designed. He found that his youngest age group of children tested (4.5 to 6.5 years of age) performed at a poorer level than the next youngest group (6.5 to 8 years), and both these groups performed more poorly than his oldest group (8 to 14 years), even though all the stimulus words, in a closed set, were known to the children. This finding confirms similar reports elsewhere (e.g. in the USA by Elliot et al., 1983). It seems that knowledge of stimulus words is not enough; experience of the words is an important factor also, and such experience needs to be considered in devising speech audiometry materials (cf. Bench and Bamford, 1979). Byrne commented that speech perception thresholds calculated for young children, if interpreted according to expectations of adult performance, could be interpreted as a hearing loss for speech, when their performance fell inside the usual range for their age group. The implications for patient management of making such an error are clear, as is the need for a 'normal subjective calibration' of any speech test materials. In passing, we may note that a somewhat similar error may be incurred if the data of speech audiometric tests with words are interpreted as directly reflecting everyday hearing of spoken English (cf. Hood and Poole, 1971), because word lists do not contain grammatical and contextual cues.

Sentence tests and usage

Sentence lists and other suprasegmental tests are used relatively rarely in routine speech audiometry testing in Australia (as elsewhere), largely because of constraints on clinical time. Some use is made of the SPIN test (Kalikow et al., 1977), where there is a need to control for context predictability, and the minimal auditory capabilities (MAC) test battery (Owens et al., 1980) is used in some centres (Blamey et al., 1985). As Clark (1981) has pointed out, the choice between word lists and sentences as test material for speech audiometry depends upon the intended application and test stringency. Sentences offer high-level contextual linguistic cues in their semantic and syntactic structure, enabling a listener to predict a word fairly accurately with relatively little reliance on the acoustic information from the actual stimulus material. Words, however, require more stringent perceptual skills on the part of the listener in that the listener is forced to rely heavily on the acoustic information of the test words.

The two main open set everyday sentence tests developed for use in Australia are those of Tonisson (1977) and Bench and Doyle (1979), while Plant and Moore (1992a,b) have recently produced closed set sentence tests which may be more appropriate for profoundly hearing impaired children who have difficulties with open set materials. Tonisson's lists reflect the Central Institute of the Deaf (Davis and Silverman, 1970) Everyday Sentences. They consist of nine lists, each containing 10 sentences or common phrases and 50 key words. The phraseology used and the length of the sentences makes these sentences appropriate for persons with relatively advanced linguistic abilities such as older children and adults, especially if deafened post-lingually, rather than the younger hearing impaired child. Bench and Doyle prepared an Australian version of the BKB (Bench and Bamford, 1979) sentence lists for use with hearing impaired children from age 8 years, which contains 21 sentence lists each of 16 sentences, with 50 key words per list. A standardization of the resulting BKB/A (Bamford-

Kowal-Bench/Australian version) sentence test (Bench et al., 1987) on a large sample of children with a wide range of hearing impairments showed the BKB/A test to be more sensitive than the Australian CID and CAI-PBM tests. This difference was ascribed to the more appropriate linguistic basis of the BKB/A material, which was derived from the spoken grammar and vocabulary used by hearing impaired children themselves. The BKB/A sentence test has recently become available also as a standardized test for speechreading (Bench et al., 1993).

A feature of sentence lists scored by key words is that the key words may be taken from the sentences and randomly ordered as word lists. Provided that the word lists so derived are arranged within the same listings as the original sentence lists, it is then possible to compare performance on the original sentence lists and the derived word lists, to assess the contribution of grammar and semantic associations (Bench, 1992). This feature can be clinically very useful in aural rehabilitation programmes.

The need for clarification of aims

It is puzzling (Merklein, 1981) that clinical testing with phonemically balanced word lists is so persistent worldwide in the light of recent work on speech pattern tests and sentence tests, and general clinical practice in Australia is no exception.

PB word lists are open to criticism for their often large, inappropriate vocabularies, open-response format and learning effects (cf. Byrne, 1983). Merklein argued for speech-hearing tests which took account of spectral or speech-envelope information as a way to go. He offered a short test for severely and profoundly deaf children which compared perception of speech envelope vs. spectral patterns, and suprasegmental (prosodic) vs. segmental (phonemic) aspects. As we have seen, this more focused approach to speech audiometry has been led in Australia by Plant and his colleagues.

The continuing routine clinical use of conventional PB word lists possibly endures because clinical audiologists tend to select tests that will quickly yield some overview of the patient's speech perception abilities. Further, because the PB word tests are well known and widely used, communication of results is made easy. However, this nowadays somewhat facile approach to speech audiometry falls well short of providing specific information about the acoustic particulars of speech perception in severe to profound hearing impairment, for which speech pattern tests are much more informative. Also, it can be misleading as an index of everyday speech hearing performance, which requires open-set connected speech perception testing. In short, it is difficult to see a continuing general clinical role for PB word lists.

Australian speech audiometry and cochlear implant prostheses

What follows only samples some salient aspects of Australian studies of speech perception testing of cochlear implantees. A more fulsome treatment would require a chapter of its own.

Work in the field of the cochlear implant prosthesis has proved to be multifaceted. Partly as a result, it has prompted further scrutiny of the aims of speech perception testing, especially for those patients with profound to total hearing loss, who have been the main source of candidates for implantation. Even so, it is not uncommon to find reports of speech perception by cochlear implantees using a variety of tests (e.g. Busby et al., 1989; Dawson et al., 1992), though at least part of the explanation for this situation lies in the wide range of abilities in speech perception found amongst implantees. Thus, Busby et al. (1989) employed the closed-set tests: the monosyllable-spondee-trochee-polysyllable test (Plant, 1984), the picture vocabulary test (Plant, 1984), the sound effects recognition test (Finitzo-Hieber et al., 1980), Northwestern University — children's perception of speech (NU-CHIPS) (Elliot and Katz, 1980), and the segmental speech feature test (Plant, 1984), together with the open set BKB sentence test, in assessing the speech perception of two profoundly to totally deaf children fitted with multi-electrode cochlear implants.

Open set word tests constrain the response set very lightly; practically the whole lexicon is available. Open set sentence tests scored by key words, with their grammatical and semantic associations, constrain responses more than open set words, but even so allow for some choice of words from the lexicon. On the other hand, a convenience of open set tests, which is often overlooked, is that with open set materials chance performance is virtually zero (Dowell et al., 1986). Thus, although it is all but impossible to isolate the effect of an implant and training in its use because of confounding, the benefit provided by the implant is strongly indicated when non-zero scores are obtained with no stimulus input other than the auditory signal from the device (Dawson et al., 1992).

Closed set tests have been designed which do not test speech understanding itself, but are concerned with perception of the prosthesis' electrical stimuli, transformed from restricted sets of speech sounds which can be discriminated by people with normal hearing (Millar et al., 1984). Such tests may be particularly suitable in assessing the performance of prelingual implantees, who perform relatively worse on tests of vowel and consonant perception than postlingual patients (Tong et al., 1988; Busby et al., 1991). Further, acoustic cues, at 20 dB SL above the frequency range where the subjects could detect normally amplified speech, have been used successfully to train non-implanted hearing impaired children to differentiate /s/ and /z/ sounds which they could not detect with hearing aids (Blamey et al., 1990). The cues were produced by amplitude-modulating white noise and then high-pass filtering at 5 kHz, with the modulation frequency at the fundamental frequency for /z/ and the fixed rate of 50 Hz for /s/.

Closed set sentences have been used to augment the test options described above (Millar et al., 1984) by expanding the range of cues to assess the perception of suprasegmentals, such as patterns of intonation, syllable counts and rhythm. Such tests are constructed so that the listener is required to discriminate amongst a restricted number of experimental features presented against a common speech background.

In addition to the above test materials, cochlear implantation programmes have drawn attention to the use of connected discourse tracking (De Filippo and Scott, 1978). Here the listener is required to repeat a story read in short phrases, and is scored on the number of words per minute correctly repeated. Various tactics can be used by the clinician or experimenter to prompt the listener when responses are not correct. Connected discourse tracking has proved useful in training cochlear implantees in simulations of aspects of everyday discourse, while providing a measure of performance at the same time (Millar et al., 1984).

Summary

Speech audiometry in Australia is conducted much like speech audiometry in other English-speaking countries. The same kinds of tests are used, usually adapted for Australian needs, there is a wide range of such tests in use, the same techniques are employed, and the same problems are encountered.

One area where Australia has needs, which are rather different from some other English-speaking countries, is that of designing and using speech audiometry tests for its significant ethnic population, which comes mainly from Europe (excluding the UK and Eire) and from North and South East Asia. Work in this field is just beginning.

Australia differs too, in having a major national service, the Australian Hearing Services (AHS), with a central research laboratory (NAL) in Sydney and clinical centres distributed across the country. AHS allows standardization of approaches to speech audiometry and other services. It has the potential to provide clinical information for a large number of patients over a period of many years. The following chapter by Dermody and Lee goes some way to illustrating this situation.

Chapter 15
Speech tests at the National Acoustic Laboratories

PHILLIP DERMODY and KERRIE LEE

In the time since the development and use of speech tests at the National Acoustic Laboratories (NAL) was described by Dermody and Mackie (1987) in the first edition of this book, NAL has been incorporated into an organization called the Australian Hearing Services (AHS) which continues to provide the national clinical audiological services and hearing aid provision in Australia as described by Dermody and Mackie (1987). The name NAL is now reserved for the research and engineering functions of the organization. Some the speech tests to be described in this review are used routinely in the clinical service of AHS after having been investigated by the NAL research groups while some tests are still being developed at the NAL. For simplicity the organization will be referred to as AHS/NAL throughout this review.

Speech reception assessment continues to be a major interest within AHS/NAL. Only the major developments since the last review by Dermody and Mackie (1987) will be described. The major speech assessment activities can be divided into speech database activities, developments for adult assessment and developments for child assessment methods.

Speech database development

One of the areas that has received little consideration in speech test development in audiology is speech databases that might better reflect different speaker characteristics and thereby extend the applicability of materials used in speech reception assessment. While the limitation of standardized materials has always been recognized — that results cannot be easily generalized beyond the speaker used — the full implications of this limitation have mostly been overlooked. The recognition of the differences between the Rush Hughes and W-22 recordings is an often cited example (e.g. Goetzinger, 1972) of how significantly different results can be obtained for different standardized speech test materials using similar words but different speakers/replay conditions.

Another problem is that speech tests have always been recorded in what is known as citation form. Words have been spoken carefully in isolation under ideal recording circumstances. These materials are unlikely to represent the type of speech confronted by hearing impaired listeners in everyday communication situations.

While attempting to maintain the rigour of standardized materials to be presented under controlled conditions in audiological testing but also attempting to select speech materials to provide more realistic assessments, we have begun the collection of different speech databases to provide a bigger pool of speakers and to characterize those speakers into categories of intelligibility.

To date several sets have been developed. The first of these collected under the Australian National Database of Spoken Language (ANDOSL) project (Millar, et al., 1990a,b; Milla et al., 1994) will provide a good range of Australian speakers for selection of high and low intelligibility speakers. The second database is based on four speakers chosen to represent Australian speech dialects that are used for category scaling judgements of quality. The ANDOSL speech database is a long term project and currently no materials are available for clinical application. The results of tests using the category scaling database will be described later.

Standardization of materials for performance intensity function assessment

Following more traditional aims of assessment using a carefully selected speaker and citation speech samples, a set of materials have been developed to provide assessment of performance-intensity (P-I) functions for adult clients in AHS clinics.

The use of P-I functions for speech reception assessment is well accepted. In the initial assessment of hearing impairment P-I functions can provide a between-ear comparison which will often show significant differences in speech reception capability even for ears that do not seem to differ much in their pure-tone audiograms. Second, the use of the P-I function in initial assessments can provide an important estimate of the relative receptive communicative capability of the hearing impaired person under test. P-I functions remain the most used supra-threshold test of hearing for hearing impaired persons and the only one employing complex signals. Therefore speech tests play an important role in understanding the nature and extent of the hearing loss for communication that occurs at supra-threshold levels. Extending the use of speech tests to assessment of aided advantage might be criticized as being too inefficient for deciding between different hearing aids and also redundant for measuring hearing aid gain but the use of speech tests to evaluate the final fitting and provide an estimate of the likely receptive communicative effectiveness of the hearing aid user remains an important but under-utilized component in hearing aid audiology.

Standardization of materials for performance-intensity function measurement

The most widely used materials for measuring P-I functions were originally developed by Boothroyd in 1968. These materials include 15 lists of 'isophonemic' words that were generated to include the 10 vowels and 20 consonants that occurred most frequently in the author's vocabulary of consonant-vowel-consonant words.

Various recordings of these materials are available and standardization of different recordings have been reported (Boothroyd,1968; Markides, 1978a; Greville, 1984). In addition, data on similar material (Olsen, Van Tasell and Speaks, 1982) has also been documented. NAL began a standardization of a modified version of the original materials based on minor modifications to the vocabulary utilized by Stevenson (1975).

The NAL standardised materials are available as a compact disc (CD) recording which incorporates list orderings based on the normal hearing standardization data. Cafeteria noise is provided on the second channel to provide estimates of speech in noise performance as required.

Recording of materials

The modified AB lists were recorded by a male speaker through a high fidelity microphone and amplification system onto a computer disc (16 bit A/D with 36 K sampling rate). These materials were edited by an experienced acoustic-phonetician who marked the beginning and end of each word. The edited files were stored on computer disc for producing different randomized orders.

The files were prepared for output by changing the output order of the original lists based on previous clinical experience with the lists but all words in the modified lists described by Stevenson (1975) were maintained in each list.

All words were digitally processed through an Leq equalization program which brought all 150 words to the same level. This technique has been shown to provide a decrease in variance for responses to words presented in an adaptive test method (Dermody, Katsch and Mackie 1983a)

Preparation and presentation of listening tapes

The materials were recorded onto high quality cassette recordings so that different counterbalancing occurred for different list presentation orders. Complete counterbalancing of list presentation order was not attempted but all lists occurred in at least two different order positions with one of these being with the list presented first in the testing.

Normal listeners were chosen and presented with one of the counterbalanced tapes. Each listener heard each list but in different orders. Each counterbalanced list order was presented to 24 listeners. The listeners were recruited from various government departments and represented a reasonable cross-section of ages (from about 20 to 55 years) and educational levels. The group was reasonably homogeneous in terms of socio-economic levels.

Listeners responded by repeating the words which were written down verbatim by the experimenter on prepared answer sheets based on the counterbalanced order being presented. The written responses were also scored for number of phonemes correct at the time of test.

Listeners were tested in a hearing test booth and heard the words through TDH-39 earphones presented via a Madsen OB-822 audiometer. The level was changed after each list in a fixed order going from highest level 40 dB SPL to the lowest level (20 dB SPL) in 5 dB steps. The boundary conditions had been chosen after pilot investigations demonstrated levels between 30% and 90% correct for normal listeners. No attempt was made to measure below about 30% correct because of the increased variance usually observed at low presentation levels and because the points of interest in the P-I function are the rising portion of the function typically between 25–75% correct. Reduction of the levels also resulted in savings in test time for the standardization.

Results

The results for phoneme scores from the standardization (which are available in the test manual) indicate that the performance of the normal listeners showed good consistency at each presentation level and the scores represents approximately the theoretical minimum of variability based on a 30-item test.

Figure 15.1 shows the summary data, which compares the function obtained for each list. Variability between lists is considerably greater than the variability between the individual words in each list but appears to be less than the interlist variability reported by Greville (1984) as well as Markides (1978a).

Recording of the clinical materials

The lists were arranged to match consecutively as closely as possible. That is, the P-I function of each list was matched as closely as possible to another list and these were recorded consecutively on the final version. This was done for several reasons. First, in initial audiological assessments it is useful to measure the performance of each ear, but to

NALAB PI FUNCTIONS

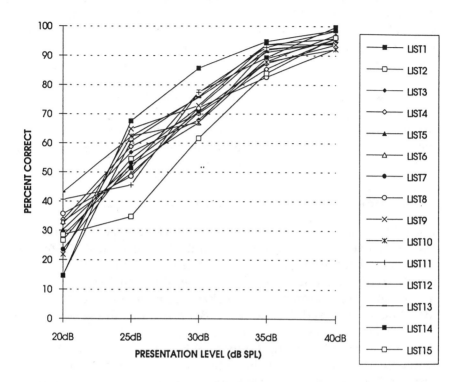

Figure 15.1 Results show the average scores in percent correct as a function of presentation level in dB SPL for the NAL recordings of the AB materials

avoid practice effects it is desirable to present a list alternatively to the left and right ear during testing. By matching consecutive lists we can improve the reliability of inter-ear comparisons. Similarly, if it is required to measure different aided conditions to compare the communicative improvement of each condition (e.g. monaural vs. binaural) it might also be useful to try to test each condition consecutively. Finally, if it is necessary to try to improve reliability of speech tests by presenting more items in evaluation it is useful to have lists that are matched for combined presentation.

The recorded digital materials were digitally transferred to produce CD masters. On the second channel of the CD a noise was recorded. The noise was the same segment of cafeteria noise that is presented against each word in each list. The duration of the noise is determined by the word duration. The noise is only presented overlapping the word so that listeners do not have to perform a vigilance task attending to speech in continuous noise. The listener is cued by approximately 500 milliseconds of noise that starts before the spoken word.

Cafeteria noise was selected based on the results in Figure 15.2. These data show that cafeteria noise produces more masking when compared to a noise proposed by Schroeder (1968) which whitens the spectral information while maintaining the same time waveform envelope of the original material. An additive four speaker babble noise was also tested for comparison and its difficulty was intermediate between the whitened temporal envelope noise and the cafeteria noise. Figure 15.3 shows that there is good correspondence between two selections of cafeteria noise. The most difficult masking condition was chosen for the final recording on the CD to provide a difficult listening environment and one that might better represent the difficulties experienced by hearing impaired listeners in typical situations.

Comparison with other AB or related materials standardization

It is difficult to provide direct comparisons with available reports of AB list performance. In the original study by Boothroyd (1968) the phoneme scores for a group of normal hearing children are presented but the scores were transformed by using the modal value to correct individual scores. Boothroyd notes that the gradient of the P-I function for adults is increased. Markides (1978a) provides a full set of P-I functions for various ages but reports the P-I function relative to the speech detection thresholds of the listeners. While it is likely that this value would be around 20 dB SPL the individual corrections that would have resulted may distort comparisons with results reported in absolute dB

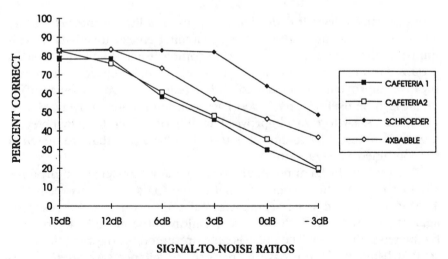

Figure 15.2 Results show the average scores in percent correct for the NALAB lists presented in four different noises at six signal-to-noise ratios

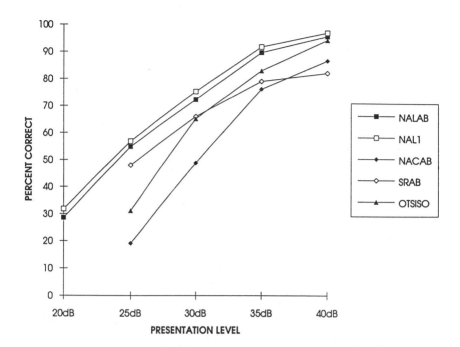

Figure 15.3 Data showing comparisons of other AB or related materials standardization results compared to the NALAB and NAL1 recordings

SPL measures. A similar problem occurs for comparison with a standardization of a new set of isophonemic words based on the Boothroyd material reported by Olsen et al., (1982). The performance of listeners on the Southhampton Recording of the AB (SRAB) lists and the Olsen, Van Tassell, and Speaks isophonemic (OVTSISO) lists are included on the graph by assuming that the sensation level of speech is approximately 8 dB less than the level at which listeners get 50% correct. A study by Greville (1984) reports data in the same form as the present results and can be used for direct comparison.

Concurrently with the AB standardization a second set of words was also standardized in the AHS/NAL study. These words had been generated to include vocabulary items that were more familiar than those used in the AB lists. Word familiarity has been noted as an important variable in word discrimination testing (Savin, 1963; Campbell, 1965; Schultz, 1964) and it was thought that inclusion of more familiar words might provide a steeper P-I function for speech reception assessment. These lists were recorded by the same speaker as the NAL AB lists (NALAB) and were prepared and presented in the same way to the same set of listeners. The results for these lists (NAL1) are also presented for comparison with the NALAB lists.

Figure 15.3 shows the results scored for phonemes correct in the Greville study (NACAB), the Markides study (SRAB), the Olsen et al. study (OTSISO) compared to the NALAB and NAL1 lists. The data indicate that there is a very close correspondence with the NALAB and NAL1 lists. In general, there is some consistency in slope between portions of the NAL recordings and the SRAB and OTSISO lists while the NACAB results show a large difference to all studies with very low performance at both the 25 and 30 dB SPL levels. Both NAL recordings show higher performance levels than all reported studies but this may be due to errors in correction of the levels in the SRAB and OTSISO studies from SL to SPL.

If the SL to SPL conversion is approximately correct the performance differences between the lists of words in each of the studies may be due to the different level equalization techniques used. In the case of the NAL lists an A-weighted Leq equalization was employed. The OVTSISO lists used a level equalization method based on peak measures. This technique provides equalization based on only the vowel level while the A-weighted Leq measures take in the whole signal by dividing the level by the duration of the signal. The A-weighting is used to bring the level closer to that of the human listener (e.g. Fuller, 1987). Dermody et al., (1983a) reported that A-weighted Leq adjustments improved recognition thresholds and reduced variance in monosyllabic adaptive testing compared to other methods of level equalization. The use of the Leq method that takes duration into account and may make low amplitude signals louder than peak level may lead to overall better performance for this normalization method. No equalization procedures are reported for the NACAB standardization and this may have contributed to the lower performance levels although the large discrepancy between this and the other studies remains unexplained.

It can be noted that phoneme scores might be expected to be about 25% greater than word scores for the same material at low presentation levels (Coles, Markides and Priede, 1973; Markides, 1978b). Given that P-I functions for word scores are typically around 5–10% correct at 20 dB SPL and around 25% correct for 25 dB SPL levels (e.g. Beattie and Raffin, 1985) then the performance levels for the NAL lists of approximately 30% and 55% correct respectively at these presentation levels is consistent with findings for other speech materials.

The slight improvement in performance for the NAL1 lists is in the expected direction given that the words had been chosen to be more familiar than the words in the NALAB lists. However, the word familiarity advantage is slight and indicates that use of the AB materials provides a good estimate of P-I functions when compared with a list with more familiar items.

Possible clinical uses of the AB recorded materials

A previous section already discussed the value of P-I functions in assessment but there may also be other possible uses for P-I in hearing aid applications.

In a study reported by Dillon (1993), insertion gain of hearing aids was compared to speech gain using the AHS/NAL AB lists. Dillon concluded from the study that speech gain could be predicted from electroacoustic measurements with only about 3 dB error. However, consideration of individual results suggests the value of considering the speech gain data to decide on overall benefit of hearing aid fitting. In Figure 7 of Dillon (1993) reproduced here as Figure 15.4, two of the 12 (or 16%) of the sample of hearing impaired listeners show very little speech gain when aided and unaided performance P-I functions are compared. A third listener also shows very little aided advantage for speech levels up to 40 dB SPL. It might be argued therefore that these two or three listeners (or 16 – 24%) of the sample were receiving little speech communication benefit through their hearing aids. These listeners were also the ones with the best unaided P-I functions of the sample. That is, while the speech gain for these listeners may have been predictable from the electroacoustic measurements the validity check of their aided benefit confirms that little practical benefit may be obtained from their use of the hearing aid in quiet conditions. Other advantages from the hearing aid fitting may be present but the results suggest that additional time might need to be spent with these persons to discuss aided benefit, at least for speech in quiet.

A second potential benefit of carrying out P-I evaluations for aided listeners is when the results cannot be predicted from simple electro-acoustic measures. Figure 15.5 shows the result of elderly listeners aged between 60 to 80 years compared to listeners aged 80 years and above. It seems clear that the elderly listeners demonstrate a roll-off at higher presentation levels that is not evident in the younger elderly listeners. While this phenomenon has been noted in previous studies of elderly listeners (e.g. Jerger and Jerger, 1971; Gang, 1976; Shrinian and Arnst, 1980, 1982; Meyer and Mishler, 1985) it is not clear yet whether the roll-over of the functions of elderly listeners has implications for hearing aid fitting. However, this result noted in the elderly may represent a subtle demonstration of effects that may occur in the situations in which elderly persons use their hearing aids.

Subjective scaling methods

Subjective scaling methods for speech quality etc. do not have a primary use for auditory function assessment but can provide important information for hearing aid evaluations as well as assessment of new speech processing strategies that might be tried with the hearing impaired.

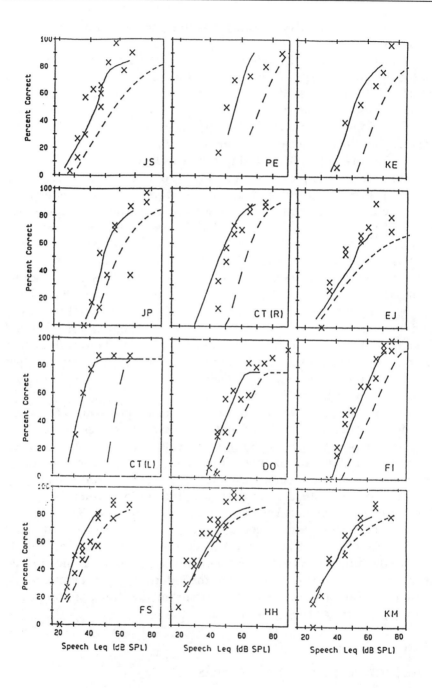

Figure 15.4 Results reprinted from Dillon (1993; Figure 7) showing smoothed functions of AB unaided (– – –); aided free-field AB results × and PI functions predicted from unaided score (————) as percent correct as a function of presentation level for individual hearing impaired listeners

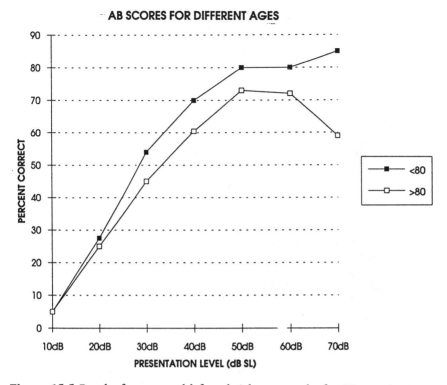

Figure 15.5 Results for averaged left and right ear results for AB tests in percent correct as a function of presentation level in dB sensation level

Two techniques are under investigation at NAL. The first is based on category scaling methods in which listeners are asked to rate the quality (or any attribute of the signal) on a scale. We have implemented a 12-person test system in an audiometric booth which uses touch-screens on which subjects record their judgements about the speech stimuli under test. The data is automatically analysed (the same system has been used to automate loudness category scaling for hearing assessment).

One potential problem with category scaling methods is that they may not be sensitive enough to demonstrate subtle differences between processing strategies or hearing aids. We have carried out investigations of listeners' ability to judge the quality of five different speech conditions that all have near perfect speech identification scores but differ in degree of harmonic distortion added to the signal.

Listeners heard 100 sentences each spoken by four talkers processed under the five different listening conditions. The listeners rated the overall quality of the materials on a 1–7 scale. The results are presented in Figure 15.6 which shows that after % normalization, the results demonstrate a clear differentiation of the speech processing conditions. These results indicate that very subtle processing differences might be measurable using category scaling methods.

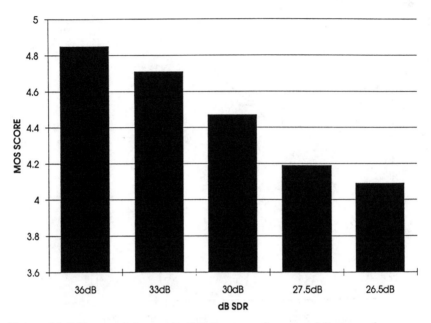

Figure 15.6 Mean opinion scale (MOS) scores for normal listeners for sentence material as a function of harmonic distortion in the signal measured in dB signal distortion ratio

Paired comparisons

Paired comparison methods have been proposed by Dillon (1984) and Byrne (1991) at NAL as a useful adjunct to hearing aid selection procedures and a clinical procedure has been proposed. The reliability and sensitivity of the paired comparison procedure was investigated by Byrne and Parkinson (1987). The results supported previous work showing good reliability for the technique but sensitivity of the measure (defined as 'the extent to which one condition is consistently chosen over another across a series of trials of one test') varied across test conditions.

Work-related speech assessment methods

Another important area for improved speech assessment methods is in work-based assessment. Increasingly employers and employees need to demonstrate that employees are capable of performing particular duties involving speech communication if they have a demonstrated hearing loss. Current legislation in many industrial countries provides protection from discrimination in the workplace based on sensory deficit alone but permits exclusion or inclusion for certain duties depending on demonstrated competence. In this area the use of improved speech discrimination tests may be of value in providing reasonably fair criterion about capacity for duty.

While we are trialling several approaches in this area an example can be reported of the use of a method to try to predict workplace performance by the use of available audiological speech tests with noise sources arranged to try to represent the workplace environment.

The results are for a male aged 49 years of age who worked in a radio communication environment for a security firm. Despite a moderate high frequency hearing loss he did not use a hearing aid and claimed that he could handle the requirements of the radio communication because most of the communications were messages with which he was very experienced. His employer claimed that while the employee did seem to cope with much of the work his performance with unexpected inputs involving new street names etc. was not adequate.

A test environment was constructed using a NAL recording of the SPIN sentences (Kalikow, Stevens and Elliott, 1977) which includes both high and low predictable words which need to be identified at the end of sentences. The sentences were filtered to telephone bandwidth and presented from a speaker directly in front of the listener at 70 dB SPL with competing noise presented from the right (45 degrees) and behind the listener. The noise was multispeaker babble. These conditions were based on an analysis of the listening situation of the communication room in which the listener was required to operate.

The results shown in Figure 15.7 provide data for a normal hearing listener and the hearing impaired listener and indicate that the listener

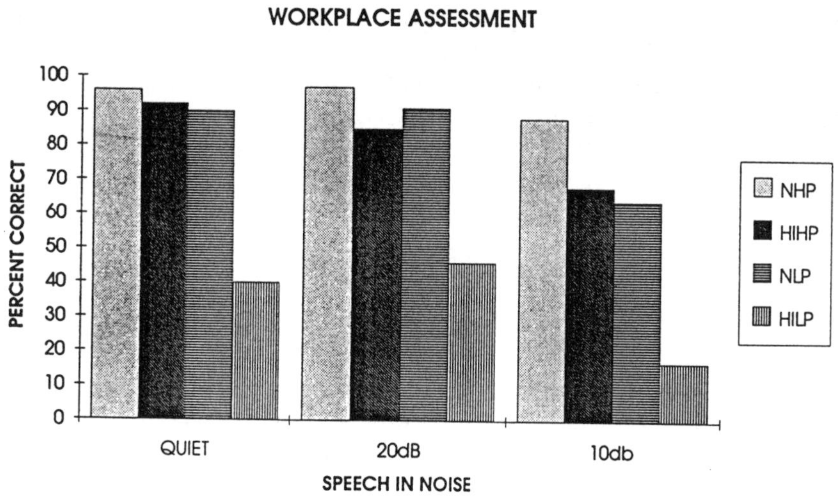

Figure 15.7 SPIN results for high and low predictable sentences in a normal hearing person (NHP and NLP) and hearing impaired person (HIHP and HILP) in percent correct as a function of signal-to-noise ratio in dB for simulation of work place assessment

could perform quite well in high predictable contexts but demonstrated poor performance relative to the normal hearing listener at signal-to-noise-ratios (SNRs) that were typical of the radio communication room (that is between +20 and +10 dB SNR).

Speech assessment for children

Paediatric speech assessment at NAL continued its use of the adaptive speech test method for children discussed by Dermody and Mackie (1987) with extensions to FM evaluations and use in non-English languages. In addition a study was reported suggesting the need to establish speech gain criteria with adaptive tests to show aided benefit from hearing aid fittings in mild hearing loss. Other developments of paediatric speech tests included extensions to the PLOTT test for severe/profoundly hearing impaired children to include both a screening test, a forced choice sentence test and a concrete object token test. During the past 2 years investigations were reported for the automation of the NAL test of auditory language learning for children in kindergarten (NALTALLCK) procedures which can be used to assess auditory receptive language function in young children with normal hearing and with mild hearing loss. Finally, an infant speech discrimination test has been evaluated and developed for potential clinical application.

Monosyllabic adaptive speech tests (MAST) for children

The monosyllabic adaptive speech test for children based on the simple up-down method proposed by Levitt and Rabiner (1967) was described in detail in Dermody and Mackie (1987). The technique presents monosyllabic words via earphones or speakers using a picture pointing response. The NU-CHIPS materials developed by Elliott and Katz, (1980) are used as the presentation materials although the same technique can be used with the Kendall test material which is suitable for younger children. The Australian standardization of the Kendall test materials was discussed in Dermody and Mackie (1987).

In the adaptive test method if a child correctly responds to the presented word the presentation level is decreased; if an incorrect response is obtained the level is increased for the next presentation. This method permits a determination of 50% correct levels in dB. Mackie and Dermody (1986) showed that the technique was reliable for children aged 3 to 7 years.

FM evaluations

As part of the speech recognition materials produced on CD at AHS/NAL the NU-CHIPS materials used in the development studies for the MAST have also been recorded with cafeteria masking noise on the other channel. These materials were also used to carry out FM evaluations (Lovegrove, Dillan and Mackie, 1991; Mackie and Cotton, 1991). That procedure, however, involves the alteration of SNRs by changing the level of the noise around a constant level speech signal to achieve a 50% recognition point.

Adaptive speech reception testing in non-English languages

The use of the adaptive speech test technique was extended by Plant (1990) for use with Aboriginal children. Words were chosen from two Aboriginal languages — Walpiri and Tiwi. Vocabulary items were chosen by Aboriginal speakers and health workers and line drawings of the nouns were made. After pilot studies to demonstrate the suitability of items 50 drawings were used to produce five randomizations of the same 25-word items. Testing demonstrated the use of the adaptive speech reception threshold to be useful for assessing hearing levels in a field test environment and demonstration of the benefit of amplification systems.

Adaptive speech reception assessment for assessing hearing aid benefit

Dermody and Mackie (1987) suggested the use of adaptive speech tests might find use in assessment of hearing aid benefit in mild hearing loss cases. This issue was also discussed earlier in terms of the use of P-I function for adults. Thorburg, et al. (1991) reported that children with less than 5 dB of speech gain (about 20% of their sample) reported little benefit from their hearing aid. Children with speech gain greater than 5 dB but less than 10 dB were mostly impartial about their hearing aids while children with greater than 10 dB speech gain were more positive about their hearing aid. Hearing loss and speech gain covary in this study, however, the results do suggest that the use of speech reception criterion to assess hearing aid benefit demonstrates a reasonable percentage of children who do not receive much speech amplification through their fitted systems. A similar percentage was noted in the adult data using monosyllabic P-I functions in adults reported by Dillon (1993) and those adults also demonstrated only mild hearing losses.

Speech assessment for severe and profound hearing loss

The PLOTT test (Plant and Westcott, 1982; Plant, 1984b) is used routinely with children with severe and profound hearing loss to provide detailed information about a child's speech reception capability. However the test takes a reasonable amount of time to administer sometimes over two or three sessions. In order to provide more compact information about abilities Plant and Moore (1992a) developed a PLOTT screening test which consists of 14 word level subtests based on the discrimination after training (DAT) test developed by Thielmeir et al. (1985). The screening PLOTT was extended to provide more detailed information about phonetic contrast discrimination and to be suitable to Australian listeners.

The PLOTT was also extended by Plant and Moore (1992a) to provide a forced choice sentence test. The sentences form a short story. The child's task is to identify which of four possible sentences were presented on a trial. The stories are about a visit to the beach or the zoo. Some of the sentences can be differentiated by use of different number of syllables in the sentences while others have the same number of syllables forcing the child to differentiate the possible sentences by discriminating phonemic differences in the words. The results of the sentence test on a group of 93 children with a range of hearing loss indicated that most children with hearing losses less than 90 dB obtained high performance levels on the test while children with average losses from 100 to 110 dB were almost evenly divided between chance and moderate levels of performance. Children with average losses of 120 dB performed at chance levels on the test.

The results of the PLOTT sentence test seemed to suggest the need for more analytic estimation of performance on a connected word test. Dermody and Mackie (1987) discussed the value of the token test for use with hearing impaired children and showed that increasing sentence length and complexity showed significant performance level differences among children with severe and profound hearing losses. Plant and Moore (1992b) attempted to extend the results on the token test reported by Dermody and Mackie (1987) to a common objects token (COT) test. The COT test provides a forced choice task similar to the original token test but uses plastic toys instead of colours in the original test and increases complexity by increasing the number of objects rather than increasing the number of attributes to be identified. The overall results of the COT test on a group of children with a range of hearing loss indicated that there is a reasonable correspondence between COT scores and PLOTT sentence test scores (Plant and Moore, 1992a). As noted by Dermody and Mackie (1987), testing speech identification of materials with increasing complexity demonstrates a significant performance decrement in children with increasing hearing loss. The COT test results support the use of sentence testing with increasing complexity to show levels of difficulty experienced by hearing impaired children in more realistic communication situations.

Speech reception assessment for normal hearing children with receptive language difficulties

Dermody and Mackie (1987) briefly described the development of the NALTALLCK procedure. This measure is designed to provide early identification of auditory receptive language problems in young normal hearing children. It is also likely that the test can also be applied effectively to assessment of auditory language development in children with mild hearing loss.

NALTALLCK consists of a set of measures to assess phonological processing (identifying the sounds in words); lexical processing (identifying the usage of words in particular contexts); and connected speech processing (deriving the meaning of phrases and sentences). These measures have been derived from a model of auditory processing and have been tested on a large group of children to provide normative data (Dermody, 1990).

Over the past several years the investigation of NALTALLCK has concentrated on the development of an automated version of the measures. The test has been implemented on a 12-person test station using touch-sensitive monitors which the children use to select a picture from four alternatives on each test. The automated version has been trialled with normal hearing 5-year-olds who are progressing normally through school or having trouble acquiring pre-reading skills. The automated results approximately match the previous group test norms and considerably speed up the test sessions. Current studies will investigate test–retest of the automated version and its application to mildly hearing impaired children.

Infant speech discrimination testing

The use of NALTALLCK measures in two longitudinal studies indicated that testing auditory language abilities at kindergarten ages provided good prediction of later receptive language abilities in normal hearing children. This raises the question of when auditory language problems begin to develop.

Infant speech discrimination tasks have been used extensively in the research literature to investigate development of linguistic skills in young children. Despite this widespread use and the suggestion by Wilson et al. in 1977 that the operant conditioning responses to speech using the head turn response could be used to develop a clinical speech discrimination test for infants most investigations have reported such a high failure and attrition rate that the method has not been adopted in routine clinical measures.

The development of a clinical speech discrimination test for infants could provide a number of potential uses and we have begun a series of studies to determine if an operant conditioned head turn response can be used routinely with young infants.

In our first study (Talay-Ongan, Dermody and Lee, in preparation) we obtained the high failure rate reported by previous investigations but found that if we could obtain at least two appointments for the testing then most infants would produce a response to at least one phonemic contrast. There was a small group of children (about 10%) who could not demonstrate a response, no matter how many appointments they attended. This study also demonstrated that testing infants at about 9 months of age produced the most efficient results.

A second study (Dermody, et al., in preparation) which utilized a refined procedure and used a two-appointment schedule to obtain a response again demonstrated that about 10% of 9-month-old infants could not demonstrate a phonemic contrast. This may be an interesting group to follow-up in a study to test a large number of infants during the first years of language development. The infant speech discrimination test has now been automated on a PC and will also be applied to children who are fitted with hearing aids by 9 months of age.

Conclusions

Speech communication abilities are the major focus of audiological assessment and rehabilitation programmes but speech reception testing remains a difficult area because of the inherent variability of human performance for speech processing and the limited applicability of most techniques that utilize clinical controls for repeatability. Nevertheless, speech test developments are occurring and speech assessment can provide essential information to the clinician and researcher. The development of computer-based methods will provide increased control of testing and will speed up complicated assessment procedures that will be required as we find out more about the nature of hearing loss and the application of digital speech processing devices to overcome hearing problems.

Chapter 16
Speech tests in some languages other than English

JOHN KNIGHT

At the risk of repetition, and even occasional elaboration, on the history of speech tests in English, it is convenient to introduce this chapter with a brief recapitulation of their development in the USA and in Britain. Lately, while consideration has been given to improving speech test materials adopted earlier in parts of Europe, the demand for audiological tests has reached other European countries and the developing world. Speech audiometry in these places then becomes important as a simple routine test of hearing as it did in the USA and Britain 40 years ago.

The material that follows summarizes some of the basic procedures for the selection and recording of suitable speech material in languages other than English, according to the restrictions and variations of structure of the particular languages. In some countries adopting American procedures, the practice has been to provide both lists of highly redundant words (such as Spondees) and lists of words with far less redundancy (such as phonetically-balanced lists). In British practice there has been little use of the former test material but it emerges that recent work in other countries has produced speech material in both levels of redundancy. In many instances, priority has been given to provision of suitable speech material for testing young children.

Background

The first tests on telephone systems with live speech were reported over 85 years ago by engineers in the USA (Campbell, 1910; Fletcher, 1929, 1953). The object was to assess quantitatively the effect of various distortions on the recognition of speech sounds. Trained listeners noted on prepared lists what they heard of nonsense syllables spoken by trained speakers, and articulation scores were calculated. Similar procedures were applied during and after the Second World War (Egan, 1948) when a further application of speech tests was to assess the degree of disability of hearing impaired people. Recorded lists of Spondees and phonetically (or phonemically) balanced words were reproduced with high sound quality in a quiet background. At this time speech audiometry provided confirmation of the pure-tone audiogram, gave a measure of benefit obtained from hearing aids and was of value in subsequent auditory training.

In 1944 the first important application of recorded speech material to audiology in Britain was for research with potential hearing aid users to determine the specifications for National Health Service (NHS) hearing aids (Medical Research Council, 1947). It was decided to prepare test lists of monosyllabic words of consonant-vowel-consonant (CVC) type with the approximate distribution of speech sounds from everyday normal English speech. Much experience was available from the earlier wartime work in the Psychoacoustic Laboratory of Harvard University (later described by Egan) where a vocabulary of 1200 monosyllabic words had been grouped into 24 lists of 50 words. They were then re-ordered and adjusted so that the final 20 lists satisfied the criteria of equal average difficulty, equal phonemic balance, composition representative of English speech and containing only words in common use. Exceptionally easy words were discarded from the original 1200. It was found that the above requirements could not be satisfied with less than 50 words in each list.

In the British Medical Research Council (MRC) study, 20 word lists each of 50 monosyllabic words were chosen to be recorded, half in a male, and the other half in female voice; the words were selected for phonemic balance by Fry, who earlier had produced sentence lists for speech tests by live voice (Fry and Kerridge, 1939). These lists were used to assess the prototype NHS hearing aids. Later, in 1945, during the hearing aid research, Fry further amended the Harvard vocabulary and re-selected words for approximate phonemic balance in groups of 25 words for the third and final series of the MRC word lists. The resulting 40 lists were recorded on double-sided 78 rpm discs; 10 lists each by two male and two female speakers. A series of modified Fry–Kerridge sentence lists was recorded under the same conditions with one of the male speakers. The sentence lists were found to be invaluable in later hearing aid development for subjects with very severe hearing loss for whom the word lists proved too difficult. From tests with the word and sentence lists it was soon clear that 40% word recognition score corresponded to 90% sentence recognition and hence that a 40% word score is a critical level. Subsequently the 50% word score with the PB lists was adopted for its generality, it corresponding to practically total sentence recognition. In the USA this equivalence led to the concept of 'hearing loss for speech' (Hirsh, 1952) now termed the 'speech recognition threshold', SRT (see in particular, chapters 5 and 12). It is defined as the level in decibels at which a subject obtains a 50% word score with reference to the level required by the average normal ear to attain that score under identical conditions.

By the early 1950s speech audiometry with recorded speech material had become an established clinical procedure in Britain and the USA, to supplement pure-tone audiometry and recruitment tests as an aid to diagnosis (Watson and Tolan, 1949; Hirsh, 1952). A detailed evaluation of the MRC Series 3 word lists with male speakers, together with a design for a simple instrument for clinical use in free field was reported by Knight and Littler in 1953. In 1961, Fry revised the MRC monosyllabic PB word and sentence lists and re-issued them recorded on reel-to-reel magnetic tape. With so much careful preparation and experience incorporated in the production of the MRC Series 3 and the Fry words lists, they have stood the test of time over more than 35 years. As sound recording techniques advanced, they have been re-recorded on cassette tape and were used extensively for tests of adults — usually being presented via an audiometer headset.

The routine clinical applications of speech audiometry in British practice have diminished in the last 15 years as new audiological and imaging procedures have emerged to aid diagnosis. In some clinics the time required for a traditional speech audiometric procedure with adults has been reduced by incorrectly adopting an abbreviated form of test. Often short word lists designed for children have been employed, so introducing much uncertainty. These factors in part account for the present lack of support to make any British speech test material available digitally recorded on compact disc (CD).

Audiological expertise and practice continues to spread to developing parts of India, Africa, the Caribbean and to acquire greater importance in some European countries. The need for simple speech tests of hearing often has arisen following the introduction of pure-tone audiometry by trained personnel, and before the latest audiological, and other instrumental, diagnostic aids could be afforded. The first step in setting up speech audiometry in another language is to obtain a detailed analysis of the language structure. Precedents are cited in which the frequency of occurrence of the phonemes was estimated from written tests and articles, or by analysing recordings of national radio news bulletins. Following the selection of suitable words for the required number of lists, the arrangements for their recording must be decided.

The procedure for recording speech tests is described in chapters 5 and 6 with the need to finally adjust the level of the individual words for uniformity. Although digital recording on CD is now commonplace for entertainment purposes in developed countries (and is the obvious choice where resources allow), a good analogue recording on magnetic tape yields perfectly satisfactory speech test results at far less cost. Listening tests on the individual word lists with an adequately sized group of normally hearing subjects have to be conducted and scored to detect any differences of importance in the average of the resulting speech audiograms and to equalize the average difficulty of the lists according to Egan's criteria. It is also important to record a calibration tone on each recording for adjusting the speech audiometer to a standard condition whenever it is used. Usually 15 seconds or more of 1kHz pure tone or one third octave band of random noise centred at this frequency is recorded at a level having a specified relation to the average speech level.

Languages other than English

While the speech test material available for English speaking people is suitable for an estimated 340 million people, this represents only 8.5% of the world population who communicate using more than 3000 known living languages, the majority of which can be ascribed to 12 main language families. More than half the world's population can be reached by as few as 13 languages. Chinese is spoken by the greatest number of people followed by English, Hindi, Russian, Spanish, Japanese, German, French, Italian, Malay, Bengali and Portuguese. In many developing countries the technical and other resources needed for the preparation of test material for speech audiometry for the other 90% or more of people who do not speak English have not existed. Recently a number of foreign students in Britain to study audiology have produced speech test lists in their own languages which have led to the award of postgraduate degrees. The accounts of speech audiometry in non-English languages that follow are necessarily incomplete but those included mostly originate from projects in which the present author was connected, either as a collaborator at the University of London, or as external examiner at the Universities of Manchester or Southampton

Romanian

Romania has a population of 23 million. After the political changes of 1989, Britain, with other countries gave aid which included audiological expertise and training with amplification systems, particularly for the benefit of the deaf children. A requirement to develop speech tests for children followed. Romanian is a Romance language alongside Italian, French, Spanish, Portuguese (and several non-standard varieties, such as Catalan, Sardinian, etc.) which developed from spoken Latin. The southern form of Romanian is regarded as standard Romanian and, even though there are slight accent variations from one region to another, there are no dialects as such. There are seven vowels and 20 consonants in Romanian, which is a phonetic language (having a direct correspondence between symbols and sounds). The most common words are monosyllables (39%) with disyllables second (24%). Dante (1994) at

Manchester University was the first to develop new word lists for speech audiometry in Romanian. She constructed 12 lists of PB monosyllabic words each containing the same phonemes arranged to form nine CVC words. The two most frequent consonants were excluded so that each list contains 25 different phonemes. The lists were recorded in standard Romanian on audio tape in two versions, one with a female, the other with a male speaker. The word lists and all the words occur at regular 8 second intervals without an introductory phrase. A calibration tone of 1 kHz for 30 seconds is provided.

Thirty normally hearing Romanian subjects were tested in the usual way with the recording by the female speaker and were scored according to the number of phonemes correctly repeated. The lists were tested for inter-list differences by presenting all 12 lists to each subject in random order at or near threshold level. To establish the reference speech recognition curve, six lists were presented in random order at six different levels to each ear separately. Analysis showed there to be no statistically significant difference between the lists. The resulting reference speech recognition curve obtained by averaging the mean scores for left and right ears has a slope on the linear section of 3% per dB. This compares with an average of 3.7% per dB with the male speakers of the MRC Series 3 lists to which reference was made, 3.8% per decibel with comparable German lists (chapter 6) and 4% per decibel with American lists, whereas the American spondees are much steeper at 10% per decibel.

Spanish

Castillian is the language of over 75% of the population of Spain, which means that it is spoken by some 30 million inhabitants, while it is also the form of Spanish spoken in Mexico, Central (except in Brazil where Portuguese is used) and Southern America. Basque, Catalan and Galician are spoken in other parts of Spain. At times, translation of British, French and American English speech test materials have been employed for speech audiometry in Spain. Then in Buenos Aires, Tato (1949) from a study of written Spanish, prepared 12 phonemically-balanced lists of 25 disyllabic words that were widely adopted. The use of monosyllabic nouns was not possible as few exist in Spanish. However Poch Viñals (1958) reported that for discrimination (as distinct from threshold) tests the linguistic characteristics of disyllabic words of Spanish rendered them too redundant. Cárdenas and Marrero (1993, 1994) remarked on the inaccuracies which result from a common practice using an abbreviated form of speech test in which only 10 words of the Tato lists are presented at each level. After detailed examination of the phonetics of Castillian Spanish, they produced two lists of 24 frequently used three and four syllable words for rapid tests of SRT. The resulting audiograms have a steep slope of approximately 8% per decibel, which is comparable to that of American Spondees.

Additionally, for discrimination tests, they have produced 10 different lists of 25 familiar disyllabic words in PB lists. The latter were selected to have low redundancy (6% per decibel). They are recorded on a single CD with 42 tracks, using a female voice. Six of the tracks carry similar lists, but with 25 more difficult words for further diagnostic use, and another 11 lists designed for feature recognition tests with children from pre-school to 12 years old. Bands of 1 kHz pure tone, 1/3 octave band noise centred on 1 kHz, and 10 kHz pure tone are provided for calibration and checking. This new material is undergoing widespread evaluation in different Spanish audiological centres. From Puerto Rico, Cancel (1993) also reported on a development from the earlier word lists provided by Tato and others with new word selection criteria. These take into account the phonetic characteristics of the Spanish language as well as criteria used by the originators of the PB and multiple-choice lists in English as already detailed.

Languages of India and Pakistan

India is the second most populous country, with 853 million inhabitants in 1990 (China had 1250 million). While Hindi is the 'lingua franca' of India, English remains the other official language and 14 regional languages are also recognized for adoption as official state languages covering 90% of the Indian population. Roughly one third speak Hindi, other popular languages being Teluga, Bengali, Marathi, Tamil, Urdu, Gujrati, Kannada, Malayalam, Orriya, Punjabi, Assamese, Kashmiri and Sanskrit. Pakistan, with a population of 84 million, has Urdu and Bengali as official languages.

Speech audiometry in India was started in 1966. By 1971 the Rehabilitation Unit in Audiology and Speech Pathology at the All-India Institute of Medical Sciences, New Delhi, had prepared PB monosyllabic and spondee word lists in the Hindi local dialect. De Sa followed in 1973 by publishing further PB word lists for speech audiometry in Hindi. Kapur (1971), referred to existing lists in Malayalam, Tamil and Telugu.

Arabic test lists

Arabic, the major Semitic language, is spoken by some 75 million inhabitants south and east of the Mediterranean. Countries in which it occupies official status include Algeria, Egypt, Iraq, Israel, Jordan, Kuwait, Lebanon, Libya, Morocco, Saudi Arabia, Syria and North and South Yemen.

It can be taken that African speech audiometry began when Messouak (1956) produced word lists in Moroccan colloquial Arabic. Alusi et al. followed at London University in 1974 with a compilation and evaluation of recorded monosyllabic and disyllabic word lists in the literary or 'classical' Arabic language. Six lists each of 25 monosyllabic words were recorded in a Baghdad accent by a male speaker. The words were phonemically balanced for vowels, but the balance was not perfect for consonants due to their unevenness of distribution in Arabic. These authors introduced the concept of plotting the speech audiogram on arithmetical probability paper to give a straight-line plot rather than the usual sigmoid curve which results from use of the traditional linear co-ordinates. As yet this potential innovation has received no support in the clinical field.

There have been later productions of Arabic word lists by Ashoor and Prochazka (1982, 1985) for testing hearing of adults and children with speech in Saudi Arabia, again with modern standard (classical) Arabic. For adults this later material comprises six lists of 20 PB nouns and, for children, eight lists of 10 PB mono- and disyllabic nouns. Onsa in 1984 at Manchester University, developed the first speech test material in standard Sudanese Arabic, the dialect of central Sudan, for use in local audiology clinics. Several 20 PB word lists and ten 10 word lists were produced using monosyllabic words. The latter were tested on normally hearing Sudanese subjects and found to be satisfactory as regards inter-list consistency and sensitivity.

Other African languages

Although Arabic is used extensively in the countries of North Africa, the 'lingua franca' of Southern Africa is Swahili. However, Muyunga in 1974 working at London University on the development of speech audiometric material for Zaire (population 30 million), reported that the great majority of the Zairian languages are Bantu languages; of the four official vernacular languages, Lingala is spoken by 8.4 million, Swahili by 6.3 million, Ciluba by 4.3 million and Kikongo by 2.8 million. He applied himself to developing speech audiometry in Lingala as it is the language of Kinshasa, the capital, and of the National Army. It is also used in Congo Brazzaville and in the Central African Republic. Ciluba was included in the study as it was the mother tongue of the investigator. Twelve PB lists of 25 Lingala disyllabic words and 14 similar lists of Ciluba words were produced. Three lists for each language were tape recorded using male speakers. The usual recording and equalization procedures were applied and a 1 kHz tone was added for standardization purposes during replay.

The speech recordings were evaluated with several normally hearing groups of subjects with comparable results to those obtained with

English speech audiometry. Hinchcliffe (1968) found (with two Indian languages, Hindi and Tamil), that knowledge of the language is not an important factor in speech audiometry, providing sufficient co-operation and understanding of the test situation is obtained from the subject. This was confirmed by Muyunga by tests on subjects to whom Lingala and Ciluba were unknown languages, with results that were reliable, particularly in respect of the maximum word score and the threshold of detectability. He concluded that this finding would help to overcome the problem of speech audiometry with the many languages used in Zaire.

Chinese (Cantonese)

Mandarin as spoken in Beijing is now the national language of China's 1250 million inhabitants, and so is spoken by three times the number of people who speak English. Unlike in India and Africa, it is only in the south-eastern maritime provinces of China that several mutually intelligible dialects are spoken, and one of these is Cantonese. The population of Canton province is 5 million. and it is estimated that at least a further 22 million inhabitants of China, 6 million in Hong Kong and the many other Chinese immigrants worldwide, speak Cantonese. It is a tonal language in which information is carried by the fundamental frequency. There are six contrasting lexical tones in Cantonese and all the root words are monosyllables. There are 18 vowels and 19 consonants and over 40% of the words are of the CV type.

Kam, a postgraduate student from nearby Hong Kong (population 5 million), developed and evaluated a forced-choice Cantonese speech test in 1982 at the University of Southampton. This used monosyllabic words, and was produced specifically for audiological diagnostic purposes. The design was based on that of the four-alternative-auditory feature (FAAF) test, except that a three-alternative closed response set was necessary with the phonological constraints imposed by Cantonese. One hundred and twenty test items were chosen, to be presented in four lists of 30 words. In the recording, the tone of voice was controlled as though it was an ordinary phonetic feature.

Others, particularly Lau and So (1988), developed further test material on conventional lines for routine speech audiometry in Cantonese with Hong Kong adults. Lau and So prepared and recorded 10 lists of phonemically balanced, monosyllabic words with a male speaker on cassette tape. A 5 second interval separated the words and a 1 kHz calibration tone was recorded. The lists were evaluated on nine normally hearing subjects, scoring the phonemes according to consonants and vowels repeated correctly and compared with scoring consonants, vowels and tones of voice. The two reference speech audiograms which resulted were practically identical, each with the maximum slope of

3.0% per decibel. Kei et al. (1991) of the Special Education Services Centre in Hong Kong fulfilled the need for a short and simple speech test in Cantonese for use with 6-to 9-year-old children. Ten lists of suitably chosen, phonemically balanced monosyllables in groups of 10 words spoken by a male at 3 second intervals were recorded on tape, with the necessary 1 kHz tone for calibration. Nineteen normally hearing 9-year-old children tested the lists for equality of difficulty around the 70% score, and another 63 children provided data to define the reference speech audiogram. With phoneme scoring this has a maximum slope of 3.3% per decibel. In most respects this material is the equivalent of Boothroyd's material for children speaking English.

Thai language

The population of Thailand is approximately 50 million. The language is basically monosyllabic and tonal, forming a branch of the Indo-Chinese linguistic family. Its vocabulary has particularly been influenced by Sanskrit and Pali. It is written in an alphabetic script derived from ancient Indian scripts (Mahidol).

The Otological Centre at the Mahidol University in Bangkok has taken a lead in developing all aspects of audiology in south east Asia, and speech audiometry is well established in the Thai language (Prasansuk, 1995). As is sometimes the case, details of the current speech test material have not been published.

Aboriginal languages

Among the 16 million inhabitants of Australia there are some 150 000 Aborigines who speak at least 30 languages and many more dialects. Many live in remote parts and they are particularly prone to middle-ear disease. Up to 50% of the children have significant hearing loss caused by chronic otitis media, and amplification is necessary in their education. For many of the children, their first language is Aboriginal, and they do not experience English before going to school. With the primary object of assessing the benefit of amplification systems used by these children, Plant (1990) developed suitable recorded material for the Warlpiri and Tiwi languages. A simple test was required in order to allow testing of children down to 5 years of age by testers who might not be fluent speakers of the language. A solution was found in a picture pointing procedure using an up-down adaptive procedure to determine the level at which a 50% word score was obtained after at least 15 reversals of presentation level. Cassette tape recorded word lists were prepared using a female voice and were reproduced under the usual specified conditions in free field. Satisfactory correlations were obtained with the children's average pure-tone thresholds. For the Warlpiri language a 50-item test list was prepared consisting of 10 pseudo-randomizations of five disyllabic words. The Tiwi test described has two such lists but uses five trisyllabic words.

Conclusions

There continues to be a worldwide need for speech audiometry as a basic audiological procedure in work with hearing impaired children and adults. While relatively simple equipment is necessary for reproduction of the tests, a significant challenge remains with the selection and production of the required speech materials, which must represent particular languages adequately. By reference to the published reports of those from the five continents who have pioneered suitable procedures, and to relevant national and international standards, it is expected that the task of preparing new material in other tongues may be simpler for future investigators. Finally, it may be remarked how similar in form are the resulting speech audiograms from comparable material in quite different groups of languages.

References

Aitken S, Bianco C (1985) Computerized instruction for hearing-impaired pre-schoolers. Paper resented at the American Speech-Language-Hearing Association's Annual Convention in Washington, DC.

Alpiner J G (1978) Handbook of adult rehabilitative audiology. Baltimore: Williams and Wilkins.

Alusi HA, Hinchcliffe R, Ingham B, Knight J J and North C (1974) Arabic speech audiometry. Audiology 13, 212–220.

American National Standards Institute. (1996) American National Standard Specification for Audiometers. ANSI S3.6. New York.

American National Standards Institute (1996) American National Standard methods for the calculation of the articulation index. ANSI S3.5–1969, New York.

American National Standards Institute. (1996) American National Standard Specification for Audiometers. ANSI S3.6 V. New York.

American Speech-Language-Hearing Association (1979) Guidelines for determining the threshold level for speech. ASHA 21: 353–355.

American Speech-Language-Hearing Association (ASHA) (1988) Guidelines for determining the threshold level for speech. ASHA 3: 85–88.

Anderson CMB, Whittle LS (1971) Physiological noise and the missing 6 dB. Acoustica 24(5): 261–272.

Anderson B, Wayne, Kalb JT (1987) English verification of the STI method for estimating speech intelligibility of a communications channel. Journal of the Acoustical Society of America 81(6): 1982–1985.

Anderson I (1988) Koorie Health in Koorie Hands: An Orientation Manual. In Aboriginal Health for Health-care Providers. Melbourne: Health Department Victoria.

Aniansson G (1974) Methods for assessing high frequency hearing loss in every-day listening situations. Acta Otolaryngologica, Suppl. 320.

Antognelli P, Birtles G (1986) The Kendall foy test revisited: the development of an Australian version. Paper presented at Australian Audiological Society 7th National Conference, Ballarat, Victoria.

Aplin DY, Kane JM (1985) Variables affecting pure tone and speech audiometry in experimentally simulated hearing loss. British Journal of Audiology 19: 219–228.

Arlinger S (1993) Quality assurance in hearing aid fitting. In Recent developments in hearing instrument technology Beilin J and Jensen GR (Eds.) Proceedings of the 15th Danavox Symposium, Stougaard Jensen, Copenhagen.

Asher JW (1958) Intelligibility tests: A review of their standardization, some experiments, and a new test. Speech Monographs 25: 14–28.

Ashoor AA, Prochazka T (1982) Saudi Arabic speech audiometry. Audiology 21: 493–508.

Ashoor AA, Prochazka T (1985) Saudi Arabic speech audiometry in children. British Journal of Audiology 19: 229–238.

Australian Bureau of Statistics (1979) Hearing and the Use of Hearing Aids (Persons Aged 15 Years or More) September 1978. Canberra: Australian Bureau of Statistics.

Australian Bureau of Statistics (1980) Sight, Hearing and Dental Health (Persons Aged 2 to 14 Years) February–May 1979. Canberra: Australian Bureau of Statistics.

Australian Bureau of Statistics (1993) Disability, Ageing and Carers, Australia, 1993 — Summary of Findings, Catalogue 4430.0. Canberra: Australian Bureau of Statistics.

Andrianjatovo J (1972) Audiométrie Vocale en Langue Malgasy. Paris: Compagnie Française d'Audiologie.

Baer, T., Moore, B.C.J., Gatehouse, S. (1990) Spectral contrast enhancement of speech in noise for listeners with sensorineural hearing impairment: effects on intelligibility, quality and response times. Journal of Rehabilitation Research and Development 30: 49–72.

Baer T, Moore BCJ, Gatehouse S (1993) Spectral contrast enhancement of speech in noise for listeners with sensorineural hearing impairment: effects on intelligibility, quality and response times. Journal of Rehabilitation Research and Development 30: 49–72.

Barfod J (1973) Intelligibility scores and confidence intervals. Proceedings, Speech Intelligibility Symposium, Liege: 25–33.

Beattie RC, Raffin M (1985) Reliability of threshold, slope and PB max for monosyllabic words. Journal of Speech and Hearing Disorders 50: 166–178.

Beattie RC, Edgerton BJ (1976) Reliability of monosyllabic discrimination test in white noise for differentiating among hearing aids. Journal of Speech and Hearing Disorders 41: 464–476.

Beattie RC, Edgerton BJ, Svihovee DV (1975) An investigation of Auditec of St Louis recordings of Central Institute for the Deaf spondees. Journal of the American Audiology Society 1: 97–101.

Beattie RC, Svihovee DV, Edgerton BJ (1975) Relative intelligibility of the CID spondées as presented via monitored live voice. Journal of Speech and Hearing Disorders 40: 84–91.

Bellman S, Marcuson M (1991) A new toy test to investigate the hearing status of young children who have English as a second language: a preliminary report. British Journal of Audiology 25: 317–322.

Bellman S, Mahon M, Triggs E (1996) Evaluation of the E2L Toy Test as a screening procedure in clinical practice. British Journal of Audiology 30: 286–296.

Bench J (1992) A note on the BKB/A sentences versus the BKB/A words: a further validation report. Australian Journal of Audiology 14: 63–65.

Bench J, Bamford J (1979) Speech Hearing Tests and the Spoken Language of Hearing Impaired Children. New York: Academic Press.

Bench J, Doyle J (1979) The BKBIA (Bamford Kowal Bench) Sentence Lists for Speech Audiometry—Australian Version. Victoria: Lincoln Institute.

Bench RJ, Duerdoth JCP (1983) Victorian Demographic Study of Hearing Impairment, Vol. 1. Services and Facilities for Hearing Impaired People in Victoria. Victoria: Deafness Foundation.

Bench J, Kowal A, Bamford JM (1979) The BKB (Bamford-Kowal-Bench) sentence lists for partially hearing children. British Journal of Audiology 13: 108–112.

Bench J, Doyle J, Greenwood KM (1987) A standardisation of the BKB/A sentence test for children in comparison with the NAL-CID sentence test and CAL-PBM word test. Australian Journal of Audiology 9: 39–48.

Bench RJ, Doyle J, Daly N, Lind C (1993) The BKB/A Speechreading test (Versions A and B). Victoria: School of Communication Disorders, La Trobe University.

Berger KW (1971) Speech Audiometry. In Rose DE (Ed.) Audiological Assessment. Englewood Cliffs NJ: Prentice-Hall, Inc.

Berger KW (1976) Prescription of hearing aids: a rationale. Journal of the American Audiology Society 2: 71–78.

Berger KW (1990) The use of an articulation index to compare three hearing aid prescription methods. Audecibel 39: 16–19.

Berger K, Hagberg NS, Rane RL (1977) Prescription of Hearing Aids. Kent, OH: Herald Publishing Co.

Berkowitz, A. and Hochberg, I. (1971) Self assessment of hearing handicap in the aged. Archives of Otolaryngology 93: 25–28.

Bernard JRL (1970) A cine X-ray study of some sounds of Australian English. Phonetica 21: 138–150.

Bernstein C (1981) Use of speech discrimination in predicting hearing handicap in the elderly. Paper presented at the New York State Speech-Language-Hearing Association Convention.

Bernstein LE, Schecter MB, Goldstein MH (1985) Vibrotactile sensitivity thresholds of hearing children and of profoundly deaf children. Journal of the Acoustical Society of America 78, Suppl. 1.

Berry BF, John AJ, Shipton MS (1979) A computer controlled audiometry system. Proceedings of the Institute of Acoustics Spring Conference, Southampton.

Bess FH (1982) Basic hearing measurement. In Lass NJ, McReynolds LV, Northern JL, Yoder DE (Eds) Speech, Language and Hearing. Philadephia: W. B. Saunders Co.

Bess FH (1982) Children with unilateral hearing loss. Journal of the Academy of Rehabilitation Audiology 15: 131–144.

Bess FH (1983) Clinical assessment of speech recognition. In Konkle DF, Rintlemann WF (Eds) Principles of Speech Audiometry. Baltimore, MD: University Park Press.

Biesalski P, Leitner H, Leitner E, Gaugel D. (1974) Der Mainzer Kindersprachtest. Sprachaudiometrie im Vorschulalter (The Mainz speech test for preschool-age children). HNO (Berlin) 22: 160–161.

Bilger RC, Wang MD (1976) Consonant confusions in patients with sensorineural hearing loss. Journal of Speech and Hearing Research 19: 718–748.

Binnie CA, Montgomery AA, Jackson PL (1974) Auditory and visual contributions to the perception of consonants. Journal of Speech and Hearing Research 17: 619–630.

Birrell R, Birrell T (1981) An Issue of People: Population and Australian Society. Melbourne: Longman Cheshire.

Black JW (1952) Accompaniments of word intelligibility. Journal of Speech and Hearing Disorders 17: 409–418.

Blair D (1977) Judging the Varieties of Australian English, Working Papers, Speech and Language Research Centre, Macquarie University, Sydney: 109–111.

Blamey PJ, Dowell RC, Brown AM, Clarke GM (1985) Clinical results with a hearing aid and a single-channel vibrotactile device for profoundly deaf adults. British Journal of Audiology 19: 203–210.

Blamey PJ, Clark GM, Tong YC, Ling D (1990). Perceptual-oral training of two hearing-impaired children in the recognition and production of /s/ and /z/. British Journal of Audiology 24: 375–379.

Bocca E, Calearo C, Cassinari V (1954) A new method for testing hearing in temporal lobe tumours. Acta Otolaryngologica 44: 219–221.

Bode D, Carhart R (1973) Measurement of articulation functions using adaptive test procedures. IEEE Transactions on Audio and Electroacoustics AU21: 196–201.

Bode D, Carhart R (1974) Stability and accuracy of adaptive tests of speech discrimination. Journal of the Acoustical Society of America 56: 963–970.

Boeninghaus HG, Röser D (1973) Neue Tabellen zur Bestimmung des prozentualen Hörverlustes für das Sprachgehör (New tables for the determination of the percentage of hearing loss for speech). Zeitschrift für Laryngologie und Rhinologie 52 Suppl.: 153–161.

Bonding P (1979) Frequency selectivity and speech discrimination in sensorineural hearing loss. Scandinavian Audiology 8: 205–215.

Boothroyd A (1968) Developments in speech audiometry. Sound 2: 3–10.

Boothroyd A (1987) CASPER: Computer Assisted Speech Perception Evaluation and Training. Proceedings of the 10th Annual Conference of the Rehabilitation Society of North America. Association for the Advancement of Rehabilitation Technology, Washington, DC 734–736.

Boothroyd A (1991) CASPER: A User-friendly System for Computer Assisted Speech Perception Testing and Training. New York: City University of New York.

Boothroyd A, Hanin L, Hnath T (1985) A Sentence Test of Speech Perception: Reliability, Set Equivalence, and Short Term Learning. City University of New York Speech and Hearing Sciences Research Center, Internal Report No. RC 110.

Boothroyd A, Hnath-Chisholm T, Hanin L, Kishon-Rabin L (1988) Voice fundamental frequency as an auditory supplement to the speechreading of sentences. Ear and Hearing 9: 306–312.

Boothroyd A, Waldstein, Yeung E (1992) Investigations into the auditory F_0 speechreading enhancement using a sinusoidal replica of the F_0 contour. Proceedings of the International Conference on Spoken Language Processing. Banff: 963–966.

Borg E (1982) Correlation between auditory brainstem response (ABR) and speech discrimination scores in patients with acoustic neurinoma and in patients with cochlear hearing loss. Scandinavian Audiology 11: 245–248.

Bosatra A, Russolo M (1982) Comparison between central tonal tests and central speech tests in elderly subjects. Audiology 21: 334–341.

Boswell J, Nienhuys T, Rickards F (1994) Conductive hearing loss with otitis media in infancy: screening and diagnosis. Journal of the Audiological Society of Australia Supplement 15: 7.

Brady PT (1971) The need for standardization in the measurement of speech level. Journal of the Acoustical Society of America 50: 712–714.

Brandy, W. T. (1966) Reliability of voice tests of speech discrimination. Journal of Speech and Hearing Research 9: 461–465.

Brimacombe JA, Danhauer JL, Mecklenburg DJ, Prietto AL (1985) Cochlear implant patient performance on the MAC battery. Paper presented at the American Speech-Language-Hearing Association Annual Convention, Washington, DC.

Brinkmann K (1974a) The new recording of 'Words for Testing Hearing with Speech'. Journal of Audiological Technique 13: 12–40.

Brinkmann, K (1974b) The new recording of the Marburg sentence intelligibility test. Journal of Audiological Technique 13: 190–206.

Brinkmann K, Diestel HG (1970) Tests with the speech audiometer. Part III: The result of hearing tests. Journal of Audiological Technique 9: 114–126.

Brinkmann K, Richter U (1983) Determination of the normal threshold of hearing by bone conduction using different types of bone vibrators. Audiological Acoustics 22: 62–85 and 114–122.

Brinkmann K, Richter U (1989) Free-field sensitivity level of audiometric earphones to be used for speech audiometer calibration. Scandinavian Audiology 18: 75–81.

Brinkmann K, Diestel HG, Mrass H (1969a) Tests with the speech audiometer. Part I: Properties of the word lists. Journal of Audiological Technique 8: 38–51.

Brinkmann K, Diestel HG, Mrass H (1969b) Tests with the speech audiometer. Part II: Electro-acoustical transmission properties. Journal of Audiological Technique 8: 126–142.

British Standards (BS), London: British Standards Institution.

BS 4009 (1991) An artificial mastoid for the calibration of bone vibrators used in hearing aids and audiometers.

BS 4668 (1971) Specification for an acoustic coupler (IEC reference type) for calibration of earphones used in audiometry.

BS 4669 (1971) Specification for an artificial ear of the wide-band type for the calibration of earphones used in audiometry.

BS EN 60645-1 (1995) Audiometers Part 1. Pure-Tone audiometers.

BS EN 60645-1 (1995) Audiometers Part 2. Equipment for Speech Audiometry.

BS ISO 389-3 (1994) A countries-Reference zero for the calibration of audiometric equipment part 3. Reference equivalent threshold force levels for pure-tone and tone vibrators.

Broadbent DE (1967) Word frequency effect and response bias. Psychological Review 74: 1–15.

Brooks PL, Frost BJ, Mason JL, Gibson DM (1986) Continuing evaluation of the Queen's University Tactile Vocoder. II — Identification of open set sentences and tracking narrative. Journal of Rehabilitation Research and Development 23: 129–138.

Brunt M (1978) Chapter 23 in Handbook of Clinical Audiology 2nd edition, Katz J, (Ed.) Baltimore, MD: Williams and Wilkins.

Bryant WS (1904) A phonographic acoumeter. Archives of Otolaryngology 33: 438–443.

Busby PA, Tong YC, Roberts SA, Altidis PM, Dettman SJ, Blamey PJ, Clark GM, Warson RK, Dowell RC, Rickards FW (1989) Results for two children using a multiple-electrode intracochlear implant. Journal of the Acoustical Society of America 86: 2088–2102.

Busby PA, Roberts SA, Tong YC, Clark GM (1991) Results of speech perception and speech production training for three prelingually deaf patients using a multiple-electrode cochlear implant. British Journal of Audiology 25: 291–302.

Byrne D (1978) Selection of hearing aids for severely deaf children. British Journal of Audiology 12: 9–22.

Byrne D (1981) Selective amplification: some psychoacoustic considerations. In Bess F, Freeman B, Sinclair J (Eds) Amplification in Education, chapter 17. Washington: AG Bell Association for Deaf.

Byrne D (1983) Theoretical prescriptive approaches to selecting the gain and frequency response of a hearing aid. Monographs in Contemporary Audiology 4: No. 1.

Byrne D (1983) Word familiarity in speech perception testing of children. British Journal of Audiology 5: 77–80.

Byrne D (1991) Evaluation measures of speech intelligibility and quality. In Studebaker G, Bess F, Beck L (Eds) The Vanderbilt Hearing-Aid Report II. Maryland: York Press.

Byrne D, Tonisson W (1976) Selecting the gain of hearing aids for persons with sensorineural hearing impairments. Scandinavian Audiology 5: 51–59.

Byrne D, Dillon H (1986) The National Acoustic Laboratories' (NAL) new procedure for selecting the gain and frequency response of a hearing aid. Ear and Hearing 7: 257–265.

Cameron RJ (1985) Year Book of Australia 1985. Canberra: Australian Bureau of Statistics.

Campbell GA (1910) Telephonic intelligibility. Philosophical Magazine 19: 152–159.

Campbell R (1965) Discrimination test word difficulty. Journal of Speech and Hearing Research 8: 130–132.

Campbell RA (1974) Computer Audiometry. Journal of Speech and Hearing Research 17: 134–140.

Cancel CA (1993) Criteria for the development of audiological Spanish materials. Proceedings of the 20th International Congress of Audiology, Halifax.

Cárdenas MR, Marrero V (1993) Speech audiometry in Spanish: new recorded (Ed) lists. Proceedings of the 20th International Congress of Audiology, Halifax.

Cárdenas MR, Marrero V (1994) Cauderno de Logoaudiometria. Madrid: UNED.

Carhart R (1946a) Speech reception in relation to pattern of pure tone loss. Journal of Speech Disorders 11: 97–108.

Carhart R (1946b) Tests for selection of hearing aids. Laryngoscope 56: 780–794.

Carhart R (1951) Basic principles of speech audiometry. Acta Otolaryngologica 40: 62–71.

Carhart R (1965) Problems in the measurement of speech discrimination. Archives of Otolaryngology 82: 253–260.

Carhart R (1971) Observations on relations between thresholds for pure tones and for speech. Journal of Speech and Hearing Disorders 36: 476–483.

Carhart R, Porter LS (1971) Audiometric configuration and prediction of threshold for spondees. Journal of Speech and Hearing Research 14: 86–95.

Carhart R (1946c) Selection of hearing aids. Archives Otolaryngology 44: 1–18.

Carney AE (1985) Tactile aids: A comparison of single and multichannel devices. Journal of the Acoustical Society of America 78, Suppl. 1: S16.

Carroll JB, Davies P, Richman B (1971) Word Frequency Book. New York: American Heritage Publishing Co. Inc.

Carter N, Farrant R (1957) Australian Application of ICAO Aircrew Hearing Standards. Commonwealth Acoustic Laboratories Report No. 12. Sydney: NAL.

Castles I (1994) Year Book — Australia, 1994. Canberra: Australian Bureau of Statistics.

Chaiklin JB (1959) The relation among three selected auditory speech thresholds. Journal of Speech and Hearing Research 2: 237–243.

Chaiklin J, Ventry I (1964) Spondee threshold measurement. A comparison of 2 and 5 dB methods. Journal of Speech and Hearing Disorders 10: 141–145.

Chaiklin J, Font J, Dixon R (1967) Spondee thresholds measured in ascending 5 dB steps. Journal of Speech and Hearing Disorders 10: 141–145.

Chilla R, Gabriel P, Kozielski P, Bausch D, Kabas M (1976) Der Gottinger Kindersprachverstandnistest (The Gottingen speech test for children). HNO (Berlin) 24: 342–346.

Cholewiak RW, Sherrick CE (1986) Tracking skill of a person with long term tactile experience: a case study. Journal of Rehabilitation Research and Development 23: 20–26.

Clark JE (1981) Four PB word lists for Australian English. Australian Journal of Audiology 3: 21–31.

Clark J, Dermody P, Palethorpe S (1985) Cue enhancement by stimulus repetition: natural and synthetic speech comparisons. Journal of the Acoustical Society of America 78: 458–462.

Coles RRA (1972) Can present day audiology really help in diagnosis?–An otologist's question. Journal of Laryngology and Otology 86: 191–224.

Coles RRA (1982) Otolaryngology 1: Otology, Gibb AG, Smith MFW (Eds), Chapter 10 London: Butterworth Scientific.

Coles RRA, Priede VM (1974) Derivations of formulae for masking of the non-test ear in speech audiometry. ISVR Memorandum No 448, Institute of Sound and Vibration Research, University of Southampton.

Coles RRA, Priede VM (1975) Masking of the non-test ear in speech audiometry. Journal of Laryngology and Otology 89: 217–226.

Coles RRA, Markides A, Priede VM (1973). In Disorders of Auditory Function, Taylor W (Ed). London: Academic Press.

Commonwealth Acoustic Laboratory Audiology Training Manual (1953). Sydney: NAL.

Commonwealth Acoustic Laboratory Audiology Training Manual (1961). Sydney: NAL.

Commonwealth Acoustic Laboratory Audiology Training Manual (1969). Sydney: NAL.

Condon M (1985) Efficacy of microcomputer scoring of the staggered spondaic word test. Paper presented at the American Speech-Language-Hearing Association Annual Convention, Washington, DC.

Conklin ES (1917) A method for determination of relative skill in lip-reading. Volta Review 19, 216–220.

Connolly P, Jerger S, Williamson WD, Smith RJH, Demmler G (1992) Evaluation of higher-level auditory function in children with asymptomatic congenital cytolmegalovirus infection. The American Journal of Otology 13(2): 185–193.

Cowan RSC, Blamey PJ, Sarant JZ, Galvin KL, Alcantara J I, Whitford LA, Clark GM (1991) Role of a multichannel electrotactile speech processor in a cochlear implant program for profoundly hearing impaired adults. Journal of the Acoustical Society of America 12: 39–46.

Cox RM (1983) Using ULCL measures to find frequency-gain and SSPL90. Hearing Instruments 32(5): 16–20.

Cox RM (1985) A structured approach to hearing aid selection. Ear and Hearing 6: 226–239.

Cox RM (1988) The MSU hearing instrument prescription procedure. Hearing Instruments 39(1): 6–10.

Cox RM (1993) On the evaluation of a new generation of hearing aids. Journal of Rehabilitation Research and Development 30: 297–304.

Cox RM, Alexander GC (1991a) Hearing aid benefit in everyday environments. Ear and Hearing 12(2): 127–139.

Cox RM, Alexander GC (1991b) Preferred hearing aid gain in everyday environments. Ear and Hearing 12(2): 123–126.

Cox RM, Alexander GC (1992) Maturation of hearing aid benefit: objective and subjective measurements (maturation of benefit). Ear and Hearing 13: 131–141.

Cox RM, Alexander GC (1994) The abbreviated profile of hearing aid benefit (APHAB). Paper presented at the American Academy of Audiology Meeting, Richmond, VA.

Cox RM, McDaniel DM (1984) Intelligibility ratings of continuous discourse: application to hearing aid selection. Journal of the Acoustical Society of America 76: 758–766.

Cox RM, Moore JN (1988) Composite speech spectrum for hearing aid gain prescriptions. Journal of Speech and Hearing Research 31: 102–107.

Cox RM, Rivera IM (1992) Predictability and reliability of hearing aid benefit measured using the PHAB. Journal of the American Academy of Audiology 3: 242–254.

Cox RM, Alexander GC, Gilmore C (1987) Development of the connected speech test (CST). Ear and Hearing 8: 119S–126S.

Cox RM, Alexander GC, Gilmore C, Pusakulich (1988) Use of the connected speech test (CST) with hearing impaired listeners. Ear and Hearing 9: 198–207.

Cox RM, Goff CM, Martin SE, McLoud LL (1994a) The contour test: normative data. Paper presented at the American Academy of Audiology Meeting, Richmond, VA.

Cox RM, Taylor IM, Gray GA, Brainerd LE (1994b) The Contour Test: applications to hearing aid selection and fitting. Paper presented at the American Academy of Audiology Meeting, Richmond, VA.

Craig WN (1964) Effects of preschool training on the development of reading and lipreading skills of deaf children. American Annals of the Deaf 109: 280–296.

Creelman CD (1957) Case of the unknown talker. Journal of the Acoustical Society of America 29: 655. Cutting JA, Pisoni DB (1978) Speech and Language in the Laboratory, School and Clinic, Kavanagh JF, Strange W (Eds). Cambridge, MA: MIT Press.

Danhauer JL, Crawford S, Edgerton BJ (1984) English, Spanish and bilingual speakers' performance on a nonsense syllable test (NST) of speech sound discrimination. Journal of Speech and Hearing Disorders 49: 164–169.

Dante D (1995) Speech audiometry in Romanian. MSc thesis, University of Manchester.

Darbyshire JO (1970) A technique for the application of speech audiometry to severely hearing impaired subjects. The Teacher of the Deaf 68: 99–103.

Davis AC (1983) Hearing disorders in the population. First phase findings of the MRC National Study of Hearing. In Lutman ME, Haggard MP (Eds) Hearing Science and Hearing Disorders. London: Academic Press.

Davis H (1948) The articulation area and the Social Adequacy Index for hearing. Laryngoscope 68: 761–778.

Davis H, Silverman RS (1970) Hearing and Deafness, 3rd edition. New York: Holt, Rinehart and Winston.

Davis H, Silverman RS (1978) Hearing and Deafness, 4th edition. New York: Holt, Rinehart and Winston.

Davis RJ, Kastelanski W, Stephens SDG (1976) Some factors influencing the results of speech tests of central auditory function. Scandinavian Audiology 5: 179–186.

Dawson PW, Blamey PJ, Rowland LC, Dettman SJ, Clark GM, Busby PJ, Brown AM, Dowell RC, Rickards FW (1992) Cochlear implants in children, adolescents, and prelinguistically deafened adults: speech perception. Journal of Speech and Hearing Research 35: 401–417.

Day HE, Fusfeld IS, Pintner R (1928) A Survey of American Schools for the Deaf. Washington, DC: National Research Council.

Deafness Forum (1994) Statistics — the results you get depend on the questions you ask: 12. Deakin, ACT: Deafness Forum.

De Filippo CL (1984) Laboratory projects in tactile aids to lipreading. Ear and Hearing 5: 211–227.

De Filippo CL, Scott BL (1978) A method for training and evaluating the reception of ongoing speech. Journal of the Acoustical Society of America 63: 1186–1192.

Demorest ME, DeHaven GP (1993) Psychometric adequacy of self-assessment scales. In: Self-assessment Scales in Audiology. Seminars in Hearing 14(4): 354–362.

Dempsey JJ, Levitt H, Josephson J, Porrazzo J (1992) Computer assisted tracking simulation (CATS). Journal of the Acoustical Society of America 92: 701–710.

Denes PB (1963) On the statistics of spoken English. Journal of the Acoustical Society of America 35: 892–904.

Denes PB, Pinson EM (1963) The Speech Chain. Murray Hill, NJ: Bell Telephone Laboratories.

Department of Immigration (1978) Consolidated Statistics, 10. Canberra: Australian Government Publishing Service.

DeRenzi E, Vignolo L (1962) The Token Testøa sensitive test to detect receptive disturbances in aphasics. Brain 85: 665–678.

Dermody P (1982) Assessing and evaluating audiological assessment and evaluation. Paper presented at the Audiological Society of Australia, 5th National Conference, Leura, NSW.

Dermody P (1990) The NALTALLCK Project. In Butler S (Ed.) The Exceptional Child. Sydney: Harcourt, Brace, Jovanovich.

Dermody P, Byrne D (1975) Variability in Speech Test Performance for Binaural Hearing Aid Evaluations. National Acoustic Laboratories Report No. 62. Sydney: NAL.

Dermody P, Mackie K (1980) Auditory Memory Deficits in Language Disordered Children. National Acoustic Laboratories Report No. 81. Sydney: NAL.

Dermody P, Mackie K (1982) An initial assessment battery for measuring auditory receptive language in children. Australian Journal of Audiology, Supplement 1: 6.

Dermody P, Mackie K (1983a) Problems in establishing tympanometric screening criteria: experience with a language/learning disordered population. Australian Journal of Human Communication Disorders 11: 41–50.

Dermody P, Mackie K (1983b) Effects of mild to moderate hearing loss on educational achievement. In Milne H, Campbell C, Payne S (Eds), Proceedings of the 8th National Conference of the Australian Association of Special Education, Volume 2. Brisbane: AASE.

Dermody P, Mackie K (1987) Speech tests in audiological assessment at the National Acoustic Laboratories. In Martin M (Ed.) Speech Audiometry. London: Taylor and Francis.

Dermody P, Cowley J, Mackie K (1982) Language disorders and academic failure in kindergarten children: possible identification procedures. Paper presented at the Australian Psychological Society Conference, Melbourne.

Dermody P, Katsch R, Mackie K (1983a) Amplitude normalisation techniques for speech intelligibility testing. Proceedings of the 11th International Congress of Acoustics 4: 45–48.

Dermody P, Katsch R, Mackie K (1983b) Auditory processing limitations in low verbal children: Evidence from a two response dichotic listening task. Ear and Hearing 4, 272–277.

Dermody P, Mackie K, Katsch R (1983c) Dichotic listening in good and poor readers. Journal Speech and Hearing Research 26: 341–348.

Dermody P, Mackie K, Anderson M (1984) Investigation of an Australian recording of the AB speech lists with elderly hearing impaired persons. Paper presented at the 6th National Conference of the Australian Audiological Society, Greenmount.

De Sa N (1973) Hindi PB lists for speech audiometry and discrimination test. Indian Journal of Otolaryngology 25: 67–75.

Dewey G (1923) Relative frequency of English speech sounds. Cambridge, MA: Harvard University Press.

DiCarlo L, Kataja R (1951) An analysis of the Utley lipreading test. Journal of Speech and Hearing Disorders 16: 226–240.

Dillon H (1982) A quantitative examination of the sources of speech discrimination test score variability. Ear and Hearing 3: 51–58.

Dillon H (1983) The effect of test difficulty on the sensitivity of speech discrimination tests. Journal of the Acoustical Society of America 73: 336–344.

Dillon H (1984) A Procedure for Subjective Quality Rating of Hearing Aids. National Acoustic Laboratories Report No. 100: 1–25. Sydney: NAL.

Dillon H (1993) Hearing aid evaluation: predicting speech gain from insertion gain. Journal of Speech and Hearing Research 36: 621–633.

Dillon H, Ching T (1995) What makes a good speech test? In Plant G and Spens K-E (Eds) Profound Deafness and Speech Communication. London: Whurr Publishers. 305–349.

Deutsche Institut für Norming (DIN)

DIN 45633-2 (1969) Prazisionsschallpegelmesser; Sonderanforderungen fur die Anwendung auf kurzdauernde und impulshaltige Vorgange (Impulsschallpegelmesser) (Precision sound level meter; special requirements for the application to impulsive sounds and sounds of short duration (impulse sound level meter)).

DIN 45621 (1961, 2nd edition 1973) Worter fur Gehorprufung mit Sprache (Word lists for intelligibility test).

DIN 45624 (1976) Sprachaudiometer; Begriffe, Anforderungen, Prufung (Speech audiometers; terminology, requirements, testing).

DIN 45626 (1976) Tontrager zum Prufen des Horvermogens; besprochen mit Wortern nach DIN 45621 (Aufnahme 1969) (Sound carrier for the hearing test using speech in accordance with DIN 45621 (recording 1969)).

DIN 45626-2 (1980) Tontrager mit Sprache fur Gehorprufung; Tontrager mit Satzen nach DIN 45621-2 (Aufnahme 1973); Anforderungen (Sound recording medium for the hearing test using speech in accordance with DIN 45621-2 (recording 1973); requirements).

DIN 45621-2 (1980) Sprache fur Gehorprufung; Satze (Sentence lists for intelligibility test).

DIN 45621-3 (1985) Sprache fur Gehorprufung; Worter fur die Gehorprufung bei Kindern (Speech material used in audiology; word lists for intelligibility testing in paediatric audiology).

Dirks DD, Wilson RH (1980) Binaural hearing in sound field. In Libby E (Ed.) Binaural Hearing and Amplification. Chicago: V I Zenetron Hearing Instruments. Inc.

Dirks DD, Stream RW, Wilson RH (1972) Speech audiometry: earphone and sound field. Speech and Hearing Disorders 7: 162–176.

Dirks DD, Kamm C, Bower D, Betsworth A (1977) Use of performance intensity functions for diagnosis. Journal of Speech and Hearing Disorders 42: 408–415.

Dirks DD, Morgan D, Dubno J (1982) A procedure for quantifying the effects of noise on speech recognition. Journal of Speech and Hearing Disorders 47: 114–123.

Dix MR, Hallpike CS, Hood JD (1949) 'Nerve' deafness: its clinical criteria, old and new. Proceedings of the Royal Society of Medicine 42: 527–536.

Djupesland G, Zwislocki JJ (1972) Sound pressure distribution in the outer ear. Scandinavian Audiology 1: 197–203.

Dodds J (1972) An object puzzle as an indicator of hearing acuity in children from a mental age of three. Sound 6: 49–55.

Dowell RC, Brown AM, Seligman PM, Clark GM (1985) Patient results for a multiple-channel cochlear prosthesis. In Schindler RA, Merzenich MM (Eds) Cochlear Implants. New York: Raven Press.

Dowell RC, Mecklenberg DJ, Clark GM (1986). Speech recognition for patients receiving multichannel cochlear implants. Archives of Otolaryngology, Head and Neck Surgery 112: 1054–1059.

Dreschler WA, Plomp R (1980) Relation between psychophysical data and speech perception for hearing-impaired subjects. Journal of the Acoustical Society of America 68: 1608–1615.

Dubno JR, Dirks DD (1982) Evaluation of hearing-impaired listeners using a nonsense syllable test I — Test reliability. Journal of Speech and Hearing Research 25: 135–141.

Dubno JR, Dirks DD, Langhofer LR (1982) Evaluation of hearing impaired listeners using a nonsense-syllable test II — Syllable recognition and consonant confusion patterns. Journal of Speech and Hearing Research 25: 141–148.

Dubno JR, Dirks DD, Schaefer AB (1989) Stop-consonant recognition for normal-hearing listeners and listeners with high-frequency hearing loss. II. Articulation index predictions. Journal of the Acoustical Society of America 85(1), 355–364.

Dudley P (1968) The Development of a Speech Hearing Test Using Recorded Sentences. Commonwealth Acoustic Laboratories Report Report No. 5. Sydney: CAL.

Duquesnoy AJ, Plomp R (1983) The effect of a hearing aid on the speech reception threshold of hearing-impaired listeners in quiet and in noise. Journal of the Acoustical Society of America 73: 2166–2173.

Edgerton BJ, Danhauer JL (1979) Clinical Implications of Speech Discrimination Testing Using Nonsense Stimuli. Baltimore, MD: University Park Press.

Egan JP (1948) Articulation testing methods. Laryngoscope 58: 955–991.

Eisenberg LS, Luckley RS, Norton NB, Berlinger KI (1977) A speech discrimination task for profoundly deafened adults: HHRC Rhyme Test. Paper presented at the American Speech-Hearing-Language Association, Convention, Chicago.

Elfenbein JL, Hardin-Jones MA, Davis JM (1994) Oral communication skills of children of adult cochlear implant candidates. Journal of Speech and Hearing Research. 37(10: 216–225.

Elliott L, Katz D (1980) Development of a New Children's Test of Speech Discrimination. St. Louis, MO: Auditec.

Elliott L, Conners S, Kille E, Levin S, Ball K, Katz D (1979) Children's understanding of monosyllabic nouns in quiet and in noise. Journal of the Acoustical Society of America 66: 12–21.

Elliot ELL, Clifton LB, Servi DG (1983) Word frequency effects for a closed-set word identification test. Audiology 22: 229–240.

Elliot M, Doyle J (1994) The performance of monolingual and bilingual Australian speakers on standard tests of speech discrimination. Australian Journal of Human Communication Disorders, In press.

Elphick R (1984) Comparison of live and video presentation of a speech reading test with children. British Journal of Audiology 18: 109–116.

Erb LLV (1985) Homophonous monosyllabic words used as a lipreading test. Paper presented at the American Speech-Language-Hearing Association Convention, Washington, DC.

Erber NP (1972) Auditory, visual and auditory-visual recognition of consonants by children with normal and impaired hearing. Journal of Speech and Hearing Research 15, 413–422.

Erber NP (1974) Pure tone thresholds and word recognition abilities of hearing impaired children. Journal of Speech and Hearing Research 17: 194–202.

Erber NP (1977) Evaluating speech perception ability in hearing impaired children. In Bess FH (Ed.) Childhood Deafness: Causation, Assessment and Management. New York: Grune and Stratton.

Erber NP (1980) Use of the auditory numbers test to evaluate speech perception abilities of hearing impaired children. Journal of Speech and Hearing Disorders 45: 527–539.

Erber N, Alencewicz C (1976) Audiologic evaluation of deaf children. Journal of Speech and Hearing Disorders 41: 256–267.

Ewertsen HW (1973) Auditive, Visual and Audio-visual Perception of Speech. The State Hearing Centre, Bispebjerg Hospital, Copenhagen: The Helen Group.

Ewertsen HW (1974) Auditory and audio-visual speech perception related to hearing disorders. Scandinavian Audiology Supplement 4: 76–82.

Ewertsen HW, Birk-Nelson H (1973) Social hearing handicap index: social handicap in relation to hearing impairment. Audiology 12: 180–187.

External Pattern Input (EPI) Group (1986a) The BKB (Bamford-Kowal-Bench) standard sentence lists, female speaker, Lists 1 to 11 and 12 to 21 (video recordings). London: EPI Group, Department of Phonetics and Linguistics, University College london.

External Pattern Input (GPI) Group (1986b) The 12 Intervocalic Consonant Test. London: EPI Group Department of Phonetics and Linguistics, University College of London.

Fabry DA, Van Tasell DJ (1990) Evaluation of an articulation index based model for predicting the effects of adaptive frequency response to aids. Journal of Speech and Hearing Research 33: 676–689.

Fairbanks G (1958) Test of phonemic differentiation: The rhyme test. Journal of the Acoustical Society of America 30: 596–600.

Fant G (1960) Acoustic Theory of Speech Production. The Hague: Mouton.

Fant G (1967) Auditory patterns of speech. In Wathen-Dunn W (Ed.) Models for the Perception of Speech and the Visual Form. Cambridge Mass: MIT Press.

Farrimond T (1959) Age differences in the ability to use visual aids in auditory communications. Language and Speech 2: 179–192.

Faulkner A, Ball V, Rosen S, Moore BCJ, Fourcin A (1992) Speech pattern hearing aids for the profoundly hearing impaired: speech perception and auditory abilities. Journal of the Acoustical Society of America 91: 2136–2155.

Feldman H (1960) A history of audiology: a comprehensive report and bibliography from the earliest beginnings to the present. (Translated by Tonndorf J from: Die Geschichtliche Entwicklung der Horprufungsmethoden, kuze Darstellung und Bibliographie von der Anfongen bis zue Gegenwart). In Leicher H, Mittermaiser R, Theissing G (Eds) Zwanglose Abhandungen aus dem Gebeit der Hals-Nasen-Ohren-Heilk-unde. Stuttgart: Georg Theime Verlag. Translation: Beltone Institute of Hearing Research 22: 1–111.

Festen JM, Plomp R (1983) Relations between auditory functions in impaired hearing. Journal of the Acoustical Society of America 73: 652–662.

Fikret-Pasa S (1993) The effects of compression ratio on speech intelligibility and quality. Northwestern University Ph.D. Dissertation. Ann Arbor, MI: University Microfilms.

Finitzo-Heiber T, Gerling IJ, Matkin ND, Cherow-Skalka E (1980) A sound effects recognition test for paediatric audiological evaluation. Ear and Hearing 1: 271–276.

Fisher J, King A, Parker A, Wright R (1983) Assessment of speech production and speech perception as a basis for therapy. In Hochberg I et al. (Eds) Speech of the Hearing Impaired. Baltimore, MD: University Park Press.

Fletcher H (1929) Speech and Hearing. New York: Van Nostrand.

Fletcher H (1950) A method of calculating hearing loss for speech from an audiogram. Journal of the Acoustical Society of America 22: 1–10.

Fletcher H (1953) Speech and Hearing in Communication. New York: Van Nostrand.

Fletcher H, Steinberg JC (1929) Articulation methods. Bell Systems Technical Journal 8: 806–854.

Foster JR, Haggard MP (1979) (FAAF) An efficient analytical test of speech perception. Proceedings of the Institute of Acoustics IA3: 9–12.

Foster JR, Haggard MP (1984) Introduction and Test Manual for FAAF 11. Nottingham: MRC Institute of Hearing Research.

Foster JR, Haggard MP, Iredale FE (1981) Prescription of gain-setting and prognosis for use and benefit of post-aural hearing aids. Audiology 20: 157–176.

Foster JR, Summerfield AQ, Marshall DH, Palmer L, Ball V, Rosen S. (1993) Lipreading the BKB sentence lists: corrections for list and practice effects. British Journal of Audiology 27: 233–246.

Fourcin AJ (1976) Speech pattern tests for deaf children. In Stephens SDG (Ed.) Disorders of Auditory Function, 11. London: Academic Press.

Fourcin AJ (1979) Chapter 9. In Beagley HA (Ed.) Auditory Investigation: The Scientific and Technological Basis. Oxford: Clarendon Press.

Fourcin AJ, Stephens SDG, Hazan V, Irwin J, Ball V, Delmont J (1985) Audiological rehabilitation of patients with brainstem disorders. British Journal of Audiology 19: 29–43.

Frank T (1980) Clinical significance of the relative intelligibility of pictorially presented spondee words. Ear and Hearing 1: 46–49.

French NR, Steinberg JC (1947) Factors governing the intelligibility of speech sounds. Journal of the Acoustical Society of America 19: 90–119.

French NR, Carter CW Jr., Koenig W Jr. (1930) The words and sounds of telephone conversations. Bell Systems Technical Journal 9: 290–324.

Fry DB (1947) The frequency of occurrence of speech sounds in Southern English. Archives Neerlandaises de Phonetique Experimentale 20: 103–106.

Fry DB (1961) Word and sentence tests for use in speech audiometry. Lancet 2: 197–199.

Fry DB (1964) Modifications to speech audiometry. International Audiology 3: 227–236.

Fry DB (1979) The Physics of Speech. Cambridge: Cambridge University Press.

Fry DB, Kerridge PMT (1939) Tests for hearing of speech by deaf people. Lancet 1: 106–111.

Fuller HC (1983) Speech level standardization in audiometry. Proceedings of the 11th International Congress of Acoustics, Paris 3: 205–208.

Fuller HC (1987) Equipment for speech audiometry and its calibration. In Martin M (Ed.) Speech Audiometry. London: Taylor and Francis.

Fuller HC, Whittle LS (1982) The measurement of speech levels for audiometry. Proceedings of the Institute of Acoustics Spring Conference, Guildford.

Fuller HC, Moss IK (1985) A Survey of Speech Audiometry in the National Health Service. Teddington: NPL National Physical Laboratory, Acoustics Report AC 105.

Gang R (1976) The effects of age on the diagnostic utility of the rollover phenomenon. Journal of Speech and Hearing Disorders 41: 63–69.

Gatehouse S (1990) Determinants of Self-reported disability in older subjects. Ear and Hearing 11(5): Supp. 575–655.

Gatehouse S (1993) Hearing aid evaluation: limitations of present procedures and future requirements. Journal of Speech Language Pathology and Audiology, Suppl. 1: 50–57.

Gatehouse S (1994) Components and determinants of hearing aid benefit. Ear and Hearing 15: 30–49.

Gatehouse S, Haggard MP (1987) The effects of air–bone gap and presentation level on auditory disability. Ear and Hearing 8: 140–146.

Gatehouse S, Killion MC (1993) HABRAT: Hearing aid brain rewiring/accommodation time. Hearing Instruments 44(10): 29–30, 32.

Gelfand SA (1975) Use of the carrier phrase in live voice speech discrimination testing. Journal of Auditory Research 15: 107–110.

Gengel RW (1971) Acceptable speech-to-noise ratios for aided speech discrimination by the hearing impaired. Journal of Auditory Research 11: 219–222.

Gengel RW, Pascoe D, Shore I (1971) A frequency-response procedure for evaluating and selecting hearing aids for severely hearing impaired children. Journal Speech and Hearing Research 36: 341–353.

Gerber SE, Fisher LB (1979) Prediction of hearing aid users' satisfaction. Journal of the American Audiological Society 5(1): 35–40.

Gimson AC (1980) An Introduction to the Pronunciation of English, 3rd edition. London: Edward Arnold.

Giolas TG, Owens E, Lamb SH, Schubert ED (1979) Hearing performance inventory. Journal of Speech and Hearing Disorders 29: 215–230.

Gladstone VA, Siegenthaler BM (1971) Carrier phrase and speech intelligibility test score. Journal of Audiology Research 11: 101–103.

Gnosspelius J, Spens K-E (1992) A computer-based speech tracking procedure. STL-QPSR/1: 131–137. Stockholm: Royal Institute of Technology.

Goetzinger C (1972) Word discrimination testing. In Katz J (Ed.) Handbook of Clinical Audiology. Baltimore, MD: Williams and Wilkins.

Grant JM (1980) The CAL-PBM's a Misnomer?, Australian Journal of Audiology 2: 19–21.

Green DS, Ross M (1968) The effect of a conventional versus a non-occluding (CROS-type) earmold upon the frequency response of a hearing aid. Journal of Speech and Hearing Research 11: 638–647.

Green RJV, Day S, Bamford J (1986) A comparative investigation of four hearing aid selection procedures. Speech discrimination measures of benefit. British Journal of Audiology 23: 185–199.

Greville K (1984) Standardisation of NAC-AB speech discrimination materials. Audiology Centre Report No 2.

Gruber J (1891) A Textbook of the Diseases of the Ear. New York: D Appleton and Co.

Hagerman B (1976) Reliability in the determination of speech discrimination. Scandinavian Audiology 5: 219–228.

Hagerman B (1979) Reliability in the determination of speech reception threshold (SRT). Scandinavian Audiology 8: 195–202.

Hagerman B (1982) Sentences for testing speech intelligibility in noise. Scandinavian Audiology 11: 79–87.

Hagerman B (1984) Clinical measurements of speech reception threshold in noise. Scandinavian Audiology 13: 57–63.

Hagerman B (1993) Efficiency of speech audiometry and other tests. Scandinavian Audiology 27: 423–425.

Hagerman B, Gabrielsson A (1984) Questionnaires on Desirable Properties of Hearing Aids. Karolinska Institute Report TA109. Stockholm: Karolinska Institute.

Hagerman B, Kinnefors C (1995) Efficient adaptive methods for measuring speech reception threshold in quiet and in noise. Scandinavian Audiology 24: 71–77.

Haggard MP, Foster JR, Iredale FE (1981) Use and benefit of postaural aids in sensory hearing loss. Scandinavian Audiology 10: 45–52.

Haggard MP, Wood ES, Carroll S (1984) Speech, admittance and tone tests in school screening. Reconciling economics with pathology and disability perspectives. British Journal of Audiology 18: 133–153.

Haggard MP, Lindblad AC, Foster JR (1986) Psychoacoustical and audiometric prediction of auditory disability at listener-adjusted presentation levels. Audiology 25: 277–298.

Hahlbrock KH (1970) Sprachaudiometrie (Speech Audiometry), 2nd edition. Stuttgart: Georg Thieme Verlag.

Hanin L, Boothroyd A, Hnath-Chisholm T (1988) Tactile presentation of voice fundamental frequency as an aid to the speechreading of sentences. Ear and Hearing 9: 335–341.

Haskins HA (1949) A phonetically balanced test of speech discrimination for children. Master's Thesis. Northwestern University, Evanston, IL.

Hawley M (Ed.) (1977) Speech Intelligibility and Speaker Recognition. Stroudsburg PA: Dowden Hutchinson and Ross.

Hayes D, Jerger J (1979) Aging and hearing aid use. Scandinavian Audiology 8: 33–40.

Hawkins DB, Montgomery AA, Mueller HG, Sedge RK (1988) Assessment of speech intelligibility by hearing-impaired listeners. In Berglund B, Karlsson J, Lindvall T (Eds) Noise as a Public Health Problem, Vol. 2, 241–246. Stockholm: Swedish Council for Building Research

Hazan V (1986) Speech pattern audiometric assessment of hearing-impaired children. PhD Thesis, University of London.

Hazan V, Fourcin AJ (1985) Microprocessor controlled speech pattern audiometry. Audiology 24(5): 325–335.

Hazan V, Rosen S (1991) Individual variability in the perception of cues to place contrasts in initial stops. Perception and Psychophysics 49: 187–200.

Hazan V, Fourcin AJ, Abberton ER (1991) Development of phonetic labelling in hearing-impaired children. Ear and Hearing 12: 71–84.

Hazan V, Wilson G, Howells D, Abberton E, Fourcin A (1995) Speech pattern audiometry for clinical use. European Journal for Disorders of Communication, 30: 1–16.

Heider F, Heider G (1940) An experimental investigation of lipreading. Psychological Monograph 124–153.

Hickson F (19870 The Manchester Picture Test: A summary. British Journal of Teachers of the Deaf 11: 161–166.

High WS, Fairbanks C, Glorig A (1964) Scale of self assessment of hearing handicap. Journal of Speech and Hearing Disorders 29: 215–230.

Hinchcliffe R (1968) Report on audiology in India. Sound 2: 59–68.

Hinkle RR, Binnie CA (1979) List equivalency CID sentences presented in three sensory conditions. Paper presented at the American Speech-Language-Hearing Association Convention, Atlanta, GA.

Hirsh IJ (1952) The Measurement of Hearing. New York: McGraw-Hill.

Hirsh IJ (1964) Clinical audiometry and the perception of speech and language. Review of Laryngology 85: 453–460.

Hirsh IJ, Davis H, Silverman SR, Reynolds EG, Eldert E, Benson RW (1952) Development of materials for speech audiometry. Journal of Speech and Hearing Disorders 17: 321–337.

Hirsh IJ, Reynolds EG, Joseph M (1954) Intelligibility of different speech materials. Journal of the Acoustical Society of America 26: 530–538.

Hochberg I, Rosen S, Ball V (1989) Effect of text complexity on connected discourse tracking rate. Ear and Hearing 10: 192–199.

Hodgson WR (1986) Speech acoustics and intelligibility. In Hodgson WR (Ed) Hearing Aid Assessment and Use in Audiologic Habilitation 3rd Edn: Baltimore MA: Williams and Wilkins 109–127.

Holmes JW (1976) Water Resources of Australia and the Pattern of Population Concentrations, Research Report No. 4. Canberra: Australian Government Publishing Service.

Holsgrove G, Halden J (1984) Speech tests of hearing. Some new test material. Journal of the British Association of Teachers of the Deaf 8: 16–18.

Hood JD (1957) The principles and practice of bone conduction audiometry: A review of the present position. Proceedings of the Royal Society of Medicine 50: 689.

Hood JD (1981) Chapter 16 in Audiology and Audiological Medicine, Vol. 1, Beagley HA (Ed.). Oxford: Oxford University Press.

Hood JD (1984) Speech discrimination in bilateral and unilateral hearing loss due to Ménière's disease. British Journal of Audiology 18: 173–177.

Hood JD, Poole JP (1971) Speech audiometry in conductive and sensorineural hearing loss. Sound 5, 30–38.

Hood JD, Poole JP (1977) Improving the reliability of speech audiometry. British Journal of Audiology 11: 93–102.

House AS, Williams CE, Hecker MHL, Kryter KD (1963) Psychoacoustic Speech Tests: a Modified Rhyme Test. U.S. Air Force Systems Command. Hanscom Field, Electronics Systems Division, Technical Document Report ESD-TDR-63–403.

House AS, Williams CE, Hecker MHL, Kryter KD (1965) Articulation testing methods: consonantal differentiation with a closed-response set. Journal of the Acoustical Society of America 37: 158–166.

Howes D (1957) On the relation between the intelligibility and frequency of occurrence of English words. Journal of the Acoustical Society of America 29: 296–305.

Howes D (1966) A word count of spoken English. Journal of Verbal Hearing and Verbal Behaviour 5: 572–607.

Hudgins CV (1949) A method of appraising the speech of the deaf. Volta Review 51: 597–601.

Hudgins CV, Hawkins JE Jr., Karlin JE, Stevens SS (1947) The development of recorded auditory tests for measuring hearing loss for speech. Laryngoscope 57: 57–89.

Huff SJ, Nerbonne A (1982) Comparison of the American Speech-Language Hearing Association and revised Tillman-Olsen methods for speech threshold measurement. Ear and Hearing 3: 335–339.

Hughson W, Thompson EA (1942) Correlation of hearing acuity for speech with discrete frequency audiograms. Archives Otolaryngologica 36: 526–540.

Humes LE (1991) Understanding the speech-understanding problems of the hearing impaired. Journal of the American Academy of Audiology 2: 59–69.

Humes LE (1993) Hearing aid selection and evaluation in the year 2000. Canadian Journal of Speech-Language Pathology and Audiology 1 (Suppl.): 98–106.

Humes LE, Roberts RL (1990) Speech recognition difficulties of the hearing impaired elderly: the contributions of audibility. Journal of Speech and Hearing Research 33: 726–735.

Humes LE, Houghton R (1992) Beyond insertion gain. Hearing Instruments 43(3): 32–35.

Humes LE, Halling DC (1994) Overview, rationale and comparison of suprathreshold-based gain-prescription procedures. In Valente M (Ed.) Strategies for Selecting and Verifying Hearing Aid Fittings. New York: Thieme Medical Publishers, Inc.

Humes LE, Boney S, Ahlstrom C (1985) Comparisons of two schemes for predicting speech recognition in normals. Paper presented at the American Speech-Language-Hearing Association Convention, Washington, DC.

Humes LE, Dirks DD, Bell TS, Ahlstrom C, Kincaid GE (1986) Application of the articulation index and the speech transmission index to the recognition of speech by normal hearing and hearing impaired listeners. Journal of Speech and Hearing Research 29: 447–462.

Hurley RM (1980) Chapter 8 in Speech Protocols in Audiology, Rupp RR, Stockdell KG (Eds). New York: Grune and Stratton.

Hygge S, Rönnberg J, Larsby B, Arlinger S (1992) Normal-hearing and hearing-impaired subjects ability to just follow conversation in competing speech, reversed speech, and noise backgrounds. Journal of Speech and Hearing Research 35: 208–215.

International Civil Aviation Organisation (1955) Special Meeting on Hearing and Visual Requirements for Personnel Licensing Report. London: ICAO.

International Electrotechnical Commission (IEC): Geneva

IEC 94–3 (1990) Magnetic recording and reproducing systems.

IEC 268–7 (1984) Sound system equipment. Part 7: Headphones and headsets.

IEC 303 (1970) IEC provisional reference coupler for the calibration of earphones used in audiometry.

IEC 318 (1970) An IEC artificial ear, of the wide-band type for the calibration of earphones used in audiometry.

IEC 373 (1990) Mechanical coupler for measurements on bone vibrators.

IEC 645–1 (1992) Audiometers part 1: Pure Tone Audiometers

IEC 645–2 (1993) Audiometers part 2: Equipment for Speech Audiometry.

IEC 651 (1979) Sound level meters.

IEC 711 (1981) Occluded-ear simulator for the measurement of earphones coupled to the ear by ear inserts.

International Organization for Standardization (ISO): Geneva

ISO 389 (1991) ISO 266 ISO 389–7 Acoustics—Standard reference zero for the calibration of pure-tone audiometers.

ISO 6189 (1983) Acoustics - Pure-tone air conduction threshold audiometry for hearing conservation purposes.

ISO 7566 (1987) Acoustics - Standard reference zero for the calibration of pure tone bone-conduction audiometers.

ISO 8253–1 (1989) Acoustics - Audiometric Test Methods. Part 1: Pure Tone Audiometry.

ISO 8253–2 (1989) Acoustics - Audiometric Test Methods. Part 2:

ISO 8253-3 (1996) Acoustics - Audiometric test methods. Part 3: Speech Audiometry.

Institute of Hearing Research (1991) Protocols for Performance Tests of Auditory Reception. Internal Report.

Jakobson RC, Fant GM, Halle M (1952) Preliminaries to speech analysis: The distinctive features and their correlates. Technical Report No. 13. Cambridge, MA: Acoustics Laboratory, MIT.

James CT (1992) The application of computers to speech audiometry. PhD Thesis, University of Surrey, Department of Physics.

Jauhiainen T (1974) An experimental study of the auditory perception of isolated bi-syllable Finnish words. Academic Dissertation. The Institute of Physiology, University of Helsinki.

Jeffers J (1967) A re-evaluation of the Utley lipreading sentence test. Paper presented at the American Speech-Language-Hearing Association. Convention, Chicago, IL.

Jeffers J, Barley M (1971) Speechreading (lipreading). Springfield, IL: Charles C Thomas.

Jerger J (1973) Audiological findings in aging. Advances in Oto-Rhino-Laryngology 20: 115–124.

Jerger S (1983) Speech Audiometry. In Jerger J (Ed.) Recent Advances Series in Speech, Hearing, and Language, 71–93. San Diego, CA: College Hill Press.

Jerger S (1987) Validation of the pediatric speech intelligibility test in children with central nervous system lesions. Audiology 26: 298–311.

Jerger J, Hayes D (1976) Hearing aid evaluation: clinical experience with a new philosophy. Archives of Otolaryngology 102: 214–225.

Jerger J, Jerger S (1971) Diagnostic significance of PB word functions. Archives of Otolaryngology 93: 573–580.

Jerger S, Jerger J (1976) Estimating speech threshold from the PI-PB function. Archives of Otolaryngology 102: 487–496.

Jerger S, Jerger J (1979) Quantifying auditory handicap. A new approach. Audiology 18: 225–237.

Jerger S, Jerger J (1982) Paediatric speech intelligibility test: performance intensity characteristics. Ear and Hearing 3: 325–334.

Jerger S, Jerger J (1984) Paediatric Speech Intelligibility Test. St Louis, MD: Auditec.

Jerger S, Jerger J (1985) Paediatric hearing aid evaluation: Case reports. Ear and Hearing 6: 240–244.

Jerger S, Zeller RS (1989) Dichotic listening in a child with a cerebral lesion: the 'paradoxical' ipsilateral ear deficit. Ear and Hearing, 10: 167–172.

Jerger J, Speaks C, Malquist C (1966) Hearing-aid performance and hearing-aid selection. Journal of Speech and Hearing Research 9: 136–149.

Jerger J, Speaks C, Trammell JL (1968) A new approach to speech audiometry. Journal of Speech and Hearing Disorders 33: 318–328.

Jerger J, Weikers NJ, Sharbrough FW III et al. (1969) Bilateral lesions of the temporal lobe: A case study. Acta Otolaryngologica, Supplement 258: 1–51.

Jerger KW, Hagberg EN, Rane RL (1977) Prescription of Hearing Aids: Rationale, Procedure, and Results. Kent, UH: Herald Publishing House.

Jerger S, Lewis S, Hawkins J, Jerger J (1980) Paediatric speech intelligibility test. I. Generation of test materials. International Journal of Paediatric Otorhinolaryngology 2: 217–230.

Jerger S, Jerger J, Lewis S (1981) Paediatric speech intelligibility test. II. Effect of receptive language age and chronological age. International Journal of Paediatric Otorhinolarnygology 3: 101–118.

Jerger S, Jerger J, Abrams S (1983) Speech audiometry in the young child. Ear and Hearing 4: 56–66.

Jerger S, Jerger J, Alford B, Abrams S (1983) Development of speech intelligibility in children with current otitis media. Ear and Hearing 4: 138–145.

Jerger S, Johnson K, Loiselle L (1988) Pediatric central auditory dysfunction: Comparison of children with confirmed lesions versus suspected processing disorders. American Journal of Otology 9, Supplement: 63–71.

Jerger S, Elizondo R, Dink T, Sanchez P, Chavira E (1994) Linguistic influences on the auditory processing of speech by children with normal hearing or hearing impairment. Ear and Hearing 15(2): 138–160.

Jerevall L, Almqvist B, Ovegård A, Arlinger S (1983) Clinical trial of in-the-ear hearing aids. Scandinavian Audiology 12: 63–70.

Johnson DR (1976) Communications characteristics of a young deaf adult population: techniques for evaluating their communication skills. American Annals of the Deaf: 409–424.

Jupiter T (1982) Audiometric and speechreading correlates of hearing handicap in the elderly. Doctoral dissertation. Teachers College, Columbia University.

Kalikow DN, Stevens KN, Elliot LL (1977) Development of a test of speech intelligibility in noise using sentence materials with controlled word predictability. Journal of the Acoustical Society of America 61: 1337–1351.

Kam TPK (1982) Speech audiometric test material in Cantonese. MSc dissertation. University of Southampton.

Kamm C, Morgan D, Dirks D (1983) Accuracy of adaptive procedure estimates of PB Max level. Journal of Speech and Hearing Disorders 48: 202–209.

Kaplan H, Pickett J (1982) Differences in speech discrimination in the elderly as a function of type of competing noise: speech babble or cafeteria. Audiology 21: 325–333

Kapur YP (1971) Needs of the Speech and Hearing Handicapped in India. Vellore: Christian Medical College and Hospital.

Katz J (1962) The use of staggered spondaic words for assessing the integrity of the central auditory nervous system. Journal of Auditory Research 2: 327–337.

Katz J (1977) Central Auditory Dysfunction, Keith RW (Ed.), chapter 4. New York: Grune and Stratton.

Katz DR, Elliot LL (1978) Development of New Children's Speech Discrimination Tests. Chicago: American Speech-Language-Hearing Association.

Kei J, Chan T, Ma MC, Ng L, Lowe C, Lai DM, Ng YH, Kwan E (1991) Cantonese speech audiometry in children of Hongkong. Australian Journal Audioligy 13(2): 41–45.

Keith RW (1977) Central Auditory Dysfunction, Keith RW (Ed.), chapter 3. New York: Grune and Stratton.

Kelly B, Pillow G (1979) Nonsense syllable discrimination by picture identification with young children. Journal of the American Auditory Society 4: 170–172.

Kendall DC (1953) Audiometry for young children: Part 1. Teacher of the Deaf 51: 171–178.

Kendall DC (1954) Audiometry for young children: Part 2. Teacher of the Deaf 52: 18–23.

Kendall DC (1956) On the management of deafness in the young child. Proceedings of the Royal Society of Medicine 49: 463–467.

Kendall MG, Stuart A (1958) The Advanced Theory of Statistics. Vol. 1. London: Griffin.

Killion MC, Villchur E (1993) Kessler was right — partly: but SIN test shows some aids improve hearing in noise. The Hearing Journal 46(9): 31–35.

Killion MC, Wilbur LA,, Gudmundsen GI (1985) Insert earphones for more interaural attenuation. Hearing Instruments 36(2): 34–36.

Klein W, Plomp R, Pols LCW (1970) Vowel spectra, vowel spaces, and vowel identification. Journal of the Acoustical Society of America 48: 999–1009.

Knight JJ, Littler TS (1953) The technique of speech audiometry and a simple speech audiometer with masking generator for clinical use. Journal of Laryngology 67: 248–265.

Koike JJM (1985) The development of the Utah Vowel Imitation Test. (U-VIT). Paper presented at the American Speech-Language, Hearing Association Convention Washington, DC.

Kollmeier B (Ed) (1992) Moderne verfahrender sprachaudiometric (modern test procedures in speech audiometry) Buchreihe Altustik Median. Verlag von Killisch-Horn GMBH 21: 23–29.

Kopra LL, Dunlop RJ, Kopra MA, Abrahamson JE (1985) Laser videodisc interactive system for computer-assisted instruction in speechreading. Scientific Exhibit at American Speech-Language-Hearing Association Convention, Washington, DC.

Korsan-Bengtsen M (1973) Distorted speech audiometry. Acta Otolaryngologica Suppl. 310.

Kruel EJ, Nixon JC, Kryter KD, Bell DW, Lang JS (1968) A proposed clinical test of speech discrimination. Journal of Speech and Hearing Research 11: 536–552.

Kruel EJ, Bell DW, Nixon JC (1969) Factors affecting speech discrimination test difficulty. Journal of Speech and Hearing Research 12: 281–287.

Kruger B, Kruger FM (1994) Future trends in hearing aid fitting strategies: with a view towards 2020. In Valente M (Ed.) Strategies for Selecting and Verifying Hearing Aid Fittings. New York: Thieme Medical Publishers, Inc., 300–342.

Kruger B, Mazor R (1987) Speech Audiometry in the USA. In Martin MC (Ed.) Speech Audiometry, 207–235. London: Taylor and Francis.

Kryter KD (1962a) Methods for the calculation and use of the articulation index. Journal of the Acoustical Society of America 34: 1689–1697.

Kryter KD (1962b) Validation of the articulation index. Journal of the Acoustical Society of America 34: 1698–1702.

Kryter KD, Williams C, Green DM (1962) Auditory acuity and the perception of speech. Journal of the Acoustical Society of America 34: 1217–1223.

Kuk FK, Harper T, Doubek K (1994) Preferred real-ear insertion gain on a commercial hearing aid at different speech and noise levels. Journal of the American Academy of Audiology 5(2): 99–109.

Ladefoged P (1962) Elements of Acoustic Phonetics. Chicago, IL: University of Chicago Press.

Ladefoged P (1982) A Course in Phonetics, 2nd edition New York: Harcourt Brace Jovanovich.

Larsby B, Arlinger S (1994) Speech recognition and just-follow-conversation tasks for normal-hearing and hearing-impaired listeners with different maskers. Audiology 33: 165–176.

Lau CC, So KW (1988) Material for Cantonese audiometry constructed by appropriate phonetic principles. British Journal Audiology 22: 297–304.

Lee K, Dermody P (1994) Development of a speech information processing task for elderly listeners. Australian Journal of Audiology, Supplement 15: 38.

Lehiste I, Peterson GE (1959) Linguistic considerations in the study of speech intelligibility. Journal of the Acoustical Society of America 31: 280–286.

Lehmann R (1962) Etude psychophysique de l'intélligibilité du langage. Thèses de l'Univérsité de Paris, Editions de la Revue d'Optique Theorique et Instrumentale.

Leijon A, Lindkvist A, Ringdahl, A, Israelsson B (1990) Preferred hearing aid gain in everyday use after prescriptive fitting. Ear and Hearing 11: 299–305.

Leijon A, Lindkvist A, Ringdahl A, Israelsson B (1991) Sound quality and speech reception for prescribed hearing aid frequency responses. Ear and Hearing 12: 251.

Lerman JW, Ross M, McLaughlin RM (1965) A picture-identification test for hearing-impaired children. Journal of Audiological Research 5: 273–278.

Leshowitz B (1977) Speech intelligibility in noise for listeners with sensorineural hearing damage. IPO Annual Progress Report 12: 11–23.

Levitt H (1971) Transformed up-down methods in psychoacoustics. Journal of the Acoustical Society of America 49: 467–477.

Levitt H, Rabiner L (1967) Use of a sequential strategy in speech intelligibility testing. Journal of Acoustical Society of America 42: 609–612.

Levitt H, Resnick S (1978) Speech perception by the hearing impaired: methods of testing and the development of new tests. In Ludwigen C, Barfod J (Eds) Sensorineural Hearing Impaired and Hearing Aids. Scandinavian Audiology Supplement 6: 107–128.

Levitt H, Collins MJ, Dubno JR, Resnick SB, White REC (1978) Development of a Protocol for the Prescriptive Fitting of a Wearable Hearing Aid, Communication Sciences Laboratory Report No. 11). New York: City University of New York.

Levitt H, Waltzman SB, Shapiro WH, Cohen NL (1986) Evaluation of a cochlear prosthesis using connected discourse tracking. Journal of Rehabilitative Research and Development 23: 147–154.

Levitt H, Youdelman K, Head J (1990) Fundamental Speech Skills Test. Englewood, CO: Resource Point, Inc.

Lewis AN (1979) Educational consequences of otitis media ear disease in aboriginal children. Proceedings of the Australian Deafness Council Seminar, October, Melbourne: 17–18.

Lewis DE (1994a) Assistive devices for classroom listening. American Journal of Audiology 3(1): 58–69.

Lewis DE (1994b) Assistive devices for classroom listening. American Journal of Audiology 3(1): 70–83.

Libby ER (1985) State-of-the-art hearing aid selection procedures. Hearing Instruments 36: 30–38, 62.

Libby ER (1988) Hearing aid selection strategies and probe tube microphone measures. Hearing Instruments 39: 7, 10–15.

Lidén G (1954) Speech audiometry. Acta Otolaryngologica Supplement 14: 1–45.

Lidén G (1971) The use and limitations of the masking noise in pure-tone and speech audiometry. Audiology 10: 115–128.

Ling D (1978) Auditory coding and reading — an analysis of training procedures for hearing impaired children. In Ross M, Giolas TG (Eds) Auditory Management of Hearing Impaired Children. Baltimore, MD: University Park Press.

Ling D, Ling A (1978) Aural Habilitation: The Foundation of Verbal Learning in Hearing Impaired Children. Washington, DC: Alexander Graham Bell Association for the Deaf.

Lipsey MW (1990) 'Design Sensitivity'-Statistical power for experimental research. London: Sage Publications.

Loiselle LH (1985) Use of the PSI for paediatric hearing aid evaluations. (A mini-seminar). Paper presented at the American Speech-Language-Hearing Association Annual Convention, Washington, DC.

Lovegrove R, Dillon H, Mackie K (1991) Northwestern University Children's Perception of Speech (NU-CHIPS). National Acoustic Laboratories Audiology Circular 1991/4: 1–10. Sydney: NAL.

Lowell EL (1975) A film test of lipreading. John Tracy Research Papers II. Los Angeles, CA: John Tracy Clinic.

Lowell EL (1974) Auditory and visual perception of different units of speech. Scandinavian Audiology Supplement 4: 31–37.

Luce P, Feustel T, Pisoni D (1983) Capacity demands in short term memory for synthetic and natural word lists. Human Factors 25: 17–32.

Ludvigsen C (1974) Construction and evaluation of an audio-visual test (the Helen test). Scandinavian Audiology Supplement 4: 67–75.

Ludvigsen C (1992) Comparison of certain measures of speech and noise level. Scandinavian Audiology 21: 23–29.

Lutman ME (1987) Psychoacoustical characterisation of sensorineural hearing loss in the UK population. British Journal of Audiology 21: 325.

Lutman ME, Clark J (1986) Speech identification under simulated hearing aid frequency response characteristics in relation to sensitivity frequency resolution and temporal resolution. Journal of the Acoustical Society of America 80: 1030–1040.

Lutman ME, Brown EJ, Coles RRA (1986) Self-reported disability and handicap in the population in relation to pure-tone threshold, age, sex and type of hearing loss. British Journal of Audiology 21: 45–58.

Lybarger SF (1978) Selective amplification — a review and evaluation. Journal of the American Audiological Society 3: 258–266.

Lynn GE, Gilroy J (1977) In Keith RW (Ed.) Central Auditory Dysfunction, Chapter 6. New York: Grune and Stratton.

Lynn JM, Brotman SR (1981) Perceptual significance of the CID W22 carrier phrase. Ear and Hearing 2: 95–99.

Lyregaard PE (1973) On the Statistics of Speech Audiometry Data. National Physical Laboratory, Teddington, Acoustic Report AC 63. Teddington: NPL Acoustics Report AC 63.

Lyregaard PE (1976) On the Relation Between Recognition and Familiarity of Words. National Physical Laboratory, Teddington, Acoustic Report AC 78. Teddington: NPL.

Lyregaard PE, Robinson DW, Hinchcliffe R (1976) A Feasibility Study of Diagnostic Speech Audiometry. National Physical Laboratory, Teddington, Acoustic Report AC 73. Teddington: NPL..

MacLeod A, Summerfield Q (1987) Quantifying the contribution of vision to speech perception in noise. British Journal of Audiology 21: 131–141.

MacLeod A, Summerfield Q (1990) A procedure for measuring auditory and audio-visual speech-reception thresholds for sentences in noise: rationale, evaluation and recommendations for use. British Journal of Audiology 24, 29–43.

McCandless GA, Lyregaard P (1983) Prescription of gain/output (POGO) for hearing aids. Hearing Instruments 34: 16–21.

McCandless GA, Dankowski NK (1985) Factors which determine speech discrimination in a multichannel cochlear implant. Paper presented at the American Speech-Language-Hearing Association Annual Convention, Washington, DC.

McClymont LG, Browning GG, Gatehouse S (1991) Reliability of patient choice between hearing aid systems. British Journal of Audiology 25: 35–39.

McCormick B (1977) The toy discrimination test: an aid for the screening of hearing of children above the mental age of 2 years. Public Health, London: 67–69.

McCormick B (1979a) The skill of lipreading — a review. Hearing 34: 126–130.

McCormick B (1979b) A comparison between a two-dimensional and a three-dimensional lipreading test. IRCS Medical Sciences Journal (Biomedical Technology) 7: 324.

McGrath M (1985) An examination of cues for visual and audio-visual speech perception using natural and computer-generated faces. PhD thesis. University of Nottingham.

McGurk H, Macdonald J (1976) Hearing lips and seeing voices. Nature 264: 746–748.

McKay CM, McDermott HJ (1993) Perceptual performance of subjects with cochlear implants using the Spectral Maxima Sound Processor (SMSP) and the Mini Speech Processor (MSP). Ear and Hearing 14: 350–367.

Mackie K, Cotton S (1991) A procedure for evaluating FM advantage using adaptive speech tests in noise. National Acoustic Laboratories Audiology Circular 1991/5: 1–9. Sydney: NAL.

Mackie K, Dermody P (1981) A normative study of the token test. Australian Journal of Human Communication Disorders 9: 14–23.

Mackie K, Dermody P (1982a) Adaptive speech testing with hearing impaired adults. Paper presented at the Audiological Society of Australia, 5th National Conference, Leura, NSW.

Mackie, K. and Dermody P (1982b) Word intelligibility tests in audiology for the assessment of communication adequacy. National Acoustic Laboratories Report No. 89. Sydney: NAL.

Mackie K, Dermody P (1986) Use of a monosyllabic adaptive speech test (MAST) with young children. Journal Speech and Hearing Research 29: 275–281.

Mackie K, Romanik S, Dermody P (1983) Audiological assessment of auditory receptive language in severely and profoundly hearing impaired children. In Milne H, Campbell C, Payner S (Eds). Proceedings of the 8th National Conference of the Australian Association of Special Education, Volume 2. Brisbane: AASE.

Mackie K, Jerger S, Dermody P (1986) Results of an Australian recording of the Paediatric Speech Intelligibility Test. Paper presented at the Audiological Society of Australia, 7th National Conference, Ballarat, Victoria.

Macrae J, Brigden D (1973) Auditory threshold impairment and everyday speech reception. Audiology 12: 272–290.

Macrae J, Farrant R (1961) Standardisation of the CAL revised (33rpm) recordings of the PBN word lists nos. 2, 3, 4, 5, 8 and 9 used in testing civil aviation aircrew. Commonwealth Acoustic Laboratories Report No. 21. Sydney: CAL.

Macrae J, Woodroffe P, Farrant R (1963) Standardisation of the Commonwealth Acoustic Laboratories' recordings of phonetically balanced monosyllabic word lists. Journal of the Oto-Laryngological Society of Australia 1: 197–203.

Marincovich PJ (1987) The articulation index and hearing aid selection. Hearing Instruments 38(1): 18, 58.

Marincovich PJ, Studebaker GA (1985) Calculation of hearing aid efficiency with an Articulation Index procedure. Paper presented at the American Speech-Language-Hearing Association Annual Convention, Washington, DC.

Markides A (1978a) Speech discrimination functions for normal hearing subjects with AB isophonemic word lists. Scandinavian Audiology 7: 239–245.

Markides A (1978b) Whole-word scoring versus phoneme scoring in speech audiometry. British Journal of Audiology 12: 40–46.

Markides A (1980a) Best listening levels of hearing impaired children. Journal of the British Association of Teachers of the Deaf 6: 117–124.

Markides A (1980b) The relationship between hearing loss for pure tones and hearing loss for speech among hearing-impaired children. British Journal of Audiology 14: 115–121.

Markides, A (1980c) The Manchester speech reading (lipreading) test. In Taylor IG, Markides A (Eds.) Disorders of Auditory Function 111. London: Academic Press.

Martin FN, Pennington CD (1971) Current trends in audiometric practices. ASHA 13: 671–677.

Martin FN, Staufer MD (1975) A modification in the Tillman-Olsen methods for speech threshold measurement. Journal of Speech and Hearing Disorders 40: 25–28.

Martin FN, Forbis NK (1978) The present status of audiometric practice: a follow-up study. ASHA 20: 531–541.

Martin FN, Sides DG (1985) Survey of current audiometric practices. ASHA 27(2): 29–36.

Martin FN, Morris LJ (1989) Current audiologic practices in the United States. The Hearing Journal 42: 25–44.

Martin FN, Hawkins RR, Bailey HAT (1962) The nonessentiality of the carrier phrase in phonetically balanced (PB) word testing. Journal of Auditory Research 2: 319–322.

Martin FN, Armstrong TW, Champlin CA (1994) A survey of audiological practices in the United States. Journal of the American Academy of Audiology.

Martin J I (1978) The Migrant Presence. Sydney: George Allen and Unwin.

Martin L, Gillies K (1994) The development of a speech perception assessment protocol for severe-profoundly deaf children. Journal of the Audiological Society of Australia, Supplement 15: 8.

Martin L, Tong YC, Clark GM (1981) A multi-channel cochlear implant. Archives of Otolaryngology 107: 157–159.

Martony J (1974) On Speechreading of Swedish Consonants and Vowels. STL-QPSR Stockholm: Royal Institute of Technology 2–3: 11–33.

Mason MK (1943) A cinematographic technique for testing visual speech comprehension. Journal of Speech Disorders 8: 271–278.

Matzker J (1959) Two new methods for the assessment of central auditory functions in cases of brain disease. Annals of Otology, Rhinology and Laryngology 68: 1185–1197.

Medawar PB (1965) The great problems: a program for the natural sciences. Address given at Cornell University.

Medical Research Council (1947) Special Report Series No. 261 Hearing Aids and Audiometers. London: HM Stationery Office.

Merklein RA (1981) A short speech perception test for severely and profoundly deaf children. Volta Review 83: 36–45.

Messouak H (1956) Audiométrie Vocale en Arabic Maghrebin. Les Cahiers de la CFA No. 4. Paris: Compagnie Française d'Audiologie.

Meyer D, Mishler E. (1985) Rollover measurements with Auditec NU-6 word lists. Journal of Speech and Hearing Disorders 50: 356–360.

Middelweerd MJ, Plomp R (1987) The effects of speechreading on the speech reception threshold of sentences in noise. Journal of the Acoustical Society of America 82: 2145–2152.

Millar B, Dermody P, Harrington J, Vonwiller J (1990a) A national database of spoken language: concept, design and implementation. In Proceedings of International Conference on Spoken Language Processing (ICSLP-90), Kobe, Japan.

Millar B, Dermody P, Harrington J, Vonwiller J (1990b) A national cluster of spoken language databases for Australia. In Proceedings of 3rd International Conference on Speech Science and Technology: 440–445.

Millar, B., Vonwiller, J., Harrington, J. and Dermody, P. (1994) The Australian National Database of Spoken Language. Proceedings of an International Conference on Acoustics, Speech and Signal Processing (ICASSP-94), Adelaide, Australia.

Millar JB, Tong YC, Clark GM (1984) Speech processing for cochlear implant prostheses. Journal of Speech and Hearing Research 27: 280–296.

Miller GA, Nicely P (1955) An analysis of perceptual confusions among some English consonants. Journal of the Acoustical Society of America 27: 338–352.

Miller GA, Heise CA, Lichten D (1951) The intelligibility of speech as a function of the context of the test material. Journal of Experimental Psychology 41: 329–335.

Miller JD, Weisenberger JM (1985) The case of tactile aids. Journal of the Acoustical Society of America Supplement 78, 1: S16.

Milner P, Flevaris-Phillips C (1985) Speech reception in deaf adults using vibrotactile aids for cochlear implants. Journal of the Acoustical Society of America 78, Supplement 1: S17.

Mines MA, Hanson BF, Shoup JE (1978) Frequency of occurrence of phonemes in conversational English. Language and Speech 21: 221–241.

Mintz SL, Johnson KC, Stach BA, Jerger JF (1985) Adaptive speech audiometry for hearing evaluations. Paper presented at the American Speech-Language-Hearing Association Annual Convention, Washington, DC.

Mitchell AG, Delbridge A (1965a) The Speech of Australian Adolescents. Sydney: Angus and Robertson.

Mitchell AG, Delbridge A (1965b) The Pronounciation of English in Australia. Australia: Angus and Robertson.

Moncur JP, Dirks P (1967) Speech intelligibility in reverberation. Journal of Speech and Hearing Research 10: 186–195.

Montgomery AA, Walden BE, Schwartz DM, Prosek RA (1984) Training auditory-visual speech reception in adults with moderate sensorineural hearing loss. Ear and Hearing 5: 30–36.

Moore A (1993) The PLOTT Screening Test and the PLOTT Sentence Test. AHS Audiology Circular, 1993/3.

Moore BCJ (1989) An Introduction to the Psychology of Hearing 3rd Edn. London: Academic Press.

Morkovin B (1974) Rehabilitation of the aurally handicapped through the study of speech reading in life situations. Journal of Speech Disorders 12: 363–368.

Mueller HG, Killion MC (1990) An easy method for calculating the articulation index. Hearing Journal 43: 14–17.

Murray N (1943) Articulation Tests in Flight. ATL Informal Report No. IR-9. Sydney: CAL.

Murray N (1952) The CAL PBO Speech Perception Tests for Deaf Children. Commonwealth Acoustic Laboratory Report No. 4. Sydney: CAL.

Murray N (1955) The CAL PBP Speech Perception Tests for Deaf Children. Commonwealth Acoustic Laboratory Report No. 9. Sydney: CAL.

Murray NM, Dermody P (1986) Development of lists for auditory lexical decision tasks. Paper presented at the Audiological Society of Australia 7th National Conference, Ballarat.

Muyunga YK (1974) Development and application of speech audiometry using Lingala and Ciluba word lists. PhD Thesis. University of London.

Myatt B, Landes B (1963) Assessing discrimination loss in children. Archives of Otolaryngology 77: 359–362.

National Acoustic Laboratories (1984) Paediatric Audiological Protocols Manual. Field Services Section. Sydney: NAL.

Neuman AC, Mills RC, Schwander TJ (1985) Noise reduction: Effects on consonant perception by normal hearing listeners. Paper presented at the American Speech-Language-Hearing Association Annual Convention, Washington, DC.

Newby HA (1958) Audiology: Principles and Practice. New York: Appleton Century Crofts.

Newman CW, Jacobson GP (1993) Application of self-report scales in balance function handicap assessment and management, in self-assessment scales in audiology. Seminars in Hearing 14(4): 354–362, 363–376.

Newman CW, Weinstein BE, Jacobson GP, Hug G (1990) Test–retest reliability of the hearing handicap inventory for adults. Ear and Hearing 12: 355–357.

Newman CW, Weinstein BE, Jacobson GP, Hug G (1991) The hearing handicap inventory for adults: Psychometric adequacy and audiometric correlates. Ear and Hearing 11: 430–433.

Niemeyer W (1967) Sprachaudiometrie mit Satzen. (Speech audiometry using sentences.) HNO (Berlin) 15: 335–343.

Nilsson M, Sullivan J, Soli SD (1990) Development of a speech intelligibility test for hearing aid research. Journal of the Acoustical Society of America 88: S175.

Nilsson M, Sullivan J, Soli SD (1991) Validation of a speech intelligibility test using SRT for hearing aid research. Journal of the Acoustical Society of America 89: S1960.

Nilsson M, Soli SD, Sullivan J (1994) Development of the hearing in noise test for the measurement of speech reception thresholds in quiet and in noise. Journal of the Acoustical Society of America 95(2): 1085–1099.

Noble WG (1978) Assessment of Impaired Hearing. New York: Academic Press.

Noble WG, Atherley GRC (1970) The hearing measurement scale: A questionnaire for the assessment of auditory disability. Journal of Auditory Research 10: 229–250.

Northern JL (1992) Introduction to computerized probe-microphone real-ear measurements in hearing aid evaluation procedures. In Mueller HG, Hawkins DB, Northern JL (Eds.) Probe Microphone Measurements: Hearing Aid Selection and Assessment, 1–19. San Diego, CA: Singular Publishing Group.

Ödkvist LM, Bergholtz LM, Ahlfeldt H, Andersson B, Edling C, Strand E (1982) Otoneurological and audiological findings in workers exposed to industrial solvents. Acta Otolaryngologica Supplement 386: 249–251.

Ödkvist LM, Arlinger SD, Edling C, Larsby B, Bergholtz LM (1987) Audiological and vestibulo-oculomotor findings in workers exposed to solvents and jet fuel. Scandinavian Audiology 16: 75–81.

Ohngren G (1992) Touching Voices: Components of Tactually Supported Speechreading. Comprehensive Summaries of Uppsala Dissertations from the Faculty of Social Sciences. Uppsala: Uppsala University.

OIML R104 (1992) Pure-tone Audiometry Organisation Internationale de Métrologie Légal. Paris.

Olsen WO, Matkin ND (1979) Speech audiometry. In Rintleman WF (Ed.) Hearing Assessment. Baltimore, MD: University Park Press.

Olsen WO, Noffsinger D, Carhart R (1976) Masking level differences encountered in clinical populations. Audiology 15: 287–301.

Olsen W, Van Tassell D, Speaks C (1982) Evaluation of isophonemic word list and sentence material. Paper presented at the Annual Convention of American Speech-Hearing-Language Association, Toronto, Ontario.

O'Neill JJ, Oyer HJ (1961) Visual Communication for the Hard of Hearing. Englewood Cliffs, NJ: Prentice-Hall.

O'Neill JJ, Oyer HJ (1981) Visual Communication for the Hard of Hearing (2nd edition). Englewood Cliffs, NJ: Prentice-Hall.

Onsa SA (1984) The development of material for speech audiometry in Sudanese Arabic. MSc. Thesis. University of Manchester.

Osborn R (1985) Personal communication.

Otto SR, Tyler RS, Preece JP, Lansing CR (1985) Consonant recognition with single and multichannel cochlear implant systems. Paper presented at the American Speech-Language-Hearing Association Annual Convention, Washington, DC.

Ousey J, Sheppard S, Twomey J, Palmer AR (1989) The IHR — McCormick automated toy discrimination test — description and initial evaluation. British Journal of Audiology 23: 245–249.

Owens E (1961) Intelligibility of words varying in familiarity. Journal of Speech and Hearing Research 4: 113–129.

Owens E, Schubert ED (1968) The development of the California Consonant Test. Journal of Speech and Hearing Research 20: 463–474.

Owens E, Telleen CC (1981) Tracking as an aural rehabilitative process. Journal of the Academy of Rehabilitation Audiology 14: 259–273.

Owens E, Benedict M, Schubert ED (1972) Consonant phonemic errors associated with pure tone configurations and certain kinds of hearing impairment. Journal of Speech and Hearing Research 15: 308–322.

Owens E, Kessler DK, Telleen CC, Schubert E (1980) The Minimal Auditory Capabilities Battery. St Louis, MD: Auditec.

Owens E, Kessler DK, Telleen CC, Schubert E (1981) The minimal auditory capabilities (MAC) battery. Hearing Aid Journal 34: 9–34.

Owens E, Kessler DK, Raggio MW, Schubert ED (1985) Analysis and revision of the minimal auditory capabilities (MAC) battery. Ear and Hearing 6: 280–290.

Palmer GR, Short SD (1989). Health Care and Public Policy: An Australian Analysis. Melbourne: MacMillan.

Pascoe DP (1975) Frequency responses of hearing aids and their effects on the speech perception of hearing-impaired subjects. Annals of Otorhinolaryngology Supplement 23, 84: 1–40.

Pascoe DP (1978) An approach to hearing aid selection. Hearing Instruments 29(6): 12–16, 36.

Patterson RD, Nimmo-Smith I, Weber DL, Milroy R (1982) The deterioration of hearing with age: Frequency selectivity, the critical ratio, the audiogram and speech threshold. Journal of the Acoustical Society of America 72: 1788–1803.

Pavlovic CV (1985) Use of the articulation index for assessing residual auditory function in listeners with sensorineural hearing impairment. Journal of the Acoustical Society of America 75(4): 1253–1257.

Pavlovic CV (1987) Derivation of primary parameters and procedures for use in speech intelligibility predictions. Journal of the Acoustical Society of America 82: 413–422.

Pavlovic CV (1988) Articulation index predictions of speech intelligibility in hearing aid selection. ASHA 30 (6–7): 63–65.

Pavlovic CV (1989) Speech spectrum considerations and speech intelligibility predictions in hearing aid evaluations. Journal Speech and Hearing Disorders 54: 3–8.

Pavlovic CV (1990) Statistical distribution of speech for various languages. 120th Meeting of Acoustical Society of America. San Diego, CA. Journal of the Acoustical Society of America 88 (1): 8SP10.

Pavlovic CV (1991) Speech recognition and five articulation indexes. Hearing Instruments 412: 20–24.

Pavlovic CV, Rossi M, Espesser R (1990) Use of the magnitude estimation technique for assessing the performance of text-to-speech synthesis system. Journal of Acoustical Society of America 87(1): 373–382.

Pavlovic CV, Studebaker GA (1984) An evaluation of some assumptions underlying the articulation index. Journal of the Acoustical Society America 75: 1606–1612.

Pavlovic CV, Studebaker GA, Sherbecoe RL (1985) Method for predicting speech discrimination of the hearing impaired. Paper presented at the American Speech-Language-Hearing Association Annual Convention, Washington, DC.

Perry FR (1979) Monash Diagnostic Test of Lipreading Ability. Melbourne: Australian Council for Education Research.

Pestalozza G, Shore I (1955) Clinical evaluation on the basis of different tests of auditory function. Laryngoscope 65: 1136–1163.

Peterson GE, Lehiste I (1962) Revised CNC lists for auditory tests. Journal of Speech and Hearing Disorders 27: 62–70.

Pickett JM (1980) The Sounds of Speech Communication. Baltimore: University Park Press.

Pickett JM, Revoile SG, Danaher EM (1983) Speech-cue measures of impaired Hearing. In Tobias JV, Schubert ED (Eds) Hearing Research and Theory, Volume 2. New York: Academic Press.

Plant G (1984a) COMMTRAM — A Communication Training Program for Profoundly Deafened Adults. Sydney: National Acoustic Laboratories.

Plant G (1984b) A diagnostic speech test for severely and profoundly hearing impaired children. Australian Journal of Audiology 6: 1–9.

Plant G (1986) A single-transducer vibrotactile aid to lipreading. STL-QPSR Stockholm: Royal Institute of Technology.

Plant G (1988) Speechreading with tactile supplements. Volta Review 90: 149–160.

Plant G (1990) The development of speech tests in Aboriginal languages. Australian Journal of Audiology 13: 30–40.

Plant G, Gnosspelius J (1994) An experienced user of tactile supplements to lipreading: A study of lipreading in Swedish and English. Paper presented at the Third International Conference on Tactile Aids, Hearing Aids, and Cochlear Implants, Coral Gables, FL.

Plant G, Macrae J (1977) Visual identification of Australian consonants vowels and diphthongs. Australian Teacher of the Deaf 18: 46–50.

Plant G, Macrae J (1981) The NAL lipreading test: development standardization and validation. Australian Journal of Audiology 3: 49–57.

Plant G, Macrae J (1985) The PLOTT test. Paper presented at the National Acoustic Laboratories, Hearing Aid Conference, Sydney.

Plant G, Moore A (1992a) Two speech discrimination tests for profoundly hearing-impaired children. Australian Journal of Audiology 14: 28 –40.

Plant G, Moore A (1992b). The Common Objects Token (COT) test: a sentence test for profoundly hearing impaired children. Australian Journal of Audiology 14: 76–83.

Plant G, Spens K-E (1986) An experienced user of tactile information as a supplement to lipreading: An evaluative study. STL-QPSR 1/1986: 87–110. Stockholm: Royal Institute of Technology.

Plant G, Westcott S (1982) A diagnostic speech perception test for severely and profoundly hearing impaired children. Australian Journal of Audiology, Supplement 1, 9.

Plant G, Macrae J, Pearce J (1980) Performance on lipreading test by native and non-native speakers of English. Australian Journal of Audiology 2: 25–29.

Plant G, Phillips D, Tsembis J (1982) An auditory-visual speech test for the elderly hearing-impaired. Australian Journal of Audiology 4: 62–68.

Plant G, Macrae J, Dillon H, Pentecost F (1984) Lipreading with minimal auditory cues. Australian Journal of Audiology 6: 65–72.

Plant G, Gnosspelius J, Spens, KE (1994) Three studies using the KTH tracking procedure. STL -QPSR. Stockholm: Royal Institute of Technology 1: 103–134.

Plant G, Franklin D, Franklin L, Steele M, (1995) Lip reading with tactile supplements: A study with an experienced subject. Seminars in Hearing, 16: 296–304.

Plomp R (1994) Noise, amplification, and compression: considerations of three main issues in hearing aid design. Ear and Hearing 15: 2–12.

Plomp R, Duquesnoy AJ (1982) A model for the speech-reception threshold in noise with and without a hearing aid. Scandinavian Audiology, Supplement 15: 95–111.

Plomp R, Mimpen AM (1979) Improving the reliability of testing the speech reception threshold for sentences. Audiology 18: 43–53.

Poch Viñals (1958) La Exploraçion Funcional Auditiva. Madrid: Pz. Montalvo.

Pollack I (1959) Message uncertainty and message reception. Journal of the Acoustical Society of America 31: 1500–1508.

Pollack I, Rubenstein H, Decker L (1959) Intelligibility of known and unknown message sets. Journal of the Acoustical Society of America 31: 273–279.

Posner J, Ventry IM (1977) Relationships between comfortable loudness levels for speech and speech discrimination in sensorineural hearing loss. Journal of Speech and Hearing Disorders 42: 370–375.

Prasansuk S (1995) Personal communication.

Preston K (1991) Speech discrimination testing of non-native English speakers. Thesis, La Trobe University.

Priede VM, Coles RRA (1976) Speech discrimination tests in investigation of sensonneural hearing loss. Journal of Laryngology and Otology: 90.

Pronovost W, Dumbleton C (1954) A picture type speech sound discrimination test for children. Journal of Speech and Hearing Research 19: 360–366.

Prosek RA (1981) Some effects of training on speech recognition by hearing impaired adults. Journal of Speech and Hearing Research 24: 207–216.

Punch JL (1980) Multidimensional scaling of quality judgments of speech signals processed by hearing aids. Journal of the Acoustical Society of America 68: 458–466.

Punch JL, Beck EL (1980) Low-frequency response of hearing aids and judgments of aided speech quality. Journal of Speech and Hearing Disorders 45: 325–335.

Punch J, Chi C, Patterson J (1990) A recommended protocol for prescriptive use of target gain rules. Hearing Instruments 41(4): 12–19.

Rabinowitz WM (1981) Measurement of the acoustic input immittance of the human ear. Journal of the Acoustical Society of America 70: 1025–1035.

Rankovic CM (1991) An application of the articulation index to hearing aid fitting. Journal of Speech and Hearing Research 34: 391–402.

Reed M (1959) A verbal screening test of hearing. Proceedings of the 111 World Congress of the Deaf, Wiesbaden. Herausgegeben vom Deutschen Gehörlosen-Bund e.v, Frankfurt am Main.

Reed CM, Durlach NI, Delhorne LA (1992) Natural methods of tactile communication. In Summers IR (Ed.) Tactile Aids for the Hearing Impaired. London: Whurr.

Reder H (1990) Noise and speech levels in noisy environments. Hearing Instruments 41(4): 32–33.

Resnick DM, Becker M (1963) Hearing aid evaluation — a new approach. ASHA 5: 659–699.

Resnick SB, Dubno JR, Hoffnung S, Levitt H (1975) Phoneme errors on a nonsense syllable test. Journal of the Acoustical Society of America 58, Supplement 1: 114.

Resnick SB, Dubno JR, Howie DG, Hoffnung S, Freeman L, Slosberg M (1976) Phoneme identification on a closed response nonsense syllable test. Houston, TX: American Speech-Hearing-Language Association.

Richards DL (1973) Telecommunication by Speech. London: Butterworth.

Richter U (1976) Klirrfaktoren verschiedenartiger Schallsender (Harmonic distortion of sound sources of different kinds). Daga-Tagung 5: 479–482. Dusseldorf: VDI Verlag.

Richter U (1988) Vorgesene Maßnahmen zur Erhöhung der Meßsicherheit in der Audiometrie (Measures intended to increase measurement reliability in audiometry). PTB-Bericht PTB-MA-12, : 43–62.

Richter U (1992) Kenndaten von Schallwandlern der Audiometrie (Characteristic data of sound transducers used in audiometry). PTB-Bericht PTB-MA 27.

Richter U, Brinkmann K (1976) The sensitivity level of bone-conduction receivers. Journal of Audiological Technique 15: 2–15.

Richter U, Brinkmann K (1977) Speech audiometry via bone-conduction. Proceedings of the Ninth International Congress on Acoustics, Madrid, Volume 1: 403.

Richter U, Gössing P (1993) Zulassunsprüfungen von Reinton- und Sprachaudiometern (Pattern evaluation testing of pure-tone and speech audiometers). HNO-Mitteilungen, 3: 101–116.

Risberg A, Öhngren G (1989) How Do We Measure Speech Perception Ability? QPSR 1/1989, 141–143. Stockholm: Department of Speech Transmission and Music Acoustics, Royal Institute of Technology.

Robertson S, Plant G (1983). An analysis of error responses for the CAL-PBM word lists. Australian Journal of Audiology 5: 28–34.

Rosen JK (1978) The evaluation of handicap secondary to acquired hearing impairment. Journal of the Academy of Rehabilitative Audiology 11(2): 2–9.

Rosen S, Corcoran T (1982) A video-recorded test of lipreading for British English. British Journal of Audiology 16: 245–254.

Rosen S, Fourcin AJ (1983) When less is more: further work. University College, London. Speech, Hearing, and Language: Work in progress. 1: 1–27.

Rosen, S., Howard, P. (1990) Signals and Systems for Speech and Hearing. London: Academic Press.

Rosen S, Moore BCJ, Fourcin AJ (1979) Lipreading with fundamental frequency information. Proceedings of the Institute of Acoustics, Autumn Conference, Windermere. Paper lA2: 5–8.

Rosen S, Fourcin A, Moore B (1981) Voice pitch as an aid to lipreading. Nature 291: 150–152.

Rosen S, Faulkner A, Smith DA (1990) The psychoacoustics of profound hearing impairment. Acta Otolaryngologica (Stockholm), Supplement 469: 16–22.

Rosenzweig MR, Postman L (1958) Frequency of usage and the perception of words. Science 127: 263–266.

Ross M (1978) Hearing aid evaluation. In Katz J (Ed.) Handbook of Clinical Audiology. Baltimore, MD: Williams and Wilkins Co.

Ross M, Lerman JW (1970) A picture identification test for hearing impaired children. Journal of Speech and Hearing Research 13: 44–53.

Rowland JP, Dirks DD, Dubno JR, Bell TS (1985) Comparison of speech recognition-in-noise and subjective communication assessment. Ear and Hearing. 6: 291–296.

Rudmose W (1964) Concerning the problem of calibrating TDH-39 earphones at 6 kHz with a 9A coupler. Journal of the Acoustical Society of America 36: 1049(A).

Rupp RR (1980) In Rupp RR, Stockdell KG (Eds) Speech Protocols in Audiology, Chapter 4. New York: Grune and Stratton.

Rupp RR, Stockdell KG (1980) In Rupp RR, Stockdell KG (Eds) Speech Protocols in Audiology, Chapter 2. New York: Grune and Stratton.

Rupp RR, Higgins J, Maurer JF (1977) A feasibility scale for predicting hearing aid use (FSPHAU) with older individuals. Journal of the Academy of Rehabilitation Audiology 10: 81.

Sanderson-Leepa ME, Rintelmann WF (1976) Articulation function and test/retest performance of normal-learning children on three speech discrimination tests: WIPI, PBK50, and NU Auditory Test No. 6. Journal of Speech Disorders 41: 503–519.

Saunders FA, Franklin B (1985) Field tests of a wearable 16-channel electrotactile sensory aid in a classroom for the deaf. Journal of the Acoustical Society of America 78, Supplement 1: S17.

Savin HB (1963) Word frequency effects and errors in the perception of speech. Journal of the Acoustical Society of America 35: 200–206.

Schmitz HD (1980) Hearing aid selection for adults. In Pollack MC (Ed.) Amplification for the Hearing impaired. New York: Grune and Stratton.

Schultz M (1964) Word familiarity influences in speech discrimination. Journal of Speech and Hearing Research 7: 395–400.

Schultz MC, Schubert ED (1969) A multiple choice discrimination test (MCDT). Laryngoscope 79: 382–399.

Schum DJ, Collins MJ (1985) Test–Retest reliability of two paired-comparison hearing aid evaluations. Paper presented at the American Speech-Language-Hearing Association Annual Convention, Washington, DC.

Schum DJ, Matthews LJ (1992) SPIN test performance of elderly hearing impaired listeners. Journal of the American Academy of Audiology 3: 303–307.

Schroeder M (1968) Reference signal for signal quality studies. Journal of the Acoustical Society of America 44: 1735–1736.

Schwartz D (1982) Hearing Aid Selection Methods: An Enigma, Studebaker GA, Bess FH (Eds.) The Vanderbilt Hearing Report. Upper Darby, PA: Monographs in Contemporary Audiology.

Shannon CE (1948) A mathematical theory of communication. Bell Systems Technical Journal 27: 379–423, 623–656.

Seewald RC (1980) The desired sensation level approach for children: selection and verification. Hearing Instruments 39(7): 18–20.

Seewald RC (1992) The desired sensation level method for fitting children: Version 3.0. The Hearing Journal 45(4): 36–41.

Seewald R, Ross M (1988) Amplification for young hearing impaired children. In Pollack M (Ed.) Amplification for the Hearing Impaired, 3rd edition. New York: Grune and Stratton.

Seewald RC, Ross M, Spiro M (1985) Selecting amplification characteristics for young hearing impaired children. Ear and Hearing 6: 48–53.

Shapiro I (1976) Hearing aid fitting by prescription. Audiology 15: 163–173.

Shaw EAG (1974) Transformation of sound pressure level from the free field to the eardrum in the horizontal plane. Journal of the Acoustical Society America 56: 1848–1861.

Shaw EAG (1975) The external ear: new knowledge. In Dalsgaard SC (Ed.) Earmolds and Associated Problems. Proceedings of the Seventh Danavox Symposium, 2450. Scandinavian Audiology, Supplement 5. 1975.

Shaw EAG (1980) The acoustics of the external ear. In Studebaker GA, Hochberg I (Eds.) Acoustical Factors Affecting Hearing Aid Performance, 109–125. Baltimore, MD: University Park Press.

Sherwood TR, McNeill HA, Torr GR (1995) Differences in the performance of metal and plastic-cased TDH-39 and TDH-49 audiometric earphones and consequences for their calibration. NPL Acoustics Report RSA (EXT) 0058.

Shoop C (1978) Training effects of CV syllables instruction on the geriatric population. Paper presented at the American Speech-Language-Hearing Association Convention, San Francisco, CA.

Shoop C, Binnie CA (1979) The effect of age on the visual perception of speech. Scandinavian Audiology 8, 3–8.

Shore I, Bilger RC, Hirsh I J (1960) Hearing aid evaluations: reliability of repeated measures. Journal of Speech and Hearing Disorders 25: 152–170.

Show RL, Bolsora NR, Smedley TC, Whitcomb DJ (1993) Aural rehabilitation by ASHA audiologists: 1980–1990. American Journal of Audiology 2(3) 28–37.

Shrinian M, Arnst D (1980) PI–PB rollover in a group of aged listeners. Ear and Hearing 1: 50–53.

Shrinian M, Arnst D (1992) Patterns in the performance-intensity functions for phonetically balanced word lists and synthetic sentences in aged listeners. Archives of Otolaryngology 108: 15–20.

Siegenthaler B, Haspiel G (1966) Development of two standardized measures of hearing for speech by children. US Department of Health, Education, and Welfare. Project No. 2372. Contract No. OE-5-10-003.

Silverman SR, Hirsh I (1955) Problems related to the use of speech in clinical audiometry. Annals of Otology, Rhinology and Laryngology 64: 1234–1244.

Sims DG, Gottermeyer L (1995) Computer-assisted interactive video methods for speech reading instruction: A review. In G Plant, K-E Spens (Eds) Profound Deafness and Speech Communication. London: Whurr Publishers. pp 557–577.

Skamris N (1974) Assessment of lipreading ability of deafened persons. Scandinavian Audiology, Supplement 4: 128–135.

Skamris N (1977) Personal communication.

Smaldino J, Hoene J (1981a) A view of the state of hearing aid fitting practices. Hearing Instruments 32(1): 14–15, 38.

Skinner MW (1988) Hearing aid evaluation. Englewood Cliffs, NJ: Prentice-Hall.

Skinner MW, Miller JD (1983) Amplification bandwidth and intelligibility of speech in quiet and noise for listeners with sensorineural hearing loss. Audiology 22: 253–279.

Slosberg M (1976) Phoneme identification on a closed response nonsense syllable test. Paper presented at the American Speech-Language-Hearing Association Convention, Houston, TX..

Smaldino J, Hoene J (1981) The nature of common hearing aid fitting practices, part II. Hearing Instruments, 32(2): 8–11.

Smith J, Tipping V, Bench J (1987) Discrimination of Boothroyd words by Greek and English speakers. Australian Journal of Audiology, 9: 87–91.

Soderlund G (1992) A personal view of tactile aids. In Risberg A, Felicetti S, Plant G, Spens K-E (Eds.) Proceedings of the Second International Conference on Tactile Aids, Hearing Aids, and Cochlear Implants. Stockholm: Royal Institute of Technology.

Soli SD, Nilsson M (1994) Assessment of communication handicap with the HINT: how to use the hearing in noise test for determining speech intelligibility. Hearing Instruments 45(2): 12–16.

Sortini A, Flake C (1953) Speech audiometry testing for pre-school children. Laryngoscope 63: 991–997.

Speaks C, Jerger J (1965) Method for measurement of speech identification. Journal of Speech and Hearing Research 8: 185–194.

Spens KE (1995) Evaluation of speech tracking results: some numerical considerations. In G. Plant, KE Spens (Eds.) Profound Deafness and Speech Communication. London: Whurr Publishers. pp 417–438.

Spitzer JB (1993) Application of self-assessment in cochlear implant and profoundly hearing-impaired patients. In Self-Assessment Scales in Audiology, Seminars in Hearing 14(4): 354–362.

Spitzer JB, Leder SB, Flevaris-Phillips C, Milner P (1985) Standardization of video-taped tests of speechreading ranging in task difficulty. Paper presented at the American Speech-Language-Hearing Association Annual Convention, Washington, DC.

Spitzer JB, Leder SB, Milner P, Flevaris-Phillips C, Giolas TG (1987) Standardization of four videotaped tests of speechreading ranging in task difficulty. Ear and Hearing 8: 227–231.

Steeneken HJM, Agterhuis E, (1982) Description of STIDAS II-D: Part I, General System and Program Description, Report No. IZF 1982–20. TNO. Soesterberg: Institute for Perception.

Steeneken HJM, Houtgast T (1980) A physical method for measuring speech transmission quality. Journal of the Acoustical Society of America 67(1): 318–326.

Stein L, Zerlin S (1963) Effect of circumaural earphones and earphone cushions on auditory threshold. Journal of the Acoustical Society of America 35: 1744–1745.

Stevenson PW (1973) An automated system for speech audiometry. PhD Thesis. University of Essex.

Stevenson PW 1975 Responses to speech audiometry and phonemic discrimination patterns in the elderly. Audiology 14: 185–231.

Stevenson P, Martin M (1977) Phonemic discrimination difficulties and sensorineural hearing loss. London: Royal National Institute for the Deaf.

Stream RW, Dirks DD (1974) Effects of loudspeaker position on differences between earphones and free-field thresholds (MAP) and (MAF). Journal of Speech and Hearing Research 17: 549–568.

Studebaker GA (1980) Fifty years of hearing aid research: an evaluation of progress. Ear and Hearing 1: 57–62.

Studebaker GA (1982) Hearing aid selection: an overview. In Studebaker GA and Bess FH (Eds) The Vanderbilt Hearing Aid Report. Upper Darby, PA.

Studebaker GA, Bissett JD, Van Ort D (1982) Paired comparison judgments of relative intelligibility in noise. Journal of the Acoustical Society of America 72: 80–92.

Studebaker GA, Pavlovic CV, Sherbecoe RL (1987) A frequency importance function for continuous discourse. Journal of the Acoustical Society of America 81: 1130–1138.

Summerfield AQ (1983) Audio-visual speech perception, lipreading and artificial stimulation. In Lutman ME and Haggard MP (Eds) Hearing Science and Hearing Disorders. London: Academic Press.

Summerfield AQ, Foster J (1983) Assessing audiovisual speech-reception disability. In Perkins WJ (Ed.) High Technology Aids for the Disabled. London: Butterworth.

Summerfield AQ, Marshall DH, Foster JR (1996) A computer-based battery for predicting and measuring outcomes from cochlear implantation in adults. BSA Annual Conference, Poster Pit. p. 420.

Tait DM (1993) Video analysis: a method of assessing changes in pre-verbal and early linguistic communication after cochlear implantation. Ear and Hearing 14: 378–389.

Tato JM (1949) Caracteristicas acústicas de nuesrtro idioma. Revista Otolaringólogica (Buenos Aires) 1: 17–34.

Taylor KS (1993) Self-perceived and audiometric evaluations of hearing aid benefit in the elderly. Ear and Hearing 14: 390–394.

Taylor M, Creelman C (1967) PEST: efficient estimates on probability functions. Journal of the Acoustical Society of America 41: 782–787.

Tecca J, Binnie C (1982) The application of an adaptive procedure to the California Consonant Test for hearing aid evaluation. Ear and Hearing 3: 72–76.

Teder H (1990) Noise and speech levels in noisy enviroments. Hearing Instruments 41(4): 32–33.

Thompson G, Lassman F (1969) Relationship of auditory distortion test results to speech discrimination through flat versus selective amplification systems. Journal of Speech and Hearing Research 12: 594–686.

Thorburg J, Joyce R, Ginis J, Heinze C, Smales A, Veliou L, Reid J (1991) The evaluation of hearing aid fitting in mildly hearing impaired children. Australian Hearing and Deafness Review 8: 3–7.

Thorndike EL, Lorge I (1944) The teacher's word book of 30 000 words. New York: Bureau of Publications, Columbia University.

Thornton A, Raffin M (1978) Speech discrimination scores modelled as a binomial variable. Journal of Speech and Hearing Research 21: 507–518.

Tillman TW, Carhart R (1966) An Expanded Test for Speech Discrimination Utilizing CNC Monosyllabic Words. Northwestern University Auditory Test No. 6. Brooks Air Force Base, TX: USAF School of Aerospace Medicine.

Tillman TW, Gish KD (1964) Comments on the effect of circumaural earphones on auditory thresholds. Journal of the Acoustical Society of America 36: 969–970.

Tillman TW, Olsen WO (1973) Speech audiometry. In Jerger J (Ed.) Modern Developments in Audiology: 37–74. New York: Academic Press.

Tillman TW, Carhart R, Wilber L (1963) A Test for Speech Discrimination Composed of CNC Monosyllabic Words. Northwestern University Auditory Test No 4. Technical Documentary Report No. SAM-TDR-62–135. Brooks Air Force Base, TX: USAF School of Aerospace Medicine.

Tillman TW, Johnson R, Olsen W (1966) Earphones versus soundfield threshold sound pressure levels for spondée words. Journal of the Acoustical Society of America 39: 125–133.

Tong YC, Busby PA, Clark GM (1988) Perceptual studies on cochlear implant patients with early onset of profound hearing impairment prior to normal development of auditory, speech, and language skills. Journal of the Acoustical Society of America 84: 951–962.

Tonnisson W (1976) Australian Standardisation of CID Everyday Sentence Test. Proceedings of the 2nd National Conference of the Audiological Society of Australia. Melbourne: ASA.

Tonisson W (1977) Australian Standardisation of CID Everyday Sentence Test. Annual Report 1976–77. Sydney: National Acoustic Laboratories.

Trammel J, Farrar C, Owens S, Schepard D, Thies T, Witlen R (1976) Test of Auditory Comprehension. North Hollywood: Foreworks.

Traynor RM, Smaldino JJ, Kopra LL, Dunlop RJ, Kopra M, Abrahamson J, Garstecki DC, Rax I (1985) High technology in aural rehabilitation. A miniseminar. Paper presented at the American Speech-Language-Hearing Association Annual Convention, Washington, DC.

Tye-Murray N, Tyler RS (1988) A critique of continuous discourse tracking as a test procedure. Journal of Speech and Hearing Disorders 53: 226–231.

Tye-Murray N, Knutson JF, Lemke JH (1993) Assessment of communication — strategies use: Questionnaires and daily diaries. Self-Assessment Scales in Audiology, Seminars in Hearing 14(4): 338–353.

Tyler RS (1993) Tinnitus disability and handicap questionnaires. Self-Assessment Scales in Audiology, Seminars in Hearing 14(4): 377–384.

Tyler RS, Smith PA (1983) Sentence identification in noise and hearing handicap questionnaires. Scandinavian Audiology 12: 285–292.

Tyler RS, Summerfield Q, Wood ES, Fernandes MA (1982) Psychoacoustic and phonetic temporal processing in normal and hearing-impaired listeners. Journal of the Acoustical Society of America 72: 740–752.

Tyler RS, Preece JP, Tye-Murray N (1987) Iowa Audiovisual Speech-Perception Tests. Iowa City, IA: The University of Iowa.

Ulrich JH (1957) An experimental study of the acquisition of information from three types of recorded television presentation. Speech Monographs: 2439–2445.

Upfold LJ, Smither MF (1981) Hearing aid fitting protocol. British Journal of Audiology 15: 181–188.

Urbantschitsch V (1985) Auditory Training for Deaf Mutism and for Deafness Acquired in Later Life. Vienna: Urban and Schwarzenberg.

Utley J (1946) A test of lipreading ability. Journal of Speech Disorders 11: 109–116.

Valente M (1994) Strategies for Selecting and Verifying Hearing Aid Fittings. New York: Thieme Medical Publishers, Inc.

Ventry IM (1976) Pure tone-spondee threshold relationship in functional hearing loss: a hypothesis. Journal of Speech and Hearing Disorders 41: 16–22.

Ventry IM (1979) Comment on Guidelines (Letter to Editor). ASHA 6: 639.

Ventry IM, Weinstein BE (1982) The hearing handicap inventory for the elderly: A new tool. Ear and Hearing 3: 128.

Victoreen JA (1973) Basic Principles of Otometry. Springfield, IL.: Charles C Thomas.

Voiers WD (1977) Diagnostic Evaluation of Speech Intelligibility. In Hawley M (Ed.) Speech Intelligibility and Speaker Recognition. Stroudsburg, PA: Dowden Hutchinson and Ross.

Walden BE, Montgomery AA (1975) Dimensions of consonant perception in normal and hearing impaired listeners. Journal of Speech and Hearing Research 18: 444–455.

Walden BE, Prosek RA, Montogomery AA, Scherr CK, Jones CJ (1977) Effects of training on the visual recognition of consonants. Journal of Speech and Hearing Research 20: 130–145.

Walden BE, Erdman SA, Montgomery AA, Schwartz DH, Prosek RA (1981) Some effects of training on speech recognition by hearing impaired adults. Journal of Speech and Hearing Research 24: 207–216.

Walden BE, Demorest ME, Helper EL (1984) Self-report approach to assessing benefit derived from amplification. Journal of Speech and Hearing Research 27: 49–56.

Walker G, Byrne D, Dillon H (1982) Learning effects with a closed set nonsense syllable test. Australian Journal of Audiology 4: 27–31.

Wall LG, Davis LA, Myers DK (1984) Four spondee threshold procedures: a comparison. Ear and Hearing 5: 171–174.

Wang MD, Bilger RC (1973) Consonant confusions in noise: A study of perceptual features. Journal of the Acoustical Society of America 54: 1248–1266.

Wang WS-Y, Crawford J (1960) Frequency studies of English consonants. Language and Speech 3: 131–139.

Watson LA, Tolan T (1949) Hearing Tests and Hearing Instruments. Baltimore, MD: Williams and Wilkins.

Watson TJ (1957) Speech audiometry in children. In Ewing AWG (Ed.) Educational Guidance and the Deaf Child. Manchester: Manchester University Press.

Watts MJ, Pegg KS (1977) The rehabilitation of adults with acquired hearing loss. British Journal of Audiology 11: 103–110.

Weber S, Redell RC (1976) A sentence test for measuring speech discrimination in children. Audiology, Hearing and Education 2: 25–30.

Weinstein BE (1984) A review of hearing handicap scales. Audiology 9(7): 91–109.

Weinstein BE (1993) Validation of self-assessment scales as outcome measures in hearing aid fitting. Self-Assessment Scales in Audiology, Seminars in Hearing 14(4): 326–337.

Weinstein BE, Ventry IM (1982) The assessment of hearing handicap in the elderly. Hearing Aid Journal 1(35): 17.

Weinstein BE, Ventry I (1983a) The audiologic correlates of hearing handicap in the elderly. Journal of Speech and Hearing Research 26: 148–151.

Weinstein BE, Ventry I (1983b) Audiometric correlates of the hearing handicap inventory for the elderly. Journal of Speech and Hearing Disorders 48: 379–384.

Weinstein BE, Spitzer JB, Ventry IM (1986) Test–retest reliability of the hearing handicap for the elderly. Ear and Hearing 7: 295–299.

Weisenberger JM, Miller JD, Moog JS, Geers AE (1985) Evaluation of the Siemens minifonator vibrotactile aid: testing with adults. Paper presented at the American Speech-Language-Hearing Association Annual Convention, Washington, DC.

White SC (1980) In Rupp RR and Stockwell KG (Eds) Speech Protocols in Audiology, chapter 7. New York: Grune and Stratton.

Wilber LA, Kruger B, Killion MC (1988) Reference thresholds for the ER-3A insert earphone. Journal of the Acoustical Society America 83(2): 669–676.

Wilde R (1985) Personal communication.

Wills R (1985) A reverberation time survey in school classrooms used by hearing impaired children with hearing aids, and in a hospital free field audiology test room. MSc. Project Report. Polytechnic of the South Bank, London.

Wilde G, Humes LE (1990) Application of the articulation index to the speech recognition of normal and impaired listeners wearing hearing protection. Journal of the Acoustical Society of America 87(3): 1192–1199.

Wilson RH, Antablin JK (1980) A picture identification task as an estimate of the word-recognition performance of non-verbal adults. Journal of Speech and Hearing Disorders 45: 223–238.

Wilson FH, Margolis RH (1983) Measurements of auditory thresholds for speech stimuli, in Konkle DF and Rintelmann WF (Eds.) Principles of Speech Audiometry, pp. 79–126 (Lloyd LL (Series Ed.), Perspectives in Audiology Series. Baltimore: University Park Press.

Wilson RH, Morgan DE, Dirks DD (1973) A proposed SRT procedure and its statistical precedent. Journal of Speech and Hearing Disorders 38, 184–191.

Wilson RH, Stream RW, Dirks DD (1973) Spread-of-masking effects on pure tones and several speech stimuli. Journal of Speech and Hearing Research 16: 385–396.

Woodward MF, Barber CG (1960) Phoneme perception in lip reading. Journal of Speech and Hearing Research 3: 212–222.

Zwicker E, Feldtkeller R (1967) Das Ohr als Nachrichtenempfanger (The human ear as a receiver of information) 2nd edition. Stuttgart: S Hirzel Verlag.

Zwislocki JJ (1953) Acoustic attenuation between the ears. Journal of the Acoustical Society of America 25: 752.

Zwislocki JJ (1971) An ear-like coupler for earphone calibration. Report LSC-S–9. Institute for Sensory Research. Syracuse University, Syracuse, New York.

Index